D0895564

Clinical Psycho-Oncology

Clinical Psycho-Oncology

An International Perspective

Luigi Grassi, MD
Professor and Chair of Psychiatry
Chairman Department of Biomedical and Specialist Surgical Sciences
University of Ferrara;
Director, Clinical & Emergency Psychiatry Unit, Department of Mental Health & Drug Abuse, Ferrara, Italy

Michelle Riba, MD, MS
Professor and Associate Chair, Integrated Medicine and Psychiatric Services
Department of Psychiatry
University of Michigan Medical School;
Director, PsychOncology
University of Michigan Comprehensive Cancer Center, MI, USA

WILEY-BLACKWELL
A John Wiley & Sons, Ltd., Publication

This edition first published 2012

Wiley-Blackwell is an imprint of John Wiley & Sons, formed by the merger of Wiley's global Scientific, Technical and Medical business with Blackwell Publishing.

Registered office: John Wiley & Sons, Ltd, The Atrium, Southern Gate, Chichester, West Sussex, PO19 8SQ, UK

Editorial offices: 9600 Garsington Road, Oxford, OX4 2DQ, UK
The Atrium, Southern Gate, Chichester, West Sussex, PO19 8SQ, UK
111 River Street, Hoboken, NJ 07030-5774, USA

For details of our global editorial offices, for customer services and for information about how to apply for permission to reuse the copyright material in this book please see our website at www.wiley.com/wiley-blackwell

Library of Congress Cataloging-in-Publication Data
Clinical psycho-oncology : an international perspective / [edited by] Luigi Grassi and Michelle Riba.
p. ; cm.
Includes bibliographical references and index.
Summary: "This international primer on psycho-oncology spans settings of care as well as regional boundaries. Designed to be easy to read, with informaton clearly displayed in concise tables and boxes accompanied by clinical vignettes, the book provides clear, practical guidance on all aspects of the psychological care of patients with cancer. Both trainees and practitioners will find it useful in the clinic as well as a resource for continued professional development"–Provided by publisher.
ISBN 978-0-470-97432-2 (hardback)
I. Grassi, Luigi. II. Riba, Michelle B.
[DNLM: 1. Neoplasms–psychology. 2. Family–psychology. 3. Needs Assessment. 4. Psychology, Medical. 5. Psychotherapy. 6. Social Support. QZ 200]
616.99′40651–dc23

2012009770

A catalogue record for this book is available from the British Library.

Wiley also publishes its books in a variety of electronic formats. Some content that appears in print may not be available in electronic books.

Set in 9/12pt Meridien by Aptara Inc., New Delhi, India
Printed and bound in Malaysia by Vivar Printing Sdn Bhd

First Impression 2012

Contents

List of Contributors

Tim Ahles, PhD
Director, Neurocognitive Research Laboratory, Department of Psychiatry and Behavioral Sciences, Memorial Sloan-Kettering Cancer Center, New York, NY, USA

Yesne Alici, MD
Attending Psychiatrist, Geriatric Psychiatry Treatment Unit, Central Regional Hospital, Butner, NC, USA

Kimlin Tam Ashing-Giwa, PhD
Professor & Founding Director, Center of Community Alliance for Research & Education (CCARE), Division of Population Sciences, City of Hope National Medical Center, Duarte, CA, USA

Lea Baider, PhD
Full Professor of Medical Psychology, Faculty of Medicine, Hebrew University Medical School, Hadassah University Hospital, Jerusalem; Director, Psycho-Oncology Unit, Sharett Institute of Oncology, Department of Radiation and Clinical Oncology, Hadassah University Hospital, Jerusalem, Israel

Walter F. Baile, MD
Professor, Departments of Behavioral Science and Faculty Development; Director, Program on Interpersonal Communication and Relationship Enhancement (I*CARE), The University of Texas MD Anderson Cancer Center, Houston, TX, USA

Susan D. Block, MD
Chair, Department of Psychosocial Oncology and Palliative Care; Co-Director, HMS Center for Palliative Care, Professor of Psychiatry and Medicine, Harvard Medical School; Dana-Farber Cancer Institute and Brigham and Women's Hospital, Boston, MA, USA

William Breitbart, MD
Chief, Psychiatry Service, Department of Psychiatry and Behavioral Sciences, and Attending Psychiatrist, Pain and Palliative Care Service, Department of Medicine, Memorial Sloan-Kettering Cancer Center; Professor of Clinical Psychiatry, Department of Psychiatry, Weill Medical College of Cornell University, New York, NY, USA

Barry D. Bultz, PhD
Director, Department of Psychosocial Resources; Program Leader: Psychosocial Oncology, Supportive, Pain and Palliative Care, Tom Baker Cancer Centre; Adjunct Professor and Chair, Division of Psychosocial Oncology, Faculty of Medicine, University of Calgary, Alberta, Canada

Phyllis Butow, BA(Hons)Dip Ed, MClinPsych, MPH, PhD
Chair in Psychology, Co-director Centre for Medical Psychology and Evidence-based Medicine (CeMPED) and Chair, Psycho-Oncology Co-operative Research Group, University of Sydney, NSW, Australia.

Santosh K. Chaturvedi, MD, FRCPsych
Professor of Psychiatry, Department of Psychiatry, National Institute of Mental Health and Neurosciences, Bangalore, India

Harvey Max Chochinov, MD, PhD, FRCPC
Director and Canada Research Chair in Palliative Medicine, Manitoba Palliative Care Research Unit, Cancer Care Manitoba; Professor of Psychiatry and Family Medicine, Departments of Psychiatry and Family Medicine, University of Manitoba, Winnipeg, Manitoba, Canada

Karen L. Clark, MS
Program Manager, Sheri & Les Biller Patient and Family Resource Center; Department of Supportive Care Medicine and Department of Population Sciences, City of Hope, Duarte, CA, USA

Anna Costantini, PhD
Director of Psychooncology Unit, Professor of Psychooncology, Sant'Andrea Hospital, Faculty of Medicine and Psychology, Sapienza University of Rome; Certified Group Psychotherapist and Member of the American Group Psychotherapy Association, President of Italian Society of Psychooncology, Italy

Matthew Cordova, PhD
Assistant Professor, Palo Alto University, Palo Alto, California Staff Psychologist, VA Northern California Health Care System, Martinez, CA

Michael Diaz
Undergraduate student, Human Biology, Stanford University, Palo Alto, CA, USA

Kristine A. Donovan, PhD, MBA
Assistant Member, Psychosocial and Palliative Care Program, Department of Health Outcomes and Behavior, Moffitt Cancer Center, Tampa, FL, USA

Jeff Dunn, PhD
Griffith Health Institute, Griffith University, Australia; School of Social Science, University of Queensland, Australia; Viertel Centre for Research in Cancer Control, Cancer Council Queensland, Australia

Laura B. Dunn, MD
Associate Professor and Director of Psycho-Oncology, Department of Psychiatry, University of California, San Francisco, San Francisco, CA, USA

Mary Jane Esplen, RN, PhD
Professor, Department of Psychiatry, Faculty of Medicine, University of Toronto; Director, de Souza Institute; Head, Program of Psychosocial & Psychotherapy Research in Cancer Genetics, University Health Network, Toronto, Canada

Richard Fielding, PhD, CPsychol, FFPH
Director, Centre for Psycho-Oncology Research & Training, Professor of Medical Psychology in Public Health, School of Public Health, The University of Hong Kong, Hong Kong, China

Peter Fitzgerald, MD MRCPysch (UK)
Fellow in Psychosocial Oncology, Princess Margaret Hospital, Toronto, Canada

Patricia A. Ganz, MD
Professor, UCLA Schools of Medicine & Public Health; Director, Division of Cancer Prevention & Control Research, Jonsson Comprehensive Cancer Center, Los Angeles (UCLA), CA, USA

Jan Geissler
Founder and CEO, Patvocates; Co-founder, CML Advocates Network; Chair, LeukaNET

Gil Goldzweig, PhD
Medical and Clinical Psychologist; Senior Lecturer, The Academic College of Tel-Aviv – Yaffo, Tel Aviv, Israel

Luigi Grassi, MD
Professor and Chair of Psychiatry, Chairman Department of Biomedical and Specialist Surgical Sciences, University of Ferrara; Director, Clinical & Emergency Psychiatry Unit, Department of Mental Health & Drug Abuse, Ferrara, Italy

Jonathan Hunter, MD, FRCPC
Associate Professor; Head, Consultation/Liaison Division, University of Toronto Department of Psychiatry; Mount Sinai Hospital, Toronto, Canada

María Elisa Irarrázaval, MD
Chief, Mental Health Unit, Fundación Arturo López Pérez Oncologic Center, Santiago, Chile

Paul B. Jacobsen, PhD
Chair, Department of Health Outcomes and Behavior, Moffitt Cancer Center, Tampa, FL, USA

Kathryn M. Kash, RN, BS, MPhil, PhD
Associate Professor, Program Director, Masters in Chronic Care Management, Jefferson School of Population Health, Thomas Jefferson University, PA, USA

Brian Kelly, BMed, PhD, FRANZCP, FAChPM
Professor of Psychiatry and Head, Discipline of Psychiatry, University of Newcastle, NSW, Australia

David W. Kissane, MD, MPM, FRANZCP, FAChPM
Jimmie C. Holland Chair of Psycho-Oncology, Attending Psychiatrist and Chairman, Department of Psychiatry and Behavioral Sciences, Memorial Sloan-Kettering Cancer Center; Professor of Psychiatry, Weill Medical College of Cornell University, New York, NY, USA

Uwe Koch, PhD, MD
Professor of Medical Psychology; Dean, Medical Faculty, Hamburg University, University Medical Center Hamburg Eppendorf, Hamburg, Germany

Wendy W.T. Lam, RN, PhD
Assistant Professor; Deputy Director, Centre for Psycho-Oncology Research & Training, School of Public Health, University of Hong Kong, Hong Kong, China

Carrie Lethborg, PhD
Senior Social Worker, Department of Oncology, St Vincent's Hospital, University of Melbourne, Victoria, Australia

Matthew J. Loscalzo, LCSW
Liliane Elkins Professor in Supportive Care Programs; Administrative Director, Sheri & Les Biller Patient and Family Resource Center; Executive Director, Department of Supportive Care Medicine; Professor, Department of Population Sciences, City of Hope, Duarte, CA, USA

Anja Mehnert, PhD
Head, Psycho-Oncology and Palliative Care Research Group, Department of Medical Psychology, University Medical Center Hamburg Eppendorf, Hamburg, Germany

Anne Merriman PhD, FRCP, MCommH
Director of Policy and International Programmes, Hospice Africa in Uganda; Honorary Professor of Palliative Medicine, Department of Internal Medicine, Makerere University, Uganda

Sue E. Morris, MPsychol (Clinical) Hons
Director of Bereavement Services, Dana-Farber/Brigham and Women's Cancer Center; Department of Psychosocial Oncology and Palliative Care, Dana-Farber Cancer Institute, Boston, MA, USA

Chiara M. Navarra, PhD
Psychooncology Unit, Sant'Andrea Hospital, Faculty of Medicine and Psychology, Sapienza University of Rome; Certified Psychotherapist, Member of Italian Society of Psychooncology, Italy

Rinat Nissim, PhD
Department of Psychosocial Oncology and Palliative Care, Princess Margaret Hospital, University Health Network, Toronto, Canada

Michelle Riba, MD, MS
Professor and Associate Chair, Integrated Medicine and Psychiatric Services, Department of Psychiatry, University of Michigan Medical School; Director, PsychOncology, University of Michigan Comprehensive Cancer Center, MI, USA

Gary Rodin, MD FRCPC
Professor of Psychiatry, University of Toronto; Head, Department of Psychosocial Oncology and Palliative Care, Princess Margaret Hospital; University of Toronto/University Health Network Chair in Psychosocial Oncology and Palliative Care; Senior Scientist, Ontario Cancer Institute, Canada

Sanne Schagen, PhD
Department of Psychosocial Research and Epidemiology, Netherlands Cancer Institute, Antoni van Leeuwenhoek Hospital, Amsterdam, the Netherlands

Ranjit Kaur Pritam Singh, AMP, MSc
Chief Executive Officer, Breast Cancer Welfare Association Malaysia, Petaling Jaya, Selangor, Malaysia

David Spiegel, MD
Willson Professor in the School of Medicine, Associate Chair, Department of Psychiatry & Behavioral Sciences, Director, Center on Stress and Health, Stanford University School of Medicine, Stanford, CA, USA

Annette L. Stanton, PhD
Professor, Psychology & Psychiatry/Biobehavioral Sciences; Member, Jonsson Comprehensive Cancer Center; Senior Research Scientist, Cousins Center for Psychoneuroimmunology, Los Angeles, CA, USA

Elizabeth M. Strom
Medical student, University of Illinois at Chicago College of Medicine, Dixon, IL, USA

Margaret L. Stuber, MD
Jane and Marc Nathanson Professor, David Geffen School of Medicine, University of California, Los Angels, CA, USA

Antonella Surbone MD, PhD, FACP
Professor of Medicine, Department of Medicine, New York University Medical School, New York, NY, USA; Faculty, Interpersonal Communication & Relationship Enhancement Program (I*CARE), M.D. Anderson Cancer Center, Houston, TX, USA; Lecturer in Clinical Bioethics and Palliative Care, Italy

Seema M. Thekdi, MD
Assistant Professor, Department of Psychiatry, MD Anderson Cancer Center, Houston, TX, USA

Kim Thiboldeaux
President & CEO, Cancer Support Community, *Uniting The Wellness Community and Gilda's Club Worldwide*, Washington DC, USA

Luzia Travado, D. Clin Psych, MSc
Clinical Psychology Unit, Central Lisbon Hospital Centre – Hospital de S. José, Lisbon, Portugal

Yosuke Uchitomi, MD, PhD
Professor and Chairman, Department of Neuropsychiatry, Okayama University Graduate School of Medicine, Dentistry and Pharmaceutical Sciences, Okayama, Japan

Janette Vardy, MD, PhD
Sydney Cancer Centre, University of Sydney, Concord Repatriation General Hospital, Concord, NSW, Australia

Maggie Watson, BSc, PhD, DipClinPsych, AFBPS
Head, Psychology Research Group, Institute of Cancer Research; Consultant Clinical Psychologist, Royal Marsden Hospital; Honorary Professor, Research Department of Clinical, Health and Educational Psychology, University College London, UK

Sophia Yeung, RN
Community Interventionist, Center of Community Alliance for Research & Education (CCARE), Division of Population Sciences, City of Hope National Medical Center, Duarte, CA, USA

Foreword

It is an honour and a privilege to write the Foreword for this book, which establishes a benchmark in the emerging field of psycho-oncology. It reflects the fact that there is now international recognition of the importance – and even necessity – of the integration of the psychosocial domain into routine cancer care in this early part of the twenty-first century. There have been significant barriers to reaching this benchmark: the fact that patients were not told their diagnosis; that the stigma attached to cancer made it a word that could not be spoken; that the psychological burden of the patient with cancer was not acknowledged by others; and that the study of patient-reported (subjective) symptoms were regarded as not quantifiable by the scientific cancer community. Progress has been quite remarkable in the past 35 years as these barriers broke down and psychological issues became the topic of scientific study and research, particularly the validation of quantitative assessment tools to measure symptoms such as pain, anxiety and depression. With the development of reliable tools, the science could move forward which allowed us to measure changes in symptoms based on interventions to reduce distressing physical and psychological symptoms. Thus, this book contains the synthesis of global state of the art research which today constitutes what we now call the 'science of care' in cancer – attention to the humanistic, ethical, psychological, social, cultural, psychiatric and behavioural issues that contribute so substantially both to the outcome of the medical treatment and the quality of the experience of the patient with cancer and the family.

The fact that this book was developed out of the Psycho-Oncology and Palliative Care Section of the World Psychiatric Association is a source of pride for me since I served as its Founding Chair. The co-editors of this book, Luigi Grassi and Michelle Riba, have carried the work of the Section forward in an impressive way, collaborating with the International Psycho-Oncology Society (IPOS), the world's leading international multidisciplinary association which addresses the psychological and social issues in cancer. IPOS has taken a lead role in establishing standards for psychological care by engaging the major global cancer organizations. The IPOS International Standard of Quality Cancer Care states that

1 Quality cancer care must integrate the psychosocial domain into routine care;

2 Distress should be measured as the Sixth Vital Sign after temperature, blood pressure, pulse, respiration and pain.

The recent endorsement by the International Union Against Cancer (UICC) and the International Pediatric Society (SIOP) speaks to the synergy that comes from these collaborative international efforts. IPOS has proposed that the World Cancer Day 2013 should call for global action on supportive care, under the banner 'Declare you care about cancer support'. These global initiatives have an immediate effect upon the potential of the national psycho-oncology societies to have an impact in their own countries, implementing the goals in ways that are culturally appropriate.

The authors of these chapters that follow are the scholars in psycho-oncology from around the globe. They have truly brought together the information that is most relevant and have synthesized it to provide an overview of the best research in the area. I am enormously proud of what our field has accomplished up to now. I am sure that the future will see major steps forward to ensure that the emotional suffering that has so long accompanied cancer will be further reduced. Francis Peabody, thoughtful physician, wrote in 1927 in the *JAMA*, 'The secret of the care of the patient is in CARING FOR the PATIENT'. The clinicians and researchers in psycho-oncology contribute that 'caring' piece to cancer, through developing the 'science of care' combined with attention to the humanistic and compassionate aspects of care.

Jimmie C. Holland, MD
Wayne E. Chapman Chair in Psychiatric Oncology
April 2012

Acknowledgements

The idea of this book originated at the World Psychiatric Association (WPA) International Congress in Florence, Italy, in April 2009, where the activity and the work done by the Section on Psycho-Oncology and Palliative Care and the Section on Psychiatry, Medicine and Primary Care, which we respectively chair, were presented. On that occasion, we decided to take the challenge to edit a book exploring, from an international perspective, the cultural aspects underlying the several areas related to psychosocial care in cancer. A fundamental concept of the book was to promote and sustain the role of our sections within the WPA and to sensitize more mental health professionals and psychiatrists to the psychosocial concomitants of cancer. Further, we hoped these collaborative efforts would give possible insights to the well-established science and discipline of psycho-oncology by stressing the role of culture, with all its complex facets, as a basic variable to be taken into account when dealing with communication, ethical, spiritual, psychological and social aspects of cancer.

We are deeply grateful to all the authors from many different parts of the world and belonging to many different cultural backgrounds who accepted to speak, as one voice, the common language of clinical psycho-oncology care, and to generously share their experiences and commitment to participate in this task. Without their enthusiasm, expertise and contributions this book would not have been possible. Our deepest thanks to the board of the World Psychiatric Association (WPA), in particular Mario Maj, Miguel Jorge and Pedro Ruiz, and Helen Herrman, for their guidance; to Jimmie Holland, founding chair of the WPA Section on Psycho-Oncology and Rodolfo Fahrer, founding chair of the WPA Section on Psychiatry, Medicine and Primary Care, for their vision and encouragement to us to persist in our efforts and to maintain the aims of the sections; to the present and the past board of the International Psycho-Oncology Society (IPOS) with whom we have collaborated and worked in many different projects over the last years, namely Elisabeth Andritsch, Lea Baider, William Breitbart, Barry Bultz, Phyllis Butow, Santosh Chaturvedi, Vicente De Carvalho, Maria Die-Trill, Sylvie Dolbeault, Jeff Dunn, Fawzy Fawzy, Richard Fielding, Lise Fillion, Thomas Hack, Elizabeth Harvey, Jimmie Holland, Takashi Hosaka, Paul Jacobsen, Christoffer Johansen, David Kissane, Uwe Koch, Katalin Muszbek, Antonella Surbone, Luzia Travado, Yosuke Uchitomi, Kazuhiro Yoshiuchi, Maggie Watson, for their friendship and constant contribution in making psycho-oncology grow year after year. We also would like to express our appreciation and acknowledgement to all the representative persons and members, most of them friends for a long time, of the several National Societies of Psycho-Oncology of different countries throughout the world, belonging to the Federation of IPOS. Their commitment and enthusiasm in founding and sustaining the Federation has been the seed for the idea of this book.

We owe a special debt of gratitude to our teachers and mentors who advocated and supported our commitment to psychosomatic medicine and collaborative models during our professional and human journey; to our families who consistently supported and encouraged us; and to all the patients and families who taught us the sense of humanity and shared their underlying suffering and pain, in all their physical, psychological, interpersonal and spiritual dimensions.

We also would like to thank the editorial staff at Wiley-Blackwell, particularly Joan Marsh, Fiona Seymour and Robyn Lyons, for their wise suggestions, help and guidance for this project.

Luigi Grassi
Ferrara, Italy

Michelle Riba
Ann Arbor, Michigan, USA
March 2012

PART 1
Clinical Issues

CHAPTER 1

Introducing Multicultural Psycho-oncology

Luigi Grassi[1] *and Michelle Riba*[2]

[1]Section of Psychiatry, Department of Medical and Surgical Disciplines of Communication and Behaviour, University of Ferrara, Italy

[2]Department of Psychiatry, University of Michigan and University of Michigan Comprehensive Cancer Center, Ann Arbor, MI, USA

> There is one short rule that should regulate human relationships. All that you see, both divine and human, is one. We are the parts of one great body. Nature created us from the same source and to the end. She imbued us with mutual affection and sociability, she taught us to be fair and just, to suffer injury rather than to inflict it. She bids us extend our hands to all in need of help. Let that well-known line be in our hearts and on our lips: *I am a man: I deem nothing pertaining to man is foreign to me (Homo sum, humani nihil a me alienum puto).*
>
> Lucius Annaeus Seneca, *Epistulae Morales ad Lucilium*, Book XV, Letter 95:52–53 (62–65 AD)

According to the World Health Organization (WHO) projections, it is estimated that the incidence of cancer will increase by the year 2030, with new cases of cancer jumping from 13.3 million in 2010 to 21.3 million in 2030 and cancer deaths rising from 7.9 million to 13.1 million. At the same time, earlier diagnoses and improvement in cancer therapies have also noted an increase in survival for about 25 million people (long-term survivors) throughout the world.[1]

It is clear that this epidemiological data has a specific value if evaluated through a global perspective which takes into account the important issues of quality of life and psychosocial needs of cancer patients. In fact, cancer is not only a series of very different diseases needing complex treatments, from many professionals, but also a devastating and 'traumatic' event with physical, emotional, interpersonal and social implications that should be constantly monitored across the disease trajectory, and into survivorship. Being affected by cancer means an overall transformation of the sense of one's own self, in which the parameters of time (the past, the present, the future), of space (one's own individual space, one's own home, one's own world context) and of existence (*Umwelt*, the biological dimension, my body; *Eigenwelt*, the relationship with myself, my-being-in-the-world; *Mitwelt*, the relational dimension with others; *Überwelt*, the spiritual dimension, the meaningfulness) are altered by the diagnosis and treatment, recovery and recurrence or transition to palliative and end-of-life care.

Starting from the work of a small group of psychiatrists,[2–6] interested in examining the psychophysiological and emotional factors implicated in cancer and cancer treatment, oncologists quickly started showing a specific need for more precise indications about the psychosocial, behavioural and rehabilitative issues in cancer care. This determined the rapid growth of the psycho-oncology discipline in the USA from the 1970s[7–10] and subsequently, from the early 1980s, in many other countries,

Clinical Psycho-Oncology: An International Perspective, First Edition. Edited by Luigi Grassi and Michelle Riba.

such as France, Germany, Italy, the Netherlands, the United Kingdom, to cite just a few.[11]

Over the last quarter of a century, a large number of psycho-oncology studies have in fact indicated that 30–40% cancer patients fail to adapt, and present emotional disorders – mainly depression, anxiety and adjustment disorders according to the ICD-10 and DSM-IV taxonomic systems – as a consequence of cancer and cancer treatments.[12] A further 15–25% present other significant psychosocial conditions, such as health anxiety, irritable mood, demoralization, or general emotional distress which are not identified by the usual categorical systems (e.g. DSM-IV and ICD-10) but by other systems (e.g. the Diagnostic Criteria for Psychosomatic Research), and which are dysfunctional and maladaptive symptoms.[13]

The implications and the impact of psychosocial disorders for patients and their families are of paramount importance in oncology with several studies demonstrating that clinically significant distress is associated with maladjustment, reduction of quality of life and impairment in social relationships, longer rehabilitation time, poor adherence to treatment and abnormal illness behaviour, and possibly shorter survival.[14] Significant levels of emotional distress have been reported also to affect family members and there is evidence that unrecognized and unmet psychosocial needs are an important predictor of psychological morbidity in caregivers in every phase of the illness.[15–18] Various types of psychosocial interventions have also been shown to be effective in reducing psychological symptoms and improving quality of life among cancer patients.[19–21]

Thus, psycho-oncology, as the specialty aiming at studying the psychological, social and spiritual factors that affect the quality of life of cancer patients and their loved ones, has today a specific and unquestionable role in the multidisciplinary approach to cancer. This role has been defined, in several countries, through the development of psycho-oncology services, programmes and/or departments with the mission of providing specific activities in terms of clinical care, education and research. Furthermore, guidelines and recommendations on psychosocial care in cancer have been developed and endorsed by national and international scientific societies of psycho-oncology as well as by advocacy movements.[22]

The *National Standards for Psychosocial Oncology* published by the Canadian Association of Psychosocial Oncology (CAPO) (1999) includes today standards of care, organizational standards, educational standards and integration of all phases of the cancer control trajectory, including prevention and survivorship.[23] Several agencies and institutions, such as the Canadian Association of Provincial Cancer Agencies, the Canadian Cancer Society, the Canadian Strategy for Cancer Control, and the Canadian Council on Health Services Accreditation, have endorsed CAPO's recommendations. Furthermore, clinical guidelines on the assessment of psychosocial needs of cancer patients and on the screening, assessment and care of psychosocial distress in cancer have also been developed (www.capo.ca).[24,25]

Comprehensive clinical guidelines are available in Australia (www.nhmrc.gov.au) where the first document, *Psychosocial clinical practice guidelines: information, support and counselling for women with breast cancer* (National Breast Cancer Centre, 1999),[26] represented the basis for the subsequent development of the *Clinical practice guidelines for the psychosocial care of adults with cancer,* published by the National Breast Cancer Centre and the National Cancer Control Initiative.[27]

In the United States, the National Comprehensive Cancer Network (NCCN) Distress Management Panel, consisting of multidisciplinary health care professionals developed the guidelines on distress, starting from 1997[28] to the most recent version I.2011.[29] The work of the panel has been recognized throughout the world, where an ultra-short tool, the distress thermometer, has rapidly become one of the 'gold standards' for the rapid screening of distress, identified as the 'sixth vital sign', with the same importance as blood pressure, temperature, heart frequency, respiratory rate and pain.[30,31]

In more recent years, at the request of the National Institutes of Health (NIH), the Institute of Medicine (IOM) of the National Academies of Sciences published the conclusions of a specific working group[32] indicating that enough evidence exists for the inclusion of psychosocial health services in cancer care, and stressing that 'Attending to psychosocial needs should be an integral part of quality cancer care [...]', since 'It is not possible to deliver good-quality cancer care without addressing patient's psychosocial health needs.'

Similarly, the conclusions of the European Council[33] clearly acknowledge the significance of psychosocial aspects in cancer care, indicating that 'to attain optimal results, a patient-centred comprehensive interdisciplinary approach and optimal psycho-social care should be implemented in routine cancer care, rehabilitation and post-treatment follow-up for all cancer'(par. 5), and emphasizing that 'cancer treatment and care is multidisciplinary, involving the cooperation of oncological surgery, medical oncology, radiotherapy, chemotherapy as well as psycho-social support and rehabilitation and, when cancer is not treatable, palliative care'(par. 11).

Thus the general results of the above-mentioned reports are that the evaluation and treatment of psychosocial consequences should be mandatory in every cancer centre. This is in accordance with the statement 'No health without mental health',[34] which sets out to guarantee the quality of life of any individual in society to receive optimal medical and psychiatric care, incorporating attention to psychosocial needs into policies, practices and standards of clinical care.[35,36]

This is also the message launched by the International Psycho-Oncology Society (IPOS) and the Federation of the Psycho-Oncology societies through the *Statement on Standards and Clinical Practice Guidelines in Cancer Care*, which indicates that 'quality cancer care must integrate the psychosocial domain into routine care' and that 'distress should be measured as the 6th Vital Sign after temperature, blood pressure, pulse, respiratory rate and pain' (www.ipos-society.org).[37] A number of organizations and associations throughout the world, including the International Union Against Cancer (UICC), the International Society of Paediatric Oncology (SIOP), the Canadian Cancer Society, the Clinical Oncological Society of Australia, the World Psychiatric Association (WPA), as well as advocacy movements, such as LIVESTRONG and Reach to Recovery International, have endorsed this statement. The webcast lectures series on psychosocial aspects of cancer care (communication, psychological assessment, distress management, anxiety, depression, family issues, bioethics, palliative care, loss and grief, psychological intervention) developed by IPOS and available online in several languages (Chinese, English, French, German, Hungarian, Italian, Japanese, Portuguese, Spanish) is also in agreement with the concept that account should be taken of multicultural and cross-cultural relevant issues.

For all these reasons, we have realized that the time has come for an international perspective on psycho-oncology, with contributions by specialists from different parts of the world, sharing their long-standing experience in the psychosocial care of patients with cancer, and their families.

More specifically, a first aim of the book is to discuss contemporary themes in psycho-oncology, such as genetic counselling, bioethics, advocacy and to provide practical suggestions for dealing with special populations, such as children, the elderly, long-term survivors, or disadvantaged or minority groups. A second aim of the book is to present the challenging clinical problems encountered when caring for cancer patients and their families, by describing the best responses to these challenges, including assessment, diagnosis and treatment, and by summarizing the evidence base and digesting clinical experience where evidence from clinical trials is lacking, and noting, through clinical examples, international and multicultural perspectives.

With respect to this, the book specifically emphasizes the possible cultural implications determined by cultural diversity, particularly where immigration and other social phenomena have influenced the creation of multiethnic and multicultural societies. Specificity and culturally relevant issues on several topics of psycho-oncology are discussed throughout the book. It is clear that language, ethnicity, race and religion have an important role in affecting patients' and families' perception of illness. We need to understand how culture may influence communication and the doctor–patient relationship (e.g. disclosure of information related to diagnosis and prognosis, role of patient and family in decision-making), coping mechanisms, psychological response and psychopathological disorders (e.g. phenomenology of anxiety or depression, abnormal illness behaviour, somatization), treatment options and acceptance of psychological intervention. We also need to better understand how the culture of the organization and health care system influence the response of patients and families to cancer and cancer treatment.

The book consists of three parts. In Part 1, clinical issues are discussed in detail by experts in the field. Butow and Baile explore in Chapter 2 how culture impacts on the relationship between patients, family members and clinicians, and how communication across cultures can be challenging, especially if language barriers are present. Chapter 3, by Jacobsen and Donovan, describes the psychosocial instruments commonly used in psycho-oncology research for the assessment of anxiety, depression and distress, including a number of brief tools that could be used for screening purposes, and summarizes evidence regarding the relative merits of these instruments. In Chapter 4, Costantini, Navarra, Ashing-Giwa and Yeung discuss the most significant aspects related to sexuality and gender in patients with cancer, by addressing the type of cancer and treatment influencing a person's appearance, body image, sexual functioning, and the role of cultural variables in different parts of the world, with comparison between Western countries, Asia and Africa. Chaturvedi and Uchitomi (Chapter 5) examine the most common psychiatric and psychosocial disorders in relation to cancer, including the challenging situation of somatization and abnormal illness behaviour in cancer patients, where cultural determinants can play a particular role, and the problem of emergency psychiatry in cancer care. Chapter 6 by Ahles, Schagen and Vardy focuses on cognitive changes associated with cancer and cancer treatments with careful analysis of the studies that have examined the role of patient characteristics and genetic factors in increasing the risk for post-treatment cognitive decline and of the problems and lack of data regarding the role racial and ethnic issues and socioeconomic factors have on this area. Bultz, Loscalzo and Clarke describe, in Chapter 7, how screening for distress, considered as the 6th vital sign, is an essential component of clinical care that facilitates the conversation within the clinical team, with positive effects in terms of better understanding of the full range of patient concerns and better integration of the different health care professionals working in an interdisciplinary fashion.

In Chapter 8, Watson provides a comprehensive overview of psychological intervention in cancer care, with particular emphasis on the best approaches to build into clinical practice, the available evidence on efficacy of psychological therapy, the differences between psychiatric and psychological models and the cost-effectiveness issues. Thekdi, Irarrázaval and Dunn (Chapter 9) examine the vast and important area of psychopharmacological intervention in cancer care carefully summarizing the role of antidepressants, antipsychotics, benzodiazepines, anticonvulsants and mood stabilizers, and exploring their clinical use, safety profile, side-effects and possible interactions, also from a cultural perspective. Chapter 10 by Mehnert and Koch review the effects of cancer rehabilitation programmes in reducing the impact of disabling conditions, in enabling people with disabilities to achieve optimal social integration and in improving quality of life, social participation and return to work.

Part 2 deals with the different approaches in psycho-oncology when applied to special populations. In Chapter 11, Stuber and Strom discuss the current situation in paediatric oncology and associated psychiatric issues by considering the normal developmental context in which children understand cancer and treatment, and examining the most common psychological and psychiatric problems of child cancer patients and their families. Fitzgerald, Nissim and Rodin (Chapter 12) examine the important theme of geriatric psycho-oncology by summarizing the main psychological and psychiatric implications of cancer on patients in the later stages of life, contrasting the problems and concerns of old age with young age and evaluating the efficacy of psycho-oncology intervention in this vulnerable segment of the population. Chapter 13, by Fielding and Lam, focuses on the significant problem of higher cancer incidence, lower knowledge of cancer risks, prevention, less screening uptake, more difficulties in access to diagnostic services and fewer or different options for treatment, and more difficulties in reintegration following treatment among underserved and minority populations.

Part 3 addresses salient topics requiring special attention in clinical psycho-oncology. The significance of cancer within the family, as a basic social and ethical unit of care, is explored in Chapter 14 by Baider and Goldzweig who discuss how individual values and beliefs and the family convergence and diversity of meaning influence the psychological response to the disease. Chapter 15 by Surbone reviews the vast and important area relative to the bioethical aspects in cancer, specifically focusing on cultural competence and culturally sensitive communication as essential instruments for ethical contemporary practice of oncology, in order to negotiate different health care related values and goals in individual therapeutic relationships with patients of different cultures, and to facilitate clinicians' ability to interact more effectively with institutions, policy-makers and various stakeholders in lower income countries. The theme related to the positive life changes secondary to cancer experience, known as post-traumatic growth, is examined by Diaz, Cordova and Spiegel in Chapter 16 by exploring similarities and differences across cultures. In Chapter 17, Esplen, Hunter and Kash provide a detailed psychological framework regarding the use of new genetic technology and discuss the genetic testing process, the potential psychological impact, and the psychotherapeutic approaches useful to augment care. Chapter 18 by Ganz and Stanton addresses the trajectories of psychosocial and physical recovery for adults after primary treatments are complete, contributors to those outcomes (i.e. medical, individual, sociocultural and developmental contexts), and considerations regarding provision of effective medical and psychosocial care during re-entry and extended survivorship. Chapter 19 by Breitbart, Chochinov and Alici focuses on the role of psycho-oncologists in helping and guiding terminally ill patients through the dying process, by presenting the most salient aspects of end-of-life care including assessment and management of a variety of possible problems, such as delirium, depression, desire for hastened death and suicide. Morris and Block describe in Chapter 20 how individual differences both within and between cultures increase the complexity of care when working with bereaved individuals and families, and how to correctly assess and provide support strategies and treatment for the bereaved. Chapter 21 is dedicated by Kissane, Lethborg and Kelly to providing a thorough description of the major religions worldwide, including studies of prayer, the power of placebo, the use of rituals, the role of meditation, in order to help clinicians to routinely make use of a spiritual assessment and integrate appropriate responses into a comprehensive and person-centred management plan. A comprehensive overview of some of the main advocacy movements is given in Chapter 22 by Travado, Geissler, Thiboldeaux, Dunn, Kaur and Merriman, who illustrate some of the actions undertaken in the five continents and how these have translated and influenced better policies in cancer care.

The book is designed to be easy to read and to reference, with information clearly displayed in concise tables and boxes accompanied by further detail within the text and clinical cases exemplifying the themes discussed in each chapter.

We hope that this book can give further insight into the multiple dimensions involved in psychosocial care of cancer patients and their families, and that it can help clinicians, teachers and researchers better understand the importance of the cultural backgrounds of patients and families as an important variable moulding the psychological response to cancer and cancer treatment.

References

1. Ferlay J, Shin HR, Bray F. *et al.* (2010) GLOBOCAN 2008 v1.2, Cancer Incidence and Mortality Worldwide: IARC CancerBase No. 10, International Agency for Research on Cancer, Lyon, France.
2. Sutherland A.M., Orbach C.E., Dyk R.B., Bard M. (1952) The psychological impact of cancer and cancer surgery. I. Adaptation to the dry colostomy: Preliminary report and summary of findings. *Cancer*, 5, 857–872.

3. Blumberg E.M., West P.M., Ellis F.W. (1954) A possible relationship between psychological factors and human cancer. *Psychosomatic Medicine*, 16, 277–286.
4. Bhanson C.B., Kissen D.M. (eds) (1966) Psychophysiological aspects of cancer. *Annals of the New York Academy of Sciences*, 125, 775–1055.
5. Bhanson C.B. (ed.) (1969) Second Conference on Psychophysiological Aspects of Cancer, May 1968. *Annals of the New York Academy of Sciences*, 164, 313–634.
6. Kübler-Ross E. (1969) *On Death and Dying*, Simon & Schuster, Touchstone.
7. Cullen J., Fox B., Isom R. (1977) *Cancer: The Behavioral Dimensions*, Raven Press, New York.
8. Cohen J., Cullen J.W., Martin L.R. (1982) *Psychosocial Aspects of Cancer*, Raven Press, New York.
9. American Cancer Society (1982) Proceedings of the Working Conference on the Psychological, Social and Behavioral Medicine Aspects of Cancer: Research and Professional Education Needs and Directions for the 1980s. *Cancer*, 50 (suppl), 1919–1978.
10. American Cancer Society (1984) Workshop Conference on Methodology in Behavioral and Psychosocial Cancer Research, 1983. *Cancer*, 54 (suppl), 2217–2384.
11. Holland J.C. (2002) History of psycho-oncology: Overcoming attitudinal and conceptual barriers. *Psychosomatic Medicine*, 64, 206–221.
12. Mitchell A.J., Chan M., Bhatti H. *et al.* (2011) Prevalence of depression, anxiety, and adjustment disorder in oncological, haematological, and palliative-care settings: A meta-analysis of 94 interview-based studies. *The Lancet Oncology*, 12, 160–174.
13. Grassi L., Biancosino B., Marmai L. *et al.* (2007) Psychological factors affecting oncology conditions. In *Psychological Factors Affecting Medical Conditions. A New Classification for DSM-V* (eds P. Porcelli, N. Sonino), Karger, Basel, vol. 28, pp. 57–71.
14. Grassi L., Riba M. (2009) New frontiers and challenges of psychiatry in oncology and palliative care. In *Advances in Psychiatry, Vol. III* (eds G.N. Christodoulou, M. Jorge, J.E. Mezzich), World Psychiatric Association, pp. 105–114.
15. Grassi L. (2007) Bereavement in families with relatives dying of cancer. *Current Opinions in Supportive and Palliative Care*, 1, 43–49.
16. Baider L., Cooper C.L., De-Nour K. (eds) (2000) *Cancer and the Family*, 2nd edn, John Wiley & Sons, Ltd, Chichester.
17. Pitceathly C., Maguire P. (2003) The psychological impact of cancer on patients' partners and other key relatives: A review. *European Journal of Cancer*, 39, 1517–1524.
18. Glajchen M. (2004) The emerging role and needs of family caregivers in cancer care. *The Journal of Supportive Oncology*, 2, 145–155.
19. Andrykowski M.A., Manne S.L. (2006) Are psychological interventions effective and accepted by cancer patients? I. Standards and levels of evidence. *Annals of Behavioral Medicine*, 32, 93–97.
20. Manne S.L., Andrykowski M.A. (2006) Are psychological interventions effective and accepted by cancer patients? II. Using empirically supported therapy guidelines to decide. *Annals of Behavioral Medicine*, 32, 98–103.
21. Osborn R.L., Demoncada A.C., Feuerstein M. (2006) Psychosocial interventions for depression, anxiety, and quality of life in cancer survivors: Meta-analyses. *International Journal of Psychiatry in Medicine*, 36, 13–34.
22. Johansen C., Grassi L. (2010) International psycho-oncology: Present and future. In *Psycho-Oncology*, 2nd edn (eds J.C. Holland, W.S. Breitbart, P.B. Jacobsen *et al.*), Oxford University Press, New York, pp. 655–659.
23. Canadian Association of Psychosocial Oncology (CAPO) (2010) *Standards of Psychosocial Health Services for Persons with Cancer and their Families* [Approved 28 May 2010], Author. (www.capo.ca)
24. Howell, D., Currie, S., Mayo, S. *et al.* (2009) *A Pan-Canadian Clinical Practice Guideline: Assessment of Psychosocial Health Care Needs of the Adult Cancer Patient*, Canadian Partnership Against Cancer (Cancer Journey Action Group) and the Canadian Association of Psychosocial Oncology, Toronto.
25. Howell D., Keller-Olaman S., Oliver T. *et al.* (2010) *A Pan-Canadian Practice Guideline: Screening, Assessment and Care of Psychosocial Distress (Depression, Anxiety) in Adults with Cancer*, Canadian Partnership Against Cancer (Cancer Journey Action Group) and the Canadian Association of Psychosocial Oncology, Toronto.
26. National Health and Medical Research Council (NHMRC), National Breast Cancer Centre Psychosocial Working Group (1999) *Psychosocial clinical practice guidelines: Information, support and counselling for women with breast cancer*, National Breast Cancer Centre, Camperdown, NSW, Australia.
27. Turner J., Zapart S., Pedersen K. et al.; National Breast Cancer Centre, Sydney, Australia; National Cancer Control Initiative, Melbourne, Australia (2005) Clinical practice guidelines for the psychosocial care of adults with cancer. *Psycho-Oncology*, 14, 159–173.

28. Holland J.C. (1997) Preliminary guidelines for the treatment of distress. *Oncology*, 11, 109–114.
29. Holland J.C., Andersen B., Breitbart W.S. *et al.* (2010) Distress management. *The Journal of the National Comprehensive Cancer Network*, 8, 448–485.
30. Bultz B.D., Carlson L.E. (2006) Emotional distress: The sixth vital sign – future directions in cancer care. *Psycho-Oncology*, 15, 93–95.
31. Bultz B., Berman B.J. (2010) Branding distress as the 6th vital sign: Policy implications, in *Handbook of Psycho-Oncology*, 2nd edn (eds J.C. Holland, W.S. Breitbart, P.B. Jacobsen *et al.*), Oxford University Press, New York, pp. 663–665.
32. Adler N.E., Page A. (eds); Institute of Medicine of the National Academies Committee on Psychosocial Services to Cancer Patients/Families in a Community Setting (2008) *Cancer Care for the Whole Patient: Meeting Psychosocial Health Needs*, National Academies Press, Washington, DC.
33. Council of the European Union (2008) Council Conclusions on reducing the burden of cancer, Luxembourg, 10 June; www.eu2008.si/en/News_and_Documents/Council_Conclusions/June/0609_EPSCO-cancer.pdf (accessed December 2011).
34. Prince M., Patel V., Saxena S. *et al.* (2007) No health without mental health. *Lancet*, 370, 859–877.
35. Holland J., Weiss T. (2008) The new standard of quality cancer care: Integrating the psychosocial aspects in routine cancer from diagnosis through survivorship. *Cancer Journal*, 14, 425–428.
36. Holland J., Watson M., Dunn J. (2011) The IPOS New International Standard of Quality Cancer Care: Integrating the psychosocial domain into routine care. *Psycho-Oncology*, 20, 677–680.
37. International Psycho-Oncology Society (IPOS) (2010) *Statement on Standards and Clinical Practice Guidelines in Cancer Care*, Author.

CHAPTER 2

Communication in Cancer Care: A Cultural Perspective

Phyllis Butow[1] *and Walter F. Baile*[2]
[1]Centre for Medical Psychology and Evidence-based Decision-Making (CeMPED) and the Psycho-Oncology Co-operative Research Group (PoCoG), University of Sydney NSW, Australia
[2]Departments of Behavioral Science and Faculty Development, University of Texas MD Anderson Cancer Center, Houston, Texas, USA

Introduction

The importance of health professional–patient communication in cancer care is now well recognized, and a large number of relevant articles are published each year. In a recent Medline search using the key words 'neoplasms and cancer' and 'communication', 9184 articles were retrieved. However, few of these articles address the particularly complex issues raised by the care of cancer patients within a multicultural society. This chapter attempts to combine a general review of communication in cancer care, with a consideration of these multicultural issues.

Why is communication important?

Communication is considered to be an essential component of good medical practice[1] and is prominently featured in medical and nursing textbooks, and clinical practice guidelines for individual tumours[2] and the psychosocial care of cancer patients.[3] Patient-centred care, most recently defined as 'a moral philosophy, which values considering patients' needs, wants and perspectives; offering patients opportunities to provide input into and participate in their care; and enhancing partnership and understanding in the doctor–patient relationship',[4] has been widely promoted as the gold standard approach. This approach is built on medical ethics that value patient autonomy and well-being.

While effective communication is essential in any medical context, the complex multidisciplinary treatment regimens with significant side-effects, and the particular horror that cancer evokes because of its association with images of extreme debility, pain and death, mean that communication is particularly significant in cancer care. Both patients and health professionals find a cancer diagnosis particularly challenging, despite progress in management turning this from an acute disease with poor prognosis to essentially a chronic disease for many patients.

Most Western countries mandate effective communication at least for information transfer and decision-making. In Australia, for example, a toolkit has been developed to assist health professionals optimize communication (see http://www.nhmrc.gov.au/guidelines/publications). The Australian Council for Safety and Quality in Health Care recently developed an *Australian Charter of Healthcare Rights*,[5] which stipulates amongst other things, that all Australians have the right to receive care that shows respect to them and their

Clinical Psycho-Oncology: An International Perspective, First Edition. Edited by Luigi Grassi and Michelle Riba.

culture, beliefs, values and personal characteristics, receive open, timely and appropriate communication about their health care in a way they can understand, and join in making decisions about their care and health service planning.

Cancer patients value effective communication highly. For example, in two studies of care at the end of life, doctor-patient communication (particularly the quality of information about prognosis and the opportunity to ask questions) dominated aspects of care rated as important by patients and families, who also identified good communication as a critical aspect of medical care.[6,7] Equally, the amount and kind of information patients should be given and the ways in which it should be delivered have been the subject of considerable debate within the medical community, suggesting that this is an issue of great concern to doctors.

There is strong evidence that communication affects cancer patient outcomes, particularly satisfaction, psychological morbidity and understanding,[8,9] although evidence regarding impact on health outcomes is still sparse. Communication challenges are also known to be a large factor in health professional stress and burnout. For example, a survey of 393 British medical oncologists found that 28% suffered from clinical levels of anxiety and depression; the clinicians themselves viewed communication difficulties as contributing significantly to their stress levels.[10]

Relevance of medical communication to psycho-oncology

While psychologists may view communication as a basic part of their therapeutic armorarium, cancer poses challenges for them also. Psychologists face particular communication challenges when they work with patients who are facing bad news, existential challenges, family conflict and end-of-life issues, which they may not encounter elsewhere in their practice. Further, psycho-oncologists are often called upon to teach communication skills to cancer health professionals and therefore need a good understanding of the issues, skills and training methods in cancer communication.

What are the critical tasks in communication?

Traditionally, communication skills training courses have focused on breaking bad news, preparing patients for aversive procedures, giving clear information, promoting shared decision-making, eliciting concerns and responding to emotion.[11–13] Interestingly, a recent Australian survey of 134 cancer specialists conducted in 2008 showed few of these topics appearing in their top 10 communication challenges.[14] The oncologists reported that their most significant challenge was 'Discussing high-cost drugs with patients I know cannot afford them', with 13% reporting having a lot of difficulty with this and 65% reporting some to quite a bit of difficulty. Other commonly experienced communication challenges included discussing treatment failure (67%), the transition from curative to palliative care (60%), a recurrence (60%) and bad test results (59%), and being completely honest about prognosis (38%). Few in fact, reported having difficulty with disclosing a cancer diagnosis, with only 4% reporting some or quite a bit of difficulty with this. It is not known whether other health professionals, or those in other countries, would rate these tasks similarly. In our experience, health professionals value more highly specific training on topics such as gaining consent to clinical trials, discussing expensive treatments, discussing prognosis and end-of-life issues and talking with people from other cultures, than generic skills training.

Cultural issues in communication

While communication is likely to be a challenge for all cancer patients, it is likely to be more so when health professional and patient do not share a cultural heritage. Migration is increasing worldwide, with the number of people who do not speak the dominant language of the country in which they live similarly increasing. In Australia, for example, the 2006 census showed that 24% of Australians were born overseas, 44% had at least one parent born overseas and over 560 000 people (3% of the total population) spoke English poorly or not at all.[15] Thus communication challenges across cultures is no longer a rare issue, but rather something health professionals are likely to face on many occasions over the course of their career.

Immigrants diagnosed with cancer have poorer cancer outcomes than comparable non-immigrant groups, with lower screening and survival rates[16] and higher rates of reported side effects.[17] In a recent systematic review of the literature on psychosocial well-being and immigrants with cancer, meta-analyses indicated significantly higher distress and depression in minority versus mainstream cancer patients not wholly accounted for by differences in socioeconomic status (SES).[18] Immigrants often report that health professionals do not understand them, which may adversely affect their psychological and physical well-being.[19] Personal or historical experiences of discrimination, violence or institutionalized racism may reduce trust in health professionals and institutions.[20] Poor outcomes may also be due to unfamiliarity with health care processes, differing beliefs and attitudes about illness, death and treatment, and language and communication barriers.[21] In a recent study involving focus groups with 73 cancer patients and 18 carers, who had migrated to Australia and spoke Chinese, Greek or Arabic, participants, especially those less acculturated, described feeling alone and misunderstood, failing to comprehend medical instructions, being unable to communicate questions and concerns and a lack of consistency in interpreters and interpretation.[19]

Culture influences most interactions and day to day behaviours. People from the same culture share common systems of symbols, gestures, language and signals that convey information and meaning. Culture also affects responses (e.g. to pain), and attitudes toward illness, disease, death and health care services.[22] Patients have culturally determined beliefs about the causes of diseases, the way the body is structured and functions, and beliefs surrounding the use of complementary and alternative therapies.[23] Religious and spiritual beliefs and practices affect how patients respond to bad news, medical treatments such as transfusions, and end-of-life issues. Thus there is ample opportunity for miscommunication and confusion between health professionals and patients from different backgrounds.

Culture is also a major factor in determining the roles played by patients and clinicians. The 'sick' are expected to behave within certain parameters, as are clinicians. For example, Chinese people have great respect for the expertise of the clinician. Any ambiguity or uncertainty in presenting the diagnosis or treatment recommendations may be viewed as reflecting a lack of expertise.[24]

In most Western countries, such as America, Australia and England, there is currently a strong emphasis on informed consent and active patient involvement in decision-making, inherent in the model of patient-centred care. However, in many other countries, such as France, Italy Japan, the Middle East and Africa, relationships with patients are much more hierarchical, protective and paternalistic. In these cultures, non-disclosure of the truth may be valued in terms of patient protection.[21]

The structure and function of family also differs markedly in different cultures.[21] In many countries, families prefer to have an input into what and when information is given to cancer patients, treatment decisions and the care of patients, particularly towards the end of life, while in some cultures men are seen as carrying the responsibility for decision-making on behalf of other family members. Family members provide key economic and emotional support for each other, and patients are seen as vulnerable and requiring protection lest they lose hope and give up. For example, in a study of Chinese cancer patients and carers living in Australia, the majority said that the family should advise the doctor how much information to give to the patient, and in what manner, as they knew the patient very well.[24] Most patients indicated a preference for the family to be fully informed about issues relating to the illness to allow each family member to contribute as much as possible to the support of the patient. Participants expressed the view that full disclosure of information was important so that that the responsibilities of the sick person could be assumed by others, and appropriate planning for the future could be undertaken.

In Japan, family members are informed of the cancer patient's diagnosis, condition and treatment, before the cancer patient is told the truth.[25] Then all family members, except the patient, discuss whether the cancer diagnosis should be disclosed and the entire family makes a final decision about the truth-telling policy. A survey in Japan of 1918 family caregivers who had recently cared for a cancer patient who died was undertaken in 1992.[25] All family caregivers reported that the physician informed them of the condition and treatment, although only 22.5% of the cancer patients were informed. Similarly, in Saudi Arabia, the patient is viewed as one member of the larger family, and the family is responsible for the patient. The consent for the patient's treatment is usually given by the family, who aims to avoid emotional disturbance to the patient.[26]

How do oncologists navigate these cultural differences? A recent study documented systematic differences in the consultations of cancer patients and oncologists when an immigrant and an interpreter are involved.[27] One hundred and forty-one oncology consultations with 78 patients (47 immigrant and 31 Anglo-Australian) and 115 family members (77 immigrant and 38 Anglo-Australian) were audio-taped and coded. Despite the fact that everything needed to be said twice through the interpreter, doctors spent significantly less time with immigrants with interpreters than with Anglo-Australians, and spent proportionally less time on cancer-related issues, summarizing and informing, and more time on other medical issues and directly advising. Thus they appeared to be taking a more paternalistic approach to immigrants, either in response to patient cues or because of the complexities of the situation. Doctors also tended to delay responses to or ignore more immigrant than Anglo-Australian cues for emotional support. Overall, this suggests that immigrants are experiencing different communication from their oncologists, and these differences may not be optimal for patient well-being and decision-making.

Whilst the provision of interpreters when patients attend medical consultations may potentially address some of these difficulties, a number of studies have revealed problems with medical interpretation, including inaccuracy, inconsistency and confusion regarding the interpreter's role.[28] Medical interpreting standards of practice developed by the International Medical Interpreters Association and Education Development Center (2007) state that interpreters must maintain accuracy, confidentiality, impartiality and professional distance at all times.[29] However, a number of studies have revealed the difficulty which interpreters experience in trying to keep to these standards. Hseih (2006) interviewed medical interpreters in the United States, who reported that they struggled to work within the definition of their role and saw themselves as an advocate for patients.[30]

Interpreters sometimes intervene in consultations in ways that their doctors may not agree with, if they were aware of such changes. For example, in a study of audio-taped oncology consultations,[31] it was found that just under half of all interpretations were not identical to the source speech, and while 70% of the changes were inconsequential or clarified information, in 30% they could have resulted in misunderstanding, non-disclosure or a poorer relationship with the doctor. Some of these changes appeared to have been deliberately made by family member interpreters trying to protect the patient from bad news; others were made by professional interpreters who had either misunderstood the source speech or were trying to navigate the difficult path of remaining culturally appropriate while faithfully interpreting.

Within the palliative care setting, Norris and colleagues[32] conducted a large qualitative study of 68 professional medical interpreters in the United States about communication on end-of-life care. These interpreters emphasized the importance of both doctor and interpreter conveying compassion when delivering bad news. They reported experiencing a tension between providing strict interpretation and being a cultural broker, finding breaking bad news difficult, feeling sometimes abandoned or abused by clinicians and finding it hard to balance the focus on patients and family. Ideally, oncologists and interpreters would work together to negotiate a shared and culturally appropriate approach to the consultation, and ensure the well-being of all parties.

Because of the importance placed on family involvement, some immigrants with cancer may be more likely to bring family members to cancer consultations, and are also likely to bring a greater number of such family members. As noted by Surbone,[33] consultations involving family members or friends tend to be more lengthy and complex than with individual patients. Patients and family members are likely to have different information and support needs, there may be conflict within family members, and between family members and the patient, and generational differences in beliefs and approaches may be apparent. Health professionals may need to provide guidance and support or specific interventions to ensure families work together to the optimal benefit of the patient. A case study demonstrating some of these cultural challenges is presented below.

Case study

Ahmed was a 74-year-old gentleman from Egypt who was brought to the United States for treatment of inoperable gastric cancer. He had been told only that he had an 'ulcer' which needed to be treated and had received front-line anticancer treatment in Egypt without much effect. On arriving at the US hospital his family, who spoke English well, had approached the first-year oncology fellow who was admitting Ahmed and told him that they did not want him told about his disease, even though it was clear to everyone that he was being admitted to a cancer centre. The fellow, who was on his second rotation, told the family that this would be 'unethical' and against hospital policy. The family became quite angry and threatened to take their father home. When the attending physician arrived he found that the nursing staff had been split with some of the staff being sympathetic to the family's wishes and others stating that they could not possibly give chemotherapy to someone who was not informed. The attending, Dr Smith, sat the family down and talked to them in a quiet conference room. He expressed regret that things had gotten to the point where they felt they needed to take their father home. He then sought to understand their concerns about their father. They said that he was a fragile man who was uneducated and that they feared that he would 'give up' if he knew he had cancer. They also remarked that they knew that this might only be superstition but that in their culture when one gives bad news it can sometimes cause such stress that the disease would progress. Dr Smith listened carefully and validated their concerns. 'I can see that this is a difficult situation for you and that you are very concerned about your father. Let me begin by asking you what you think he already knows about his illness.' He was able to discover that the family did indeed think that their father knew he had something serious going on and that he might already have heard the word cancer. Dr Smith expressed appreciation for their honesty. He acknowledged that he understood that in their culture families often do not disclose information about serious illness but also affirmed that, as they surmised, nonetheless patients often know or suspect anyway. He also pointed out that in his experience families often over-estimate the negative impact that information has on the patient and that most patients he treated appreciated the honesty of the doctor, especially when they already suspect that something is seriously amiss. He then made a suggestion that he, the attending, spend some time evaluating their dad. He proposed that during the interview, with the family present, he would ask the patient what he knew about his disease and what he wanted to know. If their father wanted to know, then he would provide information in an honest and hopeful fashion, talking frankly about his disease and the treatments available. If the father did not want to know and wanted the family to make the decisions then he would also respect that.

Dr Smith used an experienced Middle Eastern translator who pretty quickly developed a rapport with Ahmed and his family. He found out that Ahmed did indeed suspect that he was seriously ill. He said that he could see concern 'in the eyes of my family'. He said that he had had a good life and was ready to die and did not want to suffer with harsh treatments but would agree with a course of treatment for the sake of his family. One caveat he insisted on was that if his disease got worse he wanted to stop treatment and return to Egypt where he could be buried.

His family was very touched by this discourse and rallied around their father with expressions of affection and caring. Dr Smith summarized the treatment plan, which all agreed to. Several weeks later Ahmed developed renal failure and the chemotherapy was stopped. He expressed a desire to return to Egypt where he died several weeks later. Dr Smith met with his fellow who agreed that this was an effective way of approaching requests for withholding information from family but was doubtful that he could do it as smoothly. Dr Smith also explained the value of asking for an ethics consult when one is feeling uncomfortable, since often ethical issues involve serious communication challenges. The fellow thought that this might be an option for him.

Insight into the culture of the patient with cancer, their significant others, and the clinician, represents an important starting point to ensure optimal communication. However, while an understanding of culture may be of great benefit to clinicians and other health professionals, an important proviso is awareness of the diversity that exists even within the same culture context. Moreover, generalizations concerning a group linked by cultural factors can lead to stereotyping, rigid rules and a lack of tailoring to individual differences. Thus information about beliefs and practices within particular cultures and ethnic groups never obviates the need for exploring individual preferences and needs.

Ideally, all health professionals involved in cancer care would receive training in cultural competence. Cultural competence incorporates both knowledge of cultural differences and similarities in how cancer patients view their illness, treatment, death and dying, information and involvement in decision-making, and specific skills in eliciting information and involvement preferences, negotiating the potentially differing needs and values of patients, families and the health professional around these issues, and working with interpreters.[33] Lubrano di Ciccone *et al.* (2010) recently reported an evaluation of a training programme for oncologists working with interpreters.[34] This represents an important step forward; training for oncologists will likely produce as many benefits as specialized training for interpreters. Without all stakeholders participating in changed processes, they are unlikely to succeed.

Communication skills training

The notion that communication is a skill is central to the discussion of how we teach and prepare learners to improve their existing communication skills or acquire new skills. Fundamentally, communication is a set of defined verbal and non-verbal behaviours which can be observed, recorded, coded and taught. Take for example the simple behaviour of consciously trying to avoid jargon when providing important information to a patient. Jargon is not uncommon among clinicians and a source of patient dissatisfaction. But when it is pointed out to clinicians, and evidence that it is associated with patient satisfaction is provided, most clinicians are willing to make a conscious effort to practise using explanations geared to a patient's level of understanding, which can then become part of their clinical armamentarium. The same is true for some of the communication behaviours associated with cultural competency. These may include simple behaviours such as learning how to greet people from another culture, when shaking hands may not be appropriate, and how to include different members of the family in history-taking, to more complex behaviours such as how to negotiate with the family about information given to the patient when the news may be bad.

Because skills can be named, described and observed, they can also be taught. The preferred method for learning communication skills is in a simulated environment where standardized patients or actors can be programmed to take the part of patients and/or family members and scripted to present challenges to learners. For example, in Italy where the culture sometimes dictates that families are told the information about a poor prognosis before the patient, Costantini and colleagues have programmed actors to take on the role of the family member who insists that the doctor not tell the patient bad news.[35] Working in small groups, learners can then try out different strategies for addressing this issue with the assistance of a facilitator or coach. This method also promotes group participation and input and lets the learner try out different strategies in a 'stop and restart' format.[36]

Bedside teaching also presents numerous opportunities for learning how to address cultural communication challenges. Whether in the clinic or on rounds, senior physicians can create learning opportunities by setting communication goals for learners prior to patient encounters. For example if a treatment team has bad news to communicate to a family who does not speak their language, this is an opportunity to discuss how to use a translator during the encounter. Issues such as where people should sit, who should be addressed and how to deal with emotions that might arise, can be discussed ahead of time and then debriefed after the encounter. Methods of teaching these skills are only limited by the imagination, and other techniques such as spontaneous role play, case presentations, lectures and video all have a part to play in teaching culturally sensitive communication.

Conclusions

Cross-cultural encounters in medicine are increasing in association with globalization. Culture is reflected in our communications with patients and families[37] and cultural practices can present a challenge to our attitudes towards key communications. Challenges which embody sorting out issues such as 'truth-telling' may illustrate this well, since on the one hand truth-telling is a central communication challenge in cancer care, but on the other cultures define truth differently. When families or persons other than the patient have been the traditional decision-maker in illness, this may challenge attitudes which favour patient autonomy over family decision-making and suggests the need to modify our practice – to negotiate with both the patient and his or her family in regard to care planning. This may require physicians to be aware of their own beliefs and values and to develop not only an understanding but a respect for the beliefs and values of others.[38] While guidelines exist to help negotiate these differences for mutual benefit[39,40] a basic awareness of the importance of cultural difference is essential to the practice of comprehensive cancer care.

Moreover lack of attention to cultural differences can adversely affect the quality of medical care. In non-Western cultures if the details of one's cancer are not shared with family members who are the patient's surrogate decision-makers or if an adversarial relationship develops with those caregivers, important information about the patient's condition may go unheard. Likewise if a practitioner fails to respect cultural norms regarding complementary or alternative medicines, the patient or family may feel disrespected. In Western cultures this is also an important trigger for malpractice litigation.[41] In a Western country, one individual may wish to know and understand all details of their cancer to support their decision-making process, while another may rely more on emotional rapport with the physician to determine for the same process.

Taking a patient history is a routine part of medical practice. Understanding concerns patients may have about their treatment has been emphasized as a key component in providing comprehensive cancer care.[42] We propose that knowing the important areas to ask about when seeking to understand the cultural aspects of a patient and family is also a fundamental step toward comprehensive medical care. Taking such a history involves attention to key elements which result in a comprehensive survey of areas that define culture (see Box 2.1).

Box 2.1 Taking a cultural history

Beliefs, Attitudes and Values that may influence perceptions of illness and the patient's and family's definition of a life worth living. The recognition that while for some cultures illness is a state which is shared by the family and thus family members play an important part in helping decision-making is quite different from situations in which illness is a very private affair to be managed between a person and their doctor.

Language and Health Literacy (role of interpreters, accuracy of translation, metaphoric meanings, as well as understanding of the medical condition and treatment protocols). Use of jargon is an aspect of medical culture which is endemic to discussions between doctors and other health professionals but may confound and confuse patients. For example 'we're going to do a biopsy' may mean little to a person in a rural community who has scarce contact with the medical system.

Affiliations (community ties, religious and spiritual beliefs). Religious ties are extremely important for many patients and frequently religious beliefs may condition whether patients feel obligated to press ahead with treatments that have little medically determined value.

Network (social support system). Extended families, religious communities and social groups may be an important source of social support to the patient during times of navigating the cancer crisis.

Economy (socioeconomic status and community resources). Costs of illness may put significant strain on the patient and family system so that ability to undergo expensive treatments may not be an option for some patients.

Ambiance (living situation and family structure). Living in an ambiance which is satisfactory for one person may not be an option for another; for example a bone marrow patient who is exposed post-transplant to chronically ill persons or children.

Challenges (of work environment). Some work environments are supportive to patients and others may leave the patient with no alternative to retire, forcing a major decision about a life change on the patient.

Likewise it is also important to be aware of communication pitfalls that might occur when taking a cultural history: These include:

- Making assumptions about the amount of detail or information a patient may or may not want to receive;
- Being aware of our own prejudices toward certain cultures which may get in the way of providing them with optimum care;
- Disrespecting cultural norms about the role of others in the patient's illness;
- Overlooking the support of the patient's ethnic community in providing support;
- Assuming that because a patient is a part of a social or ethnic group they desire information in one way or another.

In sum it requires conscious intentionality or 'emotional labour' to adopt a strategy of openness to understanding others' cultural beliefs. Rather than finding ourselves 'reacting' to other cultures when they clash with our belief systems, one might include aspects of the cultural history in each patient evaluation. This is consistent with a recently articulated 'patient-centred' model of communication in oncology where the role of the physician is focused as much on healing the illness as treating the disease.[43] If this is so, then understanding how culture can shape coping and communication will deepen the relationship with the patient and family and improve the outcomes of care. Understanding culture can also enhance patient compliance and contribute to reducing health care disparities for minority and underserved patients. It also broadens our perspective on the human condition.[44,45]

Finally, educating clinicians as to the importance of cultural issues and the need to develop a cultural approach to patients is essential. While the Association of American Medical Colleges has recognized the importance of including training in cultural competency, its implementation has not been standardized.[46,47] In many pluralistic societies opportunities for teaching trainees cultural sensitivity and competency exist in many patient encounters. We need innovative approaches to mentoring students and doctors-in-training, sharing cultural experiences, and discussing cross-cultural differences during clinical work. Observations on the meaning of suffering in our communities of patients, and how individuals and families cope when a member is very ill or has died can provide a window on the differences that exist between cultures. Taking a cultural history can provide a tremendous amount of knowledge regarding cultural differences and similarities. Reflecting with students on how their own families cope differently with illness can complement the teaching of humanistic medicine in a way that teaches not only tolerance to various cultural practices but also how culture is woven into the very fabric of human experience.

Key points

- Effective communication is a key component of effective clinical care.
- Cultural competence is a key element within communication skills. Culture impacts on patient responses (e.g. to pain), and knowledge of and attitudes toward illness, disease, death and health care services.
- Culture impacts on the roles patients, family members and doctors expect to play, preferences for information delivery and how decisions are made.
- Communication across cultures can be challenging, especially if language barriers are present. Using an interpreter and taking a competent cultural history can be an important step in improving cross-cultural encounters.
- Communication skills training is an important tool to increase the cultural competence of cancer health professionals.

Suggested further reading

Surbone A., Baile W.F. (2010) *Pocket Guide to Cultural Competence*. Accessed at http://www.mdanderson.org/icare

Matthews-Juarez P., Weinberg A.D. (2004) *Cultural Competence in Cancer Care. A Health Care Professionals Passport*, Office of Minority Health, Health Resources and Services Administration, U.S. Department of Health and Human Services, Rockville, MD.

References

1. Donabedian A. (1988) The quality of care. How can it be assessed? *Journal of the American Medical Association*, 260, 1743–1748.
2. Australian Cancer Network Melanoma Guidelines Revision Working Party (2008) *Clinical Practice Guidelines for the Management of Melanoma in Australia and New Zealand*, Cancer Council Australia and Australian Cancer Network, Sydney and New Zealand Guidelines Group, Wellington, NZ.
3. National Breast Cancer Centre and National Cancer Control Initiative (2003) *Clinical Practice Guidelines for the Psychosocial Care of Adults with Cancer*, National Breast Cancer Centre, Camperdown, NSW.
4. Epstein R.M., Franks P., Fiscella K. *et al.* (2005) Measuring patient-centered communication in patient-physician consultations: Theoretical and practical issues. *Social Science & Medicine*, 61, 1516–1528.
5. http://www.safetyandquality.gov.au/internet/safety/publishing.nsf/Content/com-pubs_ACHR-roles/$File/17537-charter.pdf (last accessed December 2011).
6. Steinhauser K.E., Christakis N.A., Clipp E.C. *et al.* (2000) Factors considered important at the end of life by patients, family, physicians, and other care providers. *Journal of the American Medical Association*, 284, 2476–2482.
7. Wenrich M.D., Curtis J.R., Shannon S.E. *et al.* (2001) Communicating with dying patients within the spectrum of medical care from terminal diagnosis to death. *Archives of Internal Medicine*, 161, 868–874.
8. Uitterhoeve R.J., Bensing J.M., Grol R.P. *et al.* (2010) The effect of communication skills training on patient outcomes in cancer care: A systematic review of the literature. *European Journal of Cancer Care*, 19, 442–457.
9. Schofield P.E., Butow P.N., Thompson J.F. *et al.* (2003) Psychological responses of patients receiving a diagnosis of cancer. *Annals of Oncology*, 14, 48–56.
10. Ramirez A.J., Graham J., Richards M.A. *et al.* (1995) Burnout and psychiatric disorder among cancer clinicians. *British Journal of Cancer*, 71, 1263–1269.
11. Grainger M.N., Hegarty S., Schofield P. *et al.* (2010) Discussing the transition to palliative care: Evaluation of a brief communication skills training program for oncology clinicians. *Palliative and Supportive Care*, 8, 441–447.
12. Brown R., Bylund C.L., Eddington J. *et al.* (2010) Discussing prognosis in an oncology setting: Initial evaluation of a communication skills training module. *Psycho-Oncology*, 19, 408–414.
13. Fukui S., Ogawa K., Ohtsuka M., Fukui N. (2009) Effect of communication skills training on nurses' detection of patients' distress and related factors after cancer diagnosis: A randomized study. *Psycho-Oncology*, 18, 1156–1164.
14. Dimoska A., Girgis A., Hansen V. *et al.* (2008) Perceived difficulties in consulting with patients and families: A survey of Australian cancer specialists. *Medical Journal of Australia*, 189, 612–615.
15. Australian Bureau of Statistics (2006) *Australian Social Trends, 2006* (4102.0), ABS, Canberra.
16. Du X.L., Meyer T.E., Franzini L. (2007) Meta-analysis of racial disparities in survival in association with socioeconomic status among men and women with colon cancer. *Cancer*, 109, 2161–2170.
17. Krupski T.L., Sonn G., Kwan L. *et al.* (2005) Ethnic variation in health-related quality of life among low-income men with prostate cancer. *Ethnicity & Disease*, 15, 461–468.
18. Luckett T., Goldstein D., Butow P.N. *et al.* The psychological well-being and quality of life of minority cancer patients compared to the mainstream: A systematic review and meta-analysis. *The Lancet Oncology*, (in press).
19. Butow P., Sze M., Dugal-Beri P. *et al.* (2010) From inside the bubble: Migrants' perceptions of communication with the cancer team. *Supportive Care in Cancer*, DOI: 10.1007/s00520-010-0817-x.
20. Gonzalez G. (1997) Health care in the United States: A perspective from the front line, in *Communication with the Cancer Patient: Information and Truth* (eds A. Surbone, M. Zwitter), The New York Academy of Sciences, NY, pp. 211–222.
21. Moore R., Butow P. (2005) Culture and oncology: Impact of context effects, in *Cancer, Communication and Culture* (ed. D. Speigel), Kluwer Academic/Plenum Publishers, New York.
22. Cleeland C.S., Gonin R., Baez L. *et al.* (1997) Pain and treatment of pain in minority patients with cancer. The Eastern Cooperative Oncology Group Minority Outpatient Pain Study. *Annals of Internal Medicine*, 127, 813–816.

23. Kaptchuk T.J. (2002) The placebo effect in alternative medicine: Can the performance of a healing ritual have clinical significance? *Annals of Internal Medicine*, 136, 817–825.
24. Huang X., Butow P.N., Meiser M. *et al.* (1999) Communicating in a multi-cultural society: The needs of Chinese cancer patients in Australia. *Australian and New Zealand Journal of Medicine*, 29, 207–213.
25. Uchitomi Y., Yamawaki S. (1997) Truth-telling practice in cancer care in Japan, in *Communication with the Cancer Patient: Information and Truth* (eds A. Surbone, M. Zwitter), The New York Academy of Sciences, NY, pp. 290–300.
26. Younge D., Moreau P., Ezzat A., Gray A. (1997) Communicating with cancer patients in Saudi Arabia, in *Communication with the Cancer Patient: Information and Truth* (eds A. Surbone, M. Zwitter), The New York Academy of Sciences, NY, pp. 309–316.
27. Butow P.N., Bell M.L., Goldstein D. *et al.* Grappling with cultural differences; Communication between oncologists and immigrant cancer patients. *Patient Education and Counseling* (in press).
28. Flores G. (2005) The impact of medical interpreter services on the quality of health care: A systematic review. *Medical Care Research and Review*, 62, 255–299.
29. Medical Interpreting Standards of Practice Developed by the International Medical Interpreters Association & Education Development Center, Inc. Adopted October, 1995. Massachusetts Medical Interpreters Association. Copyright © 2007, 1998, 1997, 1996 by Massachusetts Medical Interpreters Association, now International Medical Interpreters Association and Education Development Center, Inc.
30. Hsieh E. (2006) Conflicts in how interpreters manage their roles in provider–patient interactions. *Social Science & Medicine*, 62, 721–730.
31. Butow P.N., Goldstein D., Bell M.L. *et al.* (2011) Interpretation in consultations with immigrant cancer patients; How accurate is it? *Journal of Clinical Oncology*, 29, 2801–2807.
32. Norris W.M., Wenrich M.D., Nielsen E.L. *et al.* (2005) Communication about end-of-life care between language-discordant patients and clinicians: Insights from medical interpreters. *Journal of Palliative Medicine*, 8, 1016–1024.
33. Surbone A. (2008) Cultural aspects of communication in cancer care. *Supportive Care in Cancer*, 16, 235–240.
34. Lubrano di Ciccone B., Brown R.F., Gueguen J.A. *et al.* (2010) Interviewing patients using interpreters in an oncology setting: Initial evaluation of a communication skills module. *Annals of Oncology*, 21, 27–32.
35. Costantini A., Baile W.F., Lenzi R. *et al.* (2009) Overcoming cultural barriers to giving bad news: Feasibility of training to promote truth-telling to cancer patients. *Journal of Cancer Education*, 24, 180–185.
36. Back A.L., Arnold R.M., Tulsky J.A. *et al.* (2003) Teaching communication skills to medical oncology fellows. *Journal of Clinical Oncology*, 21, 2433–2436.
37. Surbone A. (2006) Cultural aspects of communication in cancer care, in *Communication in Cancer Care. Recent Results Cancer Research* (ed. R Stiefel), Springer-Verlag, Heidelberg, vol. 168, pp. 91–104.
38. Dana R.H. (1993) *Multicultural Assessment Perspectives for Professional Psychology*, Allyn & Bacon, Inc., Boston, MA.
39. Surbone A., Baile W.F. (2010) *Pocket Guide to Cultural Competence*. Accessed at http://www.mdanderson.org/icare.
40. Matthews-Juarez P., Weinberg A.D. (2004) *Cultural Competence in Cancer Care. A Health Care Professionals Passport*, Office of Minority Health, Health Resources and Services Administration, U.S. Department of Health and Human Services, Rockville, MD.
41. Beckman H.B., Markakis K.M., Suchman A.L., Frankel R.M. (1994) The doctor–patient relationship and malpractice. Lessons from plaintiff depositions. *Archives of Internal Medicine*, 154, 1365–1370.
42. Baile W.F., Palmer J.L., Bruera E., Parker P.A. (2011) Assessment of palliative care patients' most important concerns. *Supportive Care in Cancer*, 19, 475–481.
43. Epstein R.M., Street R.L., Jr (2007) *Patient-Centered Communication in Cancer Care: Promoting Healing and Reducing Suffering*, National Cancer Institute, NIH Publication No. 07-6225, Bethesda, MD.
44. Surbone A. (2010) Cultural competence in oncology: Where do we stand? *Annals of Oncology*, 21, 3–5.
45. Fox R.C. (2005) Cultural competence and the culture of medicine. *New England Journal of Medicine*, 353, 1316–1319.
46. Weissman J.S., Betancourt J., Campbell E.G. *et al.* (2005) Resident physicians' preparedness to provide cross-cultural care. *Journal of the American Medical Association*, 294, 1058–1067.
47. Khanna S.K., Cheyney M., Engle M. (2009) Cultural competency in health care: Evaluating the outcomes of a cultural competency training among health care professionals. *Journal of the National Medical Association*, 101, 886–892.

CHAPTER 3

Psychosocial Assessment and Screening in Psycho-oncology

Paul B. Jacobsen and Kristine A. Donovan
Department of Health Outcomes and Behavior, Moffitt Cancer Center, Tampa, FL, USA

Introduction

Psychosocial assessment has played and continues to play a key role in the international development of psycho-oncology. This development of psycho-oncology has been spurred, in part, by research that used psychosocial assessment instruments to document the negative impact of cancer and its treatment on patients' emotional well-being. The need to address these problems led to many of the same assessment instruments also being used as outcomes in research evaluating the benefits of pharmacological and psychosocial interventions for maintaining or improving patients' emotional well-being. In both instances, the field has been advanced across cultures and countries by having instruments available that possessed good psychometric properties and were suitable for use with people with cancer. In this chapter, we identify and provide descriptions of psychosocial assessment instruments commonly used in psycho-oncology research, including multinational studies, and summarize evidence regarding the relative merits of these instruments. The focus of our review is on anxiety, depression and distress since these are among the most common ways in which emotional well-being has been assessed in psycho-oncology research.

More recently, there has been growing interest, on an international scale, in extending the use of psychosocial assessment instruments from research into everyday clinical practice. This interest has been driven, in part, by national clinical practice guidelines and consensus statements which recommend that patients' emotional well-being be routinely assessed in order to identify patients who may be in need of psychosocial care.[1,2] These recommendations have stimulated considerable research collaborations examining how well brief assessment instruments function as screening tools for detecting clinically significant problems in emotional well-being. In this chapter, we identify a number of brief psychosocial assessment instruments that could be used for screening purposes and summarize available evidence regarding how well they might function if used for this purpose.

The growth of psycho-oncology on an international scale provides exciting opportunities for expanding collaborative research and making psychosocial care available to more patients in more countries and cultures. It also presents a challenge since many psychosocial assessment instruments were not developed with international and multinational use in mind. Consequently, in this chapter we also review the issues involved in translating, adapting and validating measures that were created for use in one language or country for use in other languages and countries.

Clinical Psycho-Oncology: An International Perspective, First Edition. Edited by Luigi Grassi and Michelle Riba.

Major issues and available evidence

Judging the relative merits of available psychosocial assessment instruments for use with cancer patients in any country or culture is a complex task. Among the issues to be considered are: (1) the criteria by which to select measures to review; (2) the criteria by which to evaluate the measures; (3) the evidence to be used as part of the evaluation process; and (4) the evaluation of the available evidence. In preparing this chapter, we are fortunate to be able to draw upon two recently published systematic reviews of English language psychosocial assessment instruments used to measure anxiety, depression and distress in cancer patients.[3,4] We focus here on English language instruments because most of the existing instruments either originated in English or have been translated from their native language into English. Since the procedures used to address the issues listed above differ considerably between the two publications, a description of the methods used in each review is warranted.

Identification of instruments and relevant studies

In 2009, Vodermaier and colleagues published a systematic review designed to identify and evaluate instruments used to screen for emotional distress in cancer patients.[4] Toward this end, the authors conducted searches of MEDLINE and PsycINFO for English language studies using search terms consistent with their operational definition of distress. For purposes of this review, distress was defined as 'a state of negative affect that is suggestive of affective disorders (i.e. minor or major depressive disorder and dysthymia), anxiety disorders, and adjustment disorders (depressive, anxious, or mixed)'.[4] Studies were included in the review if they attempted to validate an interviewer-administered or standardized self-administered instrument in a sample of cancer patients. The review was further restricted to studies evaluating measures comprised of 50 or fewer items. This process led to identification of 33 instruments. Table 3.1 includes those instruments identified by the authors that were evaluated in more than one study.

In 2010 Luckett and colleagues published a systematic review designed to identify and evaluate instruments used to assess anxiety, depression and distress in randomized controlled trials (RCTs) of psychosocial interventions for people with cancer.[3] Toward this end, the authors conducted searches of MEDLINE, PsycINFO, Embase, AMED, CENTRAL, and CINAHL for RCTs of psychosocial interventions conducted with English-speaking samples of cancer patients using search terms used in previous systematic reviews of psychosocial interventions for cancer patients. The search was further limited to the previous 10 years in order to give less consideration to instruments that may have become obsolete. The authors acknowledge that distress is less well defined than anxiety or depression and is often used as an umbrella term for any unpleasant emotional experience. Consistent with this view, they included instruments assessing mood, emotion, or stress along with those explicitly described as distress measures. This process resulted in identification of 30 instruments. Table 3.1 lists those instruments identified by the authors that were evaluated in more than one RCT.

As shown in Table 3.1, a total of 35 instruments were found to have been evaluated in more than one study by Vodermaier *et al.*[4] or more than one RCT by Luckett *et al.*[3] Readers seeking more information about a particular instrument are guided to source references listed in the right-hand column. Given the different search methods, it is not surprising that only 5 of the 35 instruments were identified in both reviews. The resulting list includes measures that assess only depression, anxiety, or distress (e.g. BDI) as well as instruments that measure more than two or more of these constructs (e.g. HADS). It also includes instruments in which items assessing anxiety, depression, or distress are embedded with items measuring other constructs (e.g. POMS). Although the list is comprised mostly of self-report instruments, it also includes interviewer administered measures (e.g. HRSD). Based on the number of studies identified in either review, the 10 most frequently studied instruments in descending order

Table 3.1 Evaluated measures of anxiety, depression and distress.

Name	Acronym	Scales	No. items	No. studies (Review)[a]	Reference
Beck Depression Inventory	BDI	Dep	21	4(V)	(28)
Beck Depression Inventory II	BDI-II	Dep	21	10(L)	(29)
Beck Depression Inventory-Short Form	BDI-SF	Dep	13	2(V)	(30)
Brief Symptom Inventory	BSI	Anx, Dep, Dis	53	2(L)	(31)
Brief Symptom Inventory-18	BSI-18	Dis	18	4(V)	(32)
Calgary Symptoms of Stress Inventory	C-SOSI	Anx, Dep	56	2(L)	(33)
Center for Epidemiologic Studies Depression Scale	CES-D	Dep	20	21(L), 4(V)	(34)
Derogatis Affect Balance Scale	DABS	Anx, Dep	40	2(L)	(35)
Distress Thermometer	DT	Dis	1	2(L), 15(V)	(36)
Edmonton Symptom Assessment Scale	ESAS	Anx, Dep	9	2(V)	(37)
Edinburgh Postnatal Depression Scale	EPDS	Dep	10	4(V)	(38)
General Health Questionnaire-12	GHQ-12	Dis	12	2(V)	(39)
General Health Questionnaire-28	GHQ-28	Anx, Dep	28	1(L), 2(V)	(39)
Hamilton Depression Rating Scale	HDRS	Dep	21	2(L)	(40)
Hospital Anxiety and Depression Scale	HADS	Anx, Dep, Dis	14	20(L), 41(V)	(41)
Impact of Event Scale	IES	Dis	15	3(V)	(42)
Memorial Anxiety Scale for Prostate Cancer	MAX-PC	Anx	18	3(V)	(43)
Mental Health Inventory-18	MHI-18	Anx, Dep	18	3(L)	(44)
Mood Evaluation Questionnaire	MEQ	Dep	23	2(V)	(45)
Patient Health Questionnaire-9	PHQ-9	Dep	9	2(L), 2(V)	(8)
Positive and Negative Affect Schedule	PANAS	Dis	5	5(L)	(46)
Profile of Mood States	POMS	Anx, Dep, Dis	65	25(L)	(47)
Profile of Mood States-11	POMS-11	Dis	11	2(L)	(48)
Profile of Mood States-30	POMS-30	Anx, Dep, Dis	30	6(L)	(49)
Psychological Distress Inventory	PDI	Dis	13	2(V)	(50)
Psychosocial Screen for Cancer	PSSCAN	Anx, Dep, Dis	21	2(V)	(51)
PTSD Checklist	PCL-C	Anx	9	3(V)	(52)
Question – Single: Depressed	Q-S:D	Dep	1	6(V)	(53)
Question – Single: Lost Interest	Q-S:LI	Dep	1	2(V)	(53)
Question – Combined: Depressed and Lost Interest	Q-C:D&LI	Dep	2	3(V)	(53)
Questionnaire on Stress in Cancer Patients-Revised	QCS-R	Dis	23	2(V)	(12)
Rotterdam Symptom Checklist	RSCL	Dis	30	8(V)	(54)
State-Trait Anxiety Inventory	STAI	Anx	40	30(L)	(55)
Symptom Checklist-90-Revised	SCL-90-R	Anx, Dep, Dis	90	5(L)	(56)
Zung Self-Rating Depression Scale	ZSDS	Dep	20	6(V)	(57)

[a] L = Luckett *et al.*[3]; V = Vodermaier *et al.*[4]

were: the HADS, various versions of the POMS, the STAI, the CES-D, and the various versions of the BDI.

The review by Vodermaier *et al.*[4] evaluated the psychometric characteristics of all the instruments identified using the studies retrieved. As noted above, the current chapter considers only those instruments from this review that were evaluated in more than one study with cancer patients. Selected aspects of the psychometric evaluations of these measures conducted by the authors appear in Table 3.2.

In the review by Luckett *et al.*,[3] the instruments identified underwent another level of filtering that included elimination of measures deemed suitable for use only in specific cancer populations as well

Table 3.2 Summary of evaluative information for measures of anxiety, depression and distress.

Instrument acronym	Reliability		Validity	Availability of comparison data	Ability to identify treatment effects	Screening performance		Overall rating	
	Vodermaier *et al.*, 2009	Luckett *et al.*, 2010	Luckett *et al.*, 2010	Luckett *et al.*, 2010	Luckett *et al.*, 2010	Vodermaier *et al.*, 2009	Luckett *et al.*, 2010	Vodermaier *et al.*, 2009	Luckett *et al.*, 2010
BDI	High					High		Excellent	
BDI-SF	Low					Moderate		Poor	
BSI		0	5	10	5		0		50
BSI-18	High	0	5	10	5	High	0	Good	50
C-SOSI		5	0	0	0		0		27.5
CES-D	High	5	5	5	10	High	10	Excellent	55
DT	Moderate	0	5	5	5	Moderate	0	Fair	40
ESAS						Moderate		Fair	
EPDS	High					Moderate		Good	
GHQ-12		0	0	5	0	Moderate	5	Good	27.5
GHQ-28	High	0	0	5	0	High	5	Excellent	37.5
HADS	High	5	5	10	10	Moderate	5	Good	77.5
IES	High					Low		Poor	
MAX-PC	High							Poor	
MEQ	High					Moderate		Poor	
PHQ-9	High							Poor	
POMS		5	5	5	10		0		55
POMS-11		0	5	0	5		0		30
PDI	High					Moderate		Good	
PSSCAN	High					High		Good	
PCL-C	High					Moderate		Good	
Q-S:D						Moderate		Good	
Q-S:LI						Moderate		Moderate	
Q-C:D&LI						High		Excellent	
QCS-R	High					High		Good	
RSCL	High					Moderate		Good	
SCL-90-R		5	5	5	5		0		47.5
ZSDS	Low					Moderate		Poor	

as instruments in which one third or more of the items were considered likely to be confounded by cancer or its treatment. Searches of databases were then conducted for the remaining measures to identify additional published studies besides the RCTs that contained data regarding the reliability and validity of the measures in English-speaking cancer samples. As noted above, the current chapter considers only those instruments from this review that were evaluated in more than one RCT. Selected aspects of the psychometric evaluations of these measures conducted by the authors also appear in Table 3.2.

Reliability

Both reviews conducted evaluations of the statistical reliability of the instruments that met inclusion criteria. In the review by Vodermaier *et al.*,[4] the evaluation focused on the internal consistency reliability of the instrument. Specific cut-points for reliability statistics were used to classify an instrument's reliability as 'low', 'moderate', or 'high'. In the review by Luckett *et al.*,[3] the quality of the evidence for reliability (both internal consistency and test-retest) was assessed using a checklist adapted from other reviews. Evidence quality was then assigned one of three scores: 0 (no evidence or poor reliability), 5 (inconsistent reliability or from one or two studies only), or 10 (generally consistent evidence for reliability from several studies).

Since the two reviews used different criteria, it is not surprising that the few instruments rated in both publications received differing evaluations. For example, the CES-D received the best possible rating (high) in the Vodermaier *et al.* review,[4] but a rating indicating only limited or inconsistent evidence of reliability in the Luckett *et al.* review.[3]

More importantly, none of the instruments rated by Luckett *et al.*[3] and summarized in Table 3.2 received the highest possible rating, whereas most (83%) of the instruments rated by Vodermaier *et al.*[4] and summarized in Table 3.2 received the highest possible rating. This pattern suggests that the criteria used by Luckett *et al.*[4] were much more stringent and might discount evidence of acceptable reliability obtained in only a few studies.

Validity

Only one of the reviews evaluated validity as defined in the classic psychometric sense. Specifically, Luckett *et al.*[4] considered the quality of the evidence for each instrument's convergent, divergent, criterion and predictive validity with English-speaking cancer populations. Once again, evidence was summarized using a three-point scale: 0 (no evidence or poor validity), 5 (inconsistent validity or from one or two studies only), or 10 (generally consistent evidence for validity from several studies). None of the instruments reviewed by the authors and summarized in Table 3.2 received the highest possible rating. However, several instruments that are among the ones more widely used in RCTs in psycho-oncology research (e.g. CES-D, HADS and POMS) earned the second highest rating.

Availability of comparison data

The availability of comparison data showing how individuals in the general population and large groups of cancer patients score on a psychosocial instrument is extremely useful for both research and clinical purposes. With regard to research, these data can be used in observational studies to understand the extent to which the average patient in the sample under study is more or less anxious, depressed, or distressed than the average person in the general population or the average cancer patient in a larger reference group. The data can also be used in intervention studies to understand the extent to which participants in an intervention study were more or less anxious, depressed, or distressed than the average person in the general population or the average cancer patient in a larger reference group before and after they did or did not receive the intervention under study. With regard to clinical work, these data can be used at the level of the individual patient to understand how much more or less anxious, depressed, or distressed he/she is than the general population reference group or a cancer patient reference group. Information of this type can be very helpful for understanding the acuity of a patient's need for psychosocial care as well as the benefits a patient may or may not have derived from the psychosocial care he/she was provided. The usefulness of comparison data is further enhanced when it is also available for population subgroups based on demographic characteristics (e.g. age and gender) or disease or treatment characteristics in the case of cancer patient comparison data. These features allow for closer comparison of the sample or patient of interest to a larger group of individuals with similar characteristics.

Only one of the reviews evaluated the availability of comparison data. Specifically, Luckett *et al.*[4] considered the quality of the comparison data using a three-point scale: 0 (no or minimal comparison data available), 5 (substantial comparison data available from large-scale studies), or 10 (comparison data available for subgroups (e.g. age and gender in cancer and general populations)). Three of the instruments reviewed by the authors and summarized in Table 3.2 received the highest possible rating (i.e. BSI, BSI-18 and HADS). Six other measures reviewed by the authors and summarized in Table 3.2 received the second highest rating (i.e. CES-D, DT, GHQ-12, GHQ-28, POMS and SCL-90-R).

Screening performance

As noted previously, there is considerable interest on a national and international scale in extending the use of psychosocial assessment instruments from research into everyday clinical practice. Much of this interest has focused on the use of psychosocial assessments to routinely screen cancer patients in order to identify those individuals experiencing clinically significant anxiety, depression, or distress who should undergo evaluation and/or be referred to experts in psychosocial care. Toward this end, numerous studies have evaluated the performance characteristics of English language psychosocial assessment instruments when cut-off scores are applied for purposes of classifying the severity of cancer patients' anxiety, depression, or distress. Evaluation of performance characteristics in this regard typically involve evaluating the extent to which the classifications obtained using the instrument correspond with those that are obtained using a 'gold standard' classification instrument. For example, the utility of a cut-off score for an instrument assessing depressive symptomatology might be evaluated by performing comparisons with those classifications obtained using an established structured clinical interview to identify the presence or absence of a mood disorder based on DSM-IV criteria.[5] Evaluations are often performed by calculating the sensitivity and specificity of classifications based on the instrument under study relative to those made independently using the gold-standard measure. In this example, sensitivity would refer to the proportion of people with a mood disorder who scored at or above the cut-off score on the instrument under evaluation, and specificity would refer to the proportion of people without a mood disorder who scored below the cut-off score on the instrument under evaluation.

Both reviews conducted evaluations of the screening performance of English language psychosocial assessment instruments that met inclusion criteria. In the review by Vodermaier *et al.*,[4] specific cut-points for averaged sensitivity and specificity statistics were used to classify an instrument's validity for use in screening as 'low', 'moderate', or 'high'. The evidence reviewed included studies in which the instrument was compared to classifications (based on increasing order of strength) from clinical diagnoses to validated questionnaires to structured clinical interviews. In the review by Luckett *et al.*,[3] the quality of the evidence was evaluated in terms of the instrument's criterion validity relative to a diagnostic interview. The quality of the evidence was then assigned one of three scores: 0 (no evidence or unsatisfactory screening performance), 5 (inconsistent screening performance or from one study only), or 10 (generally consistent evidence for screening performance).

Seven measures reviewed by Vodermaier *et al.*[4] and summarized in Table 3.2 scored 'high' in screening performance. They were the BDI, BSI-18, CES-D, GHQ-28, PSSCAN, Q-C:D&LI and QCS-R23. Only one measure reviewed by Luckett *et al.*[3] earned the highest possible rating. It was the CES-D, which also earned the highest rating in the review by Vodermaier *et al.*[4] Three other measures (i.e. GHQ-12, GHQ-28 and HADS) earned the second highest rating. Of these measures, two (i.e. GHQ-12 and HADS) were rated 'moderate' and one (GHQ-28) was rated 'high' in the review by Vodermaier *et al.*[4]

In addition to identifying the instruments that scored highest among all those evaluated, it is worthwhile to consider the screening performance of brief psychosocial assessment instruments. The rationale for focusing on this subset is that the relative brevity of these instruments may more readily lend them to routine use as screeners in busy clinical settings across cultures and countries. Adopting a criterion of 10 items or less as indicative of brevity, seven brief psychosocial instruments were evaluated in one or both reviews: the DT, EPDS, PHQ-9, PCL-C, Q-S:D, Q-S:LI, Q-C:D&LI. With the exception of the DT, these measures were evaluated for their screening performance only in the review by Vodermaier *et al.*[4]

The Q-C:D&LI was the only instrument to obtain the highest possible rating. The instrument consists of two questions that correspond with DSM-IV criteria required for diagnosing Major Depressive Disorder.[5] Specifically, the questions correspond with the requirement that either depressed mood or loss of interest or pleasure in usual activities must be present along with four other symptoms for Major Depressive Disorder to be present. Evidence for the utility of this approach includes a study conducted with terminally ill cancer patients in which these two questions were found to possess good sensitivity and specificity (>90%) relative to diagnoses of major and minor depressive episodes based on a structured clinical interview.[6]

Five other measures (DT, EPDS, PCL-C, Q-S:D, Q-S:LI) obtained 'moderate' ratings. The DT was also evaluated in the review by Luckett *et al.*,[3] in which it received a rating of '0'. This low rating probably reflects a dearth of studies in which the DT was evaluated relative to a diagnostic interview, the principal evidence used to determine screening performance in this review. Additional information about the screening performance of the one-item DT comes from a systematic review by Mitchell[7] published in 2007 of the diagnostic accuracy of the DT and other very short methods in detecting cancer-related mood disorders. Of the 38 analyses identified, 19 involved the DT. This number of analyses is testament to the widespread interest in the use of the DT as a screening measure. Among the author's main conclusions is that the DT and similar very brief instruments comprised of one to four items are relatively accurate as screening measures in ruling out the presence of heightened distress relative to longer methods;[7] on the other hand, they are relatively inaccurate in ruling in the presence of heightened distress relative to longer methods.[7] In other words, among patients who score below the cut-off on the DT a relatively low proportion will be found to be experiencing heightened distress using longer established instruments; however, among patients who score above the cut-off on the DT a relatively high proportion will be found not to be experiencing heightened distress using longer established instruments. These features suggest that the DT and similar very short measures can be used by themselves to successfully identify patients not experiencing clinically significant distress. However, patients identified as experiencing clinically significant distress using the DT and similar measures may need to undergo additional evaluation to confirm these findings.

The PHQ-9 is a nine-item depression screening measure developed for use in primary care settings[8] that has demonstrated excellent properties as a screener for Major Depressive Disorder in a variety of clinical populations.[9] When the reviews by Vodermaier *et al.*[4] and Luckett *et al.*[3] were conducted, the PHQ-9 had yet to be systematically evaluated as a screening tool with cancer patients. In 2011, Thekkumpurath *et al.* published the results of a study evaluating the PHQ-9 with this population.[9] They found that it possessed good sensitivity and specificity (i.e. >80%) relative to diagnoses of Major Depressive Disorder based on a structured interview using a cut-off score derived from the study data. Assuming independent replication of these findings, the PHQ-9 is likely to be positively reviewed in future evaluations of psychosocial assessment instruments used with cancer patients.

Overall performance

In both reviews, an overall performance rating was assigned to each of the English language instruments that were evaluated. In the review by Vodermaier *et al.*,[4] the overall rating was derived using decision rules that took into account the relative merits of the instrument with regard to its reliability, the criterion measures to which its performance as a screening measure were compared, and its performance as a screening measure relative to the criterion measure(s) used. Accordingly, the overall rating primarily reflects an instrument's performance as a screener. Based on these criteria, four instruments summarized in Table 3.2 earned the highest rating of 'excellent': the BDI, CES-D, GHQ-28 and Q-C:D&LI. In the review by Luckett *et al.*,[3] the overall rating was derived based on differential weighting of the relative merits of an instrument with regard to its: validity, reliability, ability to identify treatment effects, performance as a screener relative to a diagnostic interview, available comparison data, number of constructs assessed, length, ease of administration and cognitive burden. The resulting scores (ranging from 0 to 100) thus reflect a relative broad-based evaluation of an instrument's merits. Among those instruments summarized in Table 3.2, the five most highly rated in descending order were: the HADS, the POMS and CES-D (tied), the BSI/BSI-18 (evaluated as a single instrument), and the SCL-90-R.

Cultural considerations

Given the burgeoning international practice of psycho-oncology,[10] it is important to consider psychosocial screening and assessment from a multicultural perspective. Minimally, this involves the use of existing measures to document the negative effects of cancer and its treatment and to measure the outcomes of psychosocial interventions among cancer patients in different countries and cultures. Although many of the instruments in Table 3.1 were initially published in English in predominantly English-speaking countries, this is not universally the case. For example, the RSCL[11] was developed by researchers in the Netherlands and was originally published in the Dutch language. Similarly, the QCS-R[12] originated in Germany in the German language. Before each of these instruments can be used in another country, it must be translated from the original language to the language in most common use in the other country.

Instrument translation is intended to produce different language versions of an instrument that are conceptually equivalent in another country or culture.[13] Translation from the original language should produce a foreign language version that is understandable, acceptable, and performs as close to the original version as possible.[14,15] Use of the forward-translation and back-translation procedures is a well-known and widely accepted method of translating screening and assessment instruments. This method involves several steps,[16] including forward translation, back translation, pre-testing and cognitive interviewing or committee review, and development of the final version of the foreign language version. Forward translation of an English language instrument, for example, involves a native speaker of the target language with a high fluency in English translating the measure into the target language. The emphasis should be on a conceptual translation, not a literal one. Back translation uses the same approach as forward translation, but the instrument is translated back to English by a different translator, independent of the first, who is a native English speaker and who is fluent in the language from which the instrument is being back-translated. Pre-testing of the instrument should include persons who are representative of those who will be administered the instrument. So, for example, an English language instrument designed to assess psychological distress in cancer patients and translated into Italian might be pre-tested with a sample of Italian hospital inpatients who have recently undergone surgery for newly detected cancers, as opposed to a sample of men and women from the general population in Italy. Similarly, within the United States, a Spanish language version of an instrument might be pretested with a group of individuals with cancer who identify themselves as Hispanic or Latino Americans with a preference for communicating in Spanish. Cognitive interviewing after pre-testing entails debriefing the respondents in detail about each item and exploring their qualitative responses to the items.[17] Finally, the final version of the instrument should take into account and reflect the results of each of the steps outlined above.

Researchers and clinicians who have translated a screening or assessment instrument into a language different from the original often rely on the initial validation study of the instrument to score and interpret the translated instrument.[14] This approach suggests, perhaps naively, that psychosocial aspects of cancer do not differ across countries or cultures. Before a foreign language instrument can be used in a target country it should be tested and validated for use in the population for which it is intended. Validation also is important because key words used in an instrument may not translate well or may not even exist in another language. For example, the literal translation of the word 'distress' into the French language does not have the same connotations as the English word, and according to Dolbeault *et al.*,[18] can be translated into a number of French words without or without the French translation of the adjective 'psychological'. Although the English language version of the DT refers only to 'distress', Dolbeault *et al.*[18] opted to include a reference to the psychological state in their adaptation of the DT. Another pointed, though relatively minor, example supporting the need for validating a translated measure is item nine of the HADS which includes the idiom 'butterflies in the stomach'. Literal replication of this expression in the Chinese language, for example, seems to miss the intent of the item and there is not an equivalent expression in Chinese.[19]

Validation testing also is important because different language versions of an instrument may perform differently from the original instrument.[14] Validation testing of a foreign language version may establish a different latent structure for the instrument, for example. Results of a validation study by Leung *et al.*[19] of the Chinese version of the HADS in a sample of Chinese medical students yielded three factors rather than the more commonly considered two-factor structure of the original English language instrument. According to the authors, the third factor was a 'somatic' factor reflecting a somatization tendency among Chinese people. Other validation studies of the HADS also suggest inconsistency in the factor structure of this instrument when adapted and translated into another language. See for example, studies of the Italian translations of the HADS.[20,21] Different language versions of an instrument also may have different cut-off scores for indicating clinically significant problems in emotional well-being, reflecting differences among countries and cultures.[22] Translation of the DT is one such example. The DT was first published in English in 1998.[23] It has been translated and adapted for use in a number of languages and its psychometric properties examined (see Table 3.3). An initial validation study by Jacobsen *et al.*[24] of the English language version demonstrated that a cut-off score of 4 yields optimal sensitivity and specificity relative to the HADS and BSI-18 for identifying clinically significant distress. However, as shown in Table 3.3, the optimal cut-off score varies by country; different language versions perform differently. Most studies indicate that a cut-off score of 4 maximizes sensitivity and specificity relative to an established criterion; however, cut-off scores as low as 2 and as high as 7 have been reported. The cut-off score also varies in relation to the characteristics of the patients being screened and by the setting. Costantini and colleagues[20] further suggest that a cut-off score should take into account the costs and benefits of screening; these may vary over time, by the socioeconomic status of a region or country in which care is provided, and by healthcare system.[10] Different circumstances may require different cut-off scores.

Translation, adaptation and validation studies of a foreign language version of an instrument provide some international perspective on the current state of psychosocial screening and assessment. The various translated versions of the DT, for example, are evidence of the widespread awareness of the need for psychological and social support of persons diagnosed with and treated for cancer. Validation studies of existing instruments serve to determine whether an instrument is psychometrically sound in the target language and may help to establish whether an instrument is equivalent to the original language version. Whether scores on the instrument are influenced by cultural factors is more difficult to determine; although versions of an instrument may demonstrate similar psychometric properties, scores may be different in countries with different cultural patterns of perceiving and expressing emotions as well as differences in the promotion of emotional well-being.[25] Cross-cultural validity may be challenging, if not impossible, to determine. That is, although researchers may postulate that differences in performance of an instrument may be due to cultural or linguistic influences,[16] results of a validation study for an instrument across diverse settings and samples of patients cannot always be generalized to other countries or different language versions of the instrument.

Cross-cultural validity is most accurately established with a multinational or international study, wherein multiple translations of an instrument are administered to a homogeneous study sample across multiple countries or cultures, and differences across countries or cultures are examined in systematic fashion.[26] An example of this is a study by de Haes and Olschewski,[27] which investigated the use of the RSCL as part of the 'ZEBRA' study, a multinational randomized trial comparing standard

Table 3.3 Summary of translations of the Distress Thermometer.

First author and citation	Language version	Translation process	Sample size	Position in care trajectory	Recommended cut-off score	Area under curve	Sensitivity (number and relative to what instrument)	Specificity (number and relative to what instrument)
Jacobsen[24]	English		308	Diagnosed an average of 2.5 (SD = 4.23) years previously	4	0.80 with HADS; 0.78 with BSI-18	0.77 relative to HADS; 0.70 relative to BSI-18	0.68 relative to HADS; 0.70 relative to BSI-18
Ozalp[58]	Turkish	Translated from English into Turkish by two psychiatrists. Bilingual Turkish individual blinded to original questionnaire then translated it back into English. Native English speaker also compared original and back-translated version of DT.	182	Diagnosed an average of 13.86 (SD = 12.97) months previously (range = 30 days to 132 months)	4	0.66 with HADS	0.73 relative to HADS	0.49 relative to HADS
Shim[59]	Korean	Two Koreans (a psychologist and psychiatrist) translated DT into Korean language	108	Mean number of months since diagnosis was 14.3 (SD = 20.3)	4	0.75 with HADS-T; 0.75 with HADS-A; 0.76 with HADS-D	0.83 relative to HADS-T; 0.86 relative to HADS-A; 0.79 relative to HADS-D	0.59 relative to HADS-T; 0.56 relative to HADS-A; 0.61 relative to HADS-D
Tang[60]	Chinese	Not reported	574	Not reported	4	0.803 with HADS; 0.834 with SCL-90	0.803 relative to HADS; 0.872 relative to SCL-90	0.699 relative to HADS; 0.718 relative to SCL-90
Wang[61]	Mandarin	Translated into Mandarin by two study authors. Mandarin version reviewed by the remainder of research team for editorial input. Back translation performed by another professional staff member who had not read English language version.	128	Mean number of months since diagnosis was 5.4 (SD = 16.4)	4	0.89 with psychiatric diagnoses via a clinical interview	0.98 relative to psychiatric diagnoses via a psychiatric interview	0.73 relative to psychiatric diagnoses via a psychiatric interview

Gessler[62]	English (United Kingdom)	No translation	171	Not reported	4 with HADS and BSI-18; 3 with GHQ-12	0.88 with HADS; 0.87 with BSI-18; 0.79 with GHQ-12	0.79 relative to HADS; 0.88 relative to BSI-18; 0.68 relative to GHQ-12	0.81 relative to HADS; 0.74 relative to BSI-18; 0.78 relative to GHQ-12
Bulli[63]	Italian	Unknown origin of Italian version; a back-translation into English was performed by native English speaker. This version was then compared with original English version.	290	Roughly 50% were within 1 year of diagnosis	7	0.84 with Psychological Distress Inventory	0.73 relative to Psychological Distress Inventory	0.82 relative to Psychological Distress Inventory
Gunnarsdottir[22]	Icelandic	Translated from English to Icelandic by six health care professionals and back-translated by certified translator, specialized in medical translations. Number of possible translations discussed and group agreed anonymously on translation chosen for distress.	149	≤2 months since diagnosis = 8.7%, 2–14 months = 39.6%, 15 months – 5 years = 27.5%, >5 years = 4.7%, missing = 4.7%	3	0.75 with HADS; 0.74 with GHQ-30	Cut-off score of 4: 0.72 relative to HADS; cut-off score of 3: 0.77 relative to GHQ-30	Cut-off score of 4: 0.69 relative to HADS; cut-off score of 3: 0.61 relative to GHQ-30
Bidstrup[64]	Danish	Not reported	333	<4 weeks after diagnosis	2 vs. 3	0.86 with HADS	0.99 relative to HADS	0.36 relative to HADS
SEPOS Group[65]	Italy, Spain, Portugal, Switzer-land	Not reported	312	Diagnosed with cancer between 6 months and 2 years previously	> 4	0.77 with HADS	0.65 relative to HADS	0.79 relative to HADS

(Continued)

Table 3.3 *(Continued)*

First author and citation	Language version	Translation process	Sample size	Position in care trajectory	Recommended cut-off score	Area under curve	Sensitivity (number and relative to what instrument)	Specificity (number and relative to what instrument)
Tuinman[66]	Dutch	Not reported	277	Diagnosed an average of 1.8 years before study participation (range, from 3 weeks to 17 years)	5	0.80 with HADS	0.85 relative to HADS	0.67 relative to HADS
Akizuki[67]	Japanese	Translated first from English into Japanese. Bi-lingual Japanese individual blinded to original questionnaire then translated it back into English. Native English speaker compared original and back-translated questionnaires, and after discussing translation, final Japanese version prepared.	275	Not reported	4/5	Not reported	0.84 relative to diagnostic interview based on DSM-IV criteria	0.61 relative to diagnostic interview based on DSM-IV criteria
Dolbeault[18]	French	Involved conciliation discussions between clinicians specialized in psycho-oncology; adaptation reported as Psychological Distress Scale	561	82% more than 12 months since diagnosis	3	Not reported	0.76 relative to HADS	0.82 relative to HADS
Cohen[68]	Hebrew, Arabic, Russian	Distress item given to experts who could not reach conclusive decision of optimal Hebrew or Arabic word; writing exercise with graduate students revealed two groups of synonyms closest to meaning and use of words 'emotional distress'; experts agreed to split item into 2 items; original and adapted tool translated into Russian by back-translation; Russian-speaking experts found two-item tool more suitable for use.	496	Diagnosed an average of 28 months previously	3	0.63 with HADS; 0.74 with BSI-18	0.74 relative to HADS; 0.64 relative to BSI-18	0.65 relative to HADS; 0.64 relative to BSI-18

chemotherapy or temporary ovarian ablation by hormonal treatment for the management of node positive stage II breast cancer in pre- or peri-menopausal women aged 50 years or less. Patients (n = 519) from 13 different countries divided into 6 subsamples or clusters based on language and cultural background (Eastern Europe, English-speaking, Finland, French-speaking, German and Latin) completed the RSCL at baseline and three months after the start of treatment. Significant differences between cultures at entry into the trial were observed for each of the RSCL subscales: psychological distress, physical distress, global quality of life and activity level. According to de Haes and Olschewski,[27] patients were differentially distressed based on their cultural origin. French-speaking patients, for example, reported a mean of 34.9 $\pm$ 23.0 on the subscale measuring psychological distress versus 25.8 $\pm$ 16.6 for patients from the Eastern European countries of Hungary, the Czech Republic and Slovakia. The level of change from baseline to three months was also different across cultures for psychological distress, global quality of life and activity level, but not physical distress. Patients from English-speaking countries (Australia, Ireland and the United Kingdom) reported a mean decrease of 8.5 $\pm$ 18.3 in psychological distress versus a mean decrease of 0.1 $\pm$ 18.5 for patients in the Latin cluster (Argentina, Portugal and Spain). The authors speculated that experiential differences among cultures might have accounted, at least in part, for the study findings; that perhaps, for example, patients from a more extraverted country might be more inclined to express negative experiences and that the way information is conveyed to patients might differ across countries, resulting in differences in how patients adjust to their illness. The authors suggested that, minimally, study results could not automatically be generalized across the various countries and cultures. In general, this study suggests that multinational studies of screening and assessment instruments may serve to make context-specific values available for comparison purposes, improve the instruments themselves, and help to develop revised international versions of specific screening and assessment instruments.[25,27]

Summary and conclusions

Numerous self-report instruments are available to assess the key psychosocial constructs of anxiety, depression and distress. Psycho-oncology professionals seeking to identify which measure(s) to use in their research or clinical practice are well advised to consider the relative merits of these instruments in making their selection. Important issues to consider include the reliability of the measure, as indexed by its internal consistency as well as its consistency of measurement over time. Validity is also important and can be indexed in multiple ways including convergent validity (correspondence with measures of similar constructs), divergent validity (lack of correspondence with measures of dissimilar constructs), criterion validity (correspondence with characteristics captured by a non-test measure), and predictive validity (ability to predict future behaviour or performance). Beyond the traditional considerations of reliability and validity, the availability of comparison data is of particular relevance in psycho-oncology. These data can be used to understand the extent to which an individual patient or group of patients is more or less anxious, depressed, or distressed than the average patient in the general population or the average cancer patient in a larger reference group. This chapter has provided detailed information from two recent systematic reviews about the relative merits of many commonly used English language self-report instruments on these dimensions. This information can be quite helpful in guiding clinicians and researchers to better performing measures.

Clinical case study

The following case example illustrates how psychosocial assessment instruments can contribute to the care of people with cancer. Ms Jones is a 55-year-old married female who is about to start receiving chemotherapy for treatment of stage II breast cancer. The—Cancer Centre where she is receiving treatment conducts routine screening for distress with all patients at specified intervals such as the start of chemotherapy. Ms Smith's score of 7 out of 10 on the Distress Thermometer exceeds the cut-off score of 4 used at this institution to identify distressed patients. A social worker at the centre subsequently meets with Ms Smith who reports that she has felt increasingly depressed since her breast cancer diagnosis. The social worker administers the nine-item Patient Health Questionnaire (PHQ-9) to further evaluate the extent of Ms Smith's depressive symptomatology. Ms Smith's score of 15 out of 27 strongly suggests the presence of Major Depressive Disorder. Based on this finding, the social worker refers the patient to a psychiatrist at the centre who confirms the diagnosis of Major Depressive Disorder using a structured clinical interview. Prior to starting the patient on antidepressant medication, the psychiatrist has the patient complete the Beck Depression Inventory-II (BDI-II). Ms Smith's score of 27 out of 63 on the BDI-II indicates that she has moderately severe depression and her responses to individual items show that she is experiencing a variety of somatic and non-somatic symptoms. Repeated administrations of the BDI-II at subsequent visits indicate that Ms Smith's depressive symptoms have markedly decreased following prescription of antidepressant medication. After six months of treatment, Ms Smith score of 14 on the BDI-II indicates that her symptoms are of mild severity and diagnostic interviewing confirms that she no longer meets criteria for Major Depressive Disorder.

In recent years, there has been growing interest in using psychosocial assessment measures to routinely screen cancer patients in order to identify those individuals who are experiencing clinically significant anxiety, depression and distress. These data can then be used to decide which patients might benefit from further evaluation or referral to experts in psychosocial care. Evaluation of screening performance typically involves calculating the sensitivity and specificity of classification made using the screening measure relative to those made using a longer well-established measure or another established method of classifying individuals (e.g. a diagnostic psychiatric interview). This chapter has provided detailed information from two recent systematic reviews about the screening performance of a number of relatively brief English language self-report instruments relative to 'gold standard' classifications based on established measures or clinician interviews. In addition, the chapter includes information from other sources bearing on the performance of two of the more commonly used screening measures (i.e. the DT and the PHQ-9). The information provided herein can help to guide clinicians and researchers to better performing screening measures.

The international scope of psychosocial oncology necessitates that psychosocial assessment and screening be considered from a multicultural perspective. Clinicians and researchers frequently identify a self-report instrument developed in one language that they wish to have available in another language. Although simply translating the measure from one language to another may seem sufficient, the reality is considerably more complex. Certain words and idioms may be difficult to translate from one language to another and, consequently, the wording of the original measure may need to be adapted as well as translated. In addition, one cannot assume that the validity demonstrated by a measure in its original language generalizes to the translated version of the measure. Indeed, there is considerable evidence suggesting that different language versions of a measure can perform quite differently with regard to validity. Accordingly, strong consideration should be given to collecting new validity data by administering the translated/adapted version of a measure to native speakers of the language of the newly created version. This consideration is particularly important if a measure is going to be used in a multinational study and data are going to be aggregated or compared across linguistic or cultural groups.

Key points

- Numerous self-report instruments are available to assess the key psychosocial constructs of anxiety, depression and distress.
- Psycho-oncology professionals trying to decide which instrument to use are well advised to consider the relative merits of various instruments with regard to their reliability, validity and the availability of comparison data.
- In trying to select a brief measure to be used for screening purpose, it is important to consider its performance relative to longer well-established measures or to another established method of identifying clinically significant problems (e.g. diagnostic psychiatric interview).

- The international scope of psychosocial oncology necessitates that psychosocial assessment and screening be considered from a multicultural perspective.
- Adapting a measure developed in one language for use in another language involves much more than simply translating it.

Key references

Bullinger M., Anderson R., Cella D., Aaronson N. (1993) Developing and evaluating cross-cultural instruments from minimum requirements to optimal models. *Quality of Life Research*, 2, 451–459.

Guillemin F., Bombardier C., Beaton D. (1993) Cross-cultural adaptation of health-related quality of life measures: Literature review and proposed guidelines. *Journal of Clinical Epidemiology*, 46, 1417–1432.

Institute of Medicine (2008) *Cancer Care for the Whole Patient: Meeting Psychosocial Health Needs*, National Academies Press, Washington, DC.

Luckett T., Butow P.N., King M.T. *et al.* (2010) A review and recommendations for optimal outcome measures of anxiety, depression, and general distress in studies evaluating psychosocial interventions for English-speaking adults with heterogeneous cancer diagnoses. *Supportive Care in Cancer*, 18, 1241–1262.

McNair D.M., Lorr M., Droppleman L. (1992) *Manual for the Profile of Mood States (POMS): Revised*, Educational and Industrial Testing Service, San Diego, CA.

Mitchell A.J. (2007) Pooled results from 38 analyses of the accuracy of the Distress Thermometer and other ultra-short methods of detecting cancer-related mood disorders. *Journal of Clinical Oncology*, 25, 4670–4681.

National Comprehensive Cancer Network (2010) NCCN clinical practice guidelines in oncology: Distress management. *Journal of the National Comprehensive Cancer Network*, 8, 448–485.

Van de Vijver F., Hambleton P.M. (1996) Translating tests: Some practical guidelines. *European Psychologist*, 2, 89–99.

Vodermaier A., Linden W., Siu C. (2009) Screening for emotional distress in cancer patients: A systematic review of assessment instruments. *Journal of the National Cancer Institute*, 101, 1464–1488.

Zabora J., Brintzenhofe Szoc K., Jacobsen P. *et al.* (2001) A new psychosocial screening instrument for use with cancer patients. *Psychosomatics*, 42, 241–246.

Zigmond A.S., Snaith R. (1983) The Hospital Anxiety and Depression Scale. *Acta Psychiatrica Scandinavica*, 67, 361–370.

Suggested further reading

Johansen C., Grassi, L. (2010) International psycho-oncology: Past, present, and future, in *Psycho-Oncology*, 2nd edn (eds J.C. Holland, W.S. Breitbart, P.B. Jacobsen *et al.*), Oxford University Press, New York.

Mitchell, A.J. (2010) Screening procedures for psychosocial distress, in *Psycho-Oncology*, 2nd edn (eds J.C. Holland, W.S. Breitbart, P.B. Jacobsen *et al.*), Oxford University Press, New York.

Pirl, W.F. (2010) Instruments in psycho-oncology, in *Psycho-Oncology*, 2nd edn (eds J.C. Holland, W.S. Breitbart, P.B. Jacobsen *et al.*), Oxford University Press, New York.

References

1. Institute of Medicine (2008) *Cancer Care for the Whole Patient: Meeting Psychosocial Health Needs*, National Academies Press, Washington, DC.
2. National Comprehensive Cancer Network (2010) NCCN clinical practice guidelines in oncology: Distress management. *Journal of the National Comprehensive Cancer Network*, 8, 448–485.
3. Luckett T., Butow P.N., King M.T. *et al.* (2010) A review and recommendations for optimal outcome measures of anxiety, depression, and general distress in studies evaluating psychosocial interventions for English-speaking adults with heterogeneous cancer diagnoses. *Supportive Care in Cancer*, 18, 1241–1262.
4. Vodermaier A., Linden W., Siu C. (2009) Screening for emotional distress in cancer patients: A systematic review of assessment instruments. *Journal of the National Cancer Institute*, 101, 1464–1488.
5. American Psychiatric Association (1994) *Diagnostic and Statistical Manual of Mental Disorders*, 4th edn, American Psychiatric Association, Washington, DC.
6. Chochinov H.M., Wilson K.G., Enns M., Lander S. (1997) "Are you depressed?" Screening for depression in the terminally ill. *American Journal of Psychiatry*, 154, 674–676.
7. Mitchell A.J. (2007) Pooled results from 38 analyses of the accuracy of the Distress Thermometer

and other ultra-short methods of detecting cancer-related mood disorders. *Journal of Clinical Oncology*, 25, 4670–4681.

8. Spitzer R.L., Kroenke K., Williams J. (1999) Patient Health Questionnaire primary care study group. Validation and utility of a self report version of PRIME-MD: The PHQ primary care study. *Journal of the American Medical Association*, 282, 1737–1744.
9. Thekkumpurath P., Walker J., Butcher I. *et al.* (2011) Screening for depression in cancer outpatients: The diagnostic accuracy of the 9-item Patient Health Questionnaire. *Cancer*, 117, 218–27.
10. Johansen C., Grassi L. (2010) International psycho-oncology: Present and future, in *Psycho-Oncology*, 2nd edn (eds J.C. Holland, W.S. Breitbart, P.B. Jacobsen *et al.*), Oxford University Press, New York.
11. de Haes J.C., van Knippenberg F.C., Neijt J.P. (1990) Measuring psychological and physical distress in cancer patients: Structure and application of the Rotterdam Symptom Checklist *British Journal of Cancer*, 62, 1034–1038.
12. Herschbach P., Keller M., Knight L. *et al.* (2004) Psychological problems of cancer patients: A cancer distress screening with a cancer-specific questionnaire. *British Journal of Cancer*, 91, 504–511.
13. Harkness J.A., Schoua-Glusberg A. (1998) Questionnaires in translation, in *ZUMA Nachrichten Spezial No. 3 Cross-Cultural Survey Equivalence* (ed. J.A. Harkness), ZUMA, Mannheim.
14. Sperber A.D. (2004) Translation and validation of study instruments for cross-cultural research. *Gastroenterology*, 126, S124–S128.
15. Van de Vijver F., Hambleton R.K. (1996) Translating tests: Some practical guidelines. *European Psychologist*, 1, 89–99.
16. Guillemin F., Bombardier C., Beaton D. (1993) Cross-cultural adaptation of health-related quality of life measures: Literature review and proposed guidelines. *Journal of Clinical Epidemiology*, 46, 1417–1432.
17. Willis G.B. (2005) *Cognitive Interviewing: A tool for improving questionnaire design*, Sage Publishing, Inc., Thousand Oaks.
18. Dolbeault S., Bredart A., Mignot V. *et al.* (2008) Screening for psychological distress in two French cancer centers: Feasibility and performance of the adapted distress thermometer. *Palliative and Supportive Care*, 6, 107–117.
19. Leung C.M., Ho S., Kan C.S. *et al.* (1993) Evaluation of the Chinese version of the Hospital Anxiety and Depression Scale. A cross-cultural perspective. *International Journal of Psychosomatics*, 40, 29–34.
20. Costantini M., Musso M., Viterbori P. *et al.* (1999) Detecting psychological distress in cancer patients: Validity of the Italian version of the Hospital Anxiety and Depression Scale. *Supportive Care in Cancer*, 7, 121–127.
21. Annunziata M.A., Muzzatti B., Altoe G. (2011) Defining Hospital Anxiety and Depression Scale (HADS) structure by confirmatory factor analysis: A contribution to validation for oncological settings. *Annals of Oncology*, 22, 2330–2333.
22. Gunnarsdottir S., Thorvaldsdottir G.H., Fridriksdottir N. *et al.* The psychometric properties of the Icelandic version of the Distress Thermometer and Problem List. *Psycho-Oncology* (in press).
23. Roth A.J., Kornblith A.B., Batel-Copel L. *et al.* (1998) Rapid screening for psychologic distress in men with prostate carcinoma: A pilot study. *Cancer*, 82, 1904–1908.
24. Jacobsen P.B., Donovan K.A., Trask P.C. *et al.* (2005) Screening for psychologic distress in ambulatory cancer patients. *Cancer*, 103, 1494–1502.
25. Herrmann C. (1997) International experiences with the Hospital Anxiety and Depression Scale: A review of validation data and clinical results. *Journal of Psychosomatic Research*, 42, 17–41.
26. Bullinger M., Anderson R., Cella D., Aaronson N. (1993) Developing and evaluating cross-cultural instruments from minimum requirements to optimal models. *Quality of Life Research*, 2, 451–459.
27. de Haes J.C., Olschewski M. (1998) Quality of life assessment in a cross-cultural context: Use of the Rotterdam Symptom Checklist in a multinational randomised trial comparing CMF and Zoladex (Goserlin) treatment in early breast cancer. *Annals of Oncology*, 9, 745–750.
28. Beck A.T., Ward C.H., Mendelson M. *et al.* (1961) An inventory for measuring depression. *Archives of General Psychiatry*, 4, 561–571.
29. Beck A.T., Steer R.A., Brown G.K. (1996) *BDI-II Manual*, The Psychological Corporation, San Antonio, TX.
30. Beck A.T., Rial W.Y., Rickels K. (1974) Short form of depression inventory: Cross validation. *Psychological Reports*, 34, 1184–1186.
31. Derogatis L.R., Melisaratos N. (1983) The Brief Symptom Inventory: An introductory report. *Psychological Medicine*, 13, 595–605.
32. Zabora J., Brintzenhofe Szoc K., Jacobsen P. *et al.* (2001) A new psychosocial screening instrument for use with cancer patients. *Psychosomatics*, 42, 241–246.

33. Carlson L.E., Thomas B.C. (2007) Development of the Calgary Symptoms of Stress Inventory (C-SOSI). *International Journal of Behavioral Medicine*, 14, 249–256.
34. Center for Epidemiologic Studies (1971) *Center for Epidemiologic Studies Depression Scale (CES-D)*, National Institute of Mental Health, Rockville, MD.
35. Derogatis L.R., Rutigliano P. (1996) Derogatis Affects Balance Scale (DABS), in *Quality of Life and Pharmacoeconomics in Clinical Trials* (ed. B. Spiker), Lippincott-Raven, Philadelphia, PA.
36. Roth A.J., Kornblith A., Batel-Copel L. *et al.* (1998) Rapid screening for psychologic distress in men with prostate carcinoma: A pilot study. *Cancer*, 82, 1904–1908.
37. Bruera E., Kuehn N., Miller M.J. *et al.* (1991) The Edmonton Symptom Assessment System: A simple method for the assessment of palliative care patients. *Journal of Palliative Care*, 7, 6–9.
38. Cox J.L., Holden J.M., Sagovsky R. (1987) Detection of postnatal depression: Development of the 10-item Edinburgh Postnatal Depression Scale. *British Journal of Psychiatry*, 150, 782–786.
39. Goldberg D., Williams P. (1988) *A User's Guide to the General Health Questionnaire (GHQ)*, GL Assessment, London.
40. Hamilton M. (1976) Development of a rating scale for primary depressive illness. *British Journal of Social and Clinical Psychology*, 6, 278–296.
41. Zigmond A.S, Snaith R. (1983) The Hospital Anxiety and Depression Scale. *Acta Psychiatrica Scandinavica*, 67, 361–370.
42. Horowitz M., Wilner N., Alvarez W. (1979) Impact of event scale: A measure of subjective stress. *Psychosomatic Medicine*, 41, 209–218.
43. Roth A.J., Rosenfeld B., Kornblith A.B. *et al.* (2003) The Memorial Anxiety Scale for Prostate Cancer: Validation of a new scale to measure anxiety in men with prostate cancer. *Cancer*, 97, 2910–2918.
44. Veit C.T., Ware J. (1983) The structure of psychological distress and well-being in general populations. *Journal of Consulting and Clinical Psychology*, 51, 730–42.
45. Meyer H.A., Sinnott C., Seed P.T. (2003) Depressive symptoms in advanced cancer: The Mood Evaluation Questionnaire. *Palliative Medicine*, 17, 596–603.
46. Watson D., Clark L., Tellegen A. (1988) Development and validation of brief measures of positive and negative affect: The PANAS scale. *Journal of Personality and Social Psychology*, 54, 1063–1070.
47. McNair D.M., Lorr M., Droppleman L. (1992) *Manual for the Profile of Mood States (POMS): Revised*, Educational and Industrial Testing Service, San Diego, CA.
48. Cella D.F., Jacobsen P., Orav E. *et al.* (1987) A brief POMS measure of distress for cancer patients. *Journal of Chronic Diseases*, 40, 939–942.
49. McNair D.M., Heuchert J. (2003) *Profile of Mood States Technical Update*, MHS, North Tonawanda.
50. Morasso G., Costantini M., Baracco G. *et al.* (1996) Assessing psychological distress in cancer patients: Validation of a self-administered questionnaire. *Oncology*, 53, 295–302.
51. Linden W., Yi D., Barroetavena M.C. *et al.* (2005) Development and validation of a psychosocial screeing instrument for cancer. *Health and Quality of Life Outcomes*, 3, 54.
52. Weathers F.W., Huska J.A., Keane T.M. (1991) *PCL-C for DSM-IV*, National Center for PTSD – Behavioral Science Division, Boston, MA.
53. Spitzer R.L., Williams J.B., Gibbon M., First M.B. (1992) The Structured Clinical Interview for DSM-III-R (SCID): I. History, rationale, and description. *Archives of General Psychiatry*, 49, 624–629.
54. de Haes J.C.J.M., van Knippenberg F.C.E., Neijt J.P. (1990) Measuring psychological and physical distress in cancer patients: Structure and application of the Rotterdam Symptom Checklist. *British Journal of Cancer*, 62, 1034–1038.
55. Spielberger C.D., Gorsuch R., Lushene R. *et al.* (1983) *Manual for the State-Trait Anxiety Inventory*, Consulting Psychologists, Palo Alto, CA.
56. Derogatis L.R., Lipman R., Covi L. (1973) SCL-90: An outpatient psychiatric rating scale. Preliminary report. *Psychopharmacology Bulletin*, 9, 13–28.
57. Zung W.W. (1965) A self-rating depression scale. *Archives of General Psychiatry*, 12, 63–70.
58. Ozalp E., Cankurtaran E.S., Soygur H. *et al.* (2007) Screening for psychological distress in Turkish cancer patients. *Psycho-Oncology*, 16, 304–311.
59. Shim E.J., Shin Y.W., Jeon H.J., Hahm B.J. (2008) Distress and its correlates in Korean cancer patients: Pilot use of the distress thermometer and the problem list. *Psycho-Oncology*, 17, 548–555.
60. Tang L., Zhang Y., Pang Y. *et al.* (2011) Validation and Reliability of Distress Thermometer in Chinese Cancer Patients. *Clinical Journal of Cancer Research*, 23, 54–58.
61. Wang G.L., Hsu S.H., Feng A.C. *et al.* (2011) The HADS and the DT for screening psychosocial distress of cancer patients in Taiwan. *Psycho-Oncology*, 20, 639–646.

62. Gessler S., Low J., Daniells E. *et al.* (2008) Screening for distress in cancer patients: Is the distress thermometer a valid measure in the UK and does it measure change over time? A prospective validation study. *Psycho-Oncology*, 17, 538–547.
63. Bulli F., Miccinesi G., Maruelli A. *et al.* (2009) The measure of psychological distress in cancer patients: The use of Distress Thermometer in the Oncological Rehabilitation Center of Florence. *Supportive Care in Cancer*, 17, 771–779.
64. Bidstrup P.E., Mertz B.G., Dalton S.O. *et al.* Accuracy of the Danish version of the 'distress thermometer'. *Psycho-Oncology* (in press).
65. The SEPOS Group, Gil F., Grassi L. *et al.* (2005) Use of distress and depression thermometers to measure psychosocial morbidity among southern European cancer patients. *Supportive Care in Cancer*, 13, 600–606.
66. Tuinman M.A., Gazendam-Donofrio S.M., Hoekstra-Weebers J.E. (2008) Screening and referral for psychosocial distress in oncologic practice: Use of the Distress Thermometer. *Cancer*, 113, 870–878.
67. Akizuki N., Akechi T., Nakanishi T. *et al.* (2003) Development of a brief screening interview for adjustment disorders and major depression in patients with cancer. *Cancer*, 97, 2605–2613.
68. Cohen, M., Gagin, R., Cinamon, T. *et al.* Translating 'distress' and screening for emotional distress in multicultural cancer patients in Israel. *Quality of Life Research* (in press).

CHAPTER 4

Sexuality and Gender: Psychosocial Implications in Cancer Patients: A Multicultural Perspective

Anna Costantini[1], *Chiara M. Navarra*[1], *Kimlin Tam Ashing-Giwa*[2] *and Sophia Yeung*[2]

[1]Psychoncology Unit, Department of Oncological Sciences, Sant'Andrea Hospital, Sapienza University of Rome, Italy
[2]Center of Community Alliance for Research & Education, Department of Population Sciences, City of Hope National Medical Center, Duarte, CA, USA

Introduction

The World Health Organization (WHO) 2006[1] defines sexual health as a crucial aspect in the life of a human being which includes sexuality, gender identity and role, sexual orientation, eroticism, pleasure, intimacy and reproduction. It is experienced and expressed in thoughts, fantasies, desires, convictions, attitudes, values, behaviours, practices and relations. Sexuality affects almost every aspect of human life: from the way one perceives oneself as male or female to how we structure our self-image, our relations with others and even some aspects of our very sense of self or who we are as persons. Therefore, the experience of a life-threatening disease like cancer is accompanied by deleterious and often permanent repercussions on sexuality.

Cancer treatments include primary surgical therapies and adjunctive chemotherapies and radiotherapies resulting in hormonal and sometimes physical changes to sexual organs. The sexual sequelae of cancer and cancer therapies affect sexual health (e.g. functioning, fertility) and sexual well-being (e.g. desire, pleasure, sexuality). These physical and emotional insults on sexual health often entail changes to our body image and to our sense of personal identity, thus influencing the patients' perception of themselves and their family. These changes make it difficult for individuals to engage in gender roles and social practices that prior to cancer, defined their lives.

Cancer, for many, has increasingly become a chronic disease. Therefore, the impact of cancer and its treatments varies depending on the phase of the illness. During the active treatment phase, patients may even come to consider their intimate relationships mainly in connection to their treatment needs and their concerns about their survival. However, following active treatment and into the early survivorship phase sexual problems may persist and sexuality may be reduced to a focus on sexual functioning or performance. This maladaptive approach to sexual health is often shared by patients, caregivers and providers and can lead to lack of attention towards early sexual health assessment and intervention. Thus, there is a

Clinical Psycho-Oncology: An International Perspective, First Edition. Edited by Luigi Grassi and Michelle Riba.

failure to collect information and tackling sexually related problems in clinical practice in a timely manner to reduce the risk of poor sexual outcomes. More specifically, the patient considers their sex life from the point of view of 'performance', thus neglecting the comprehensive and dynamic impact of associated relational aspects. The inherent complexity of the suffering that arises from the loss of sex-linked and multi-factoriality aspects of life can cause a profoundly altered and disaffected sense of one's masculinity or femininity.

Sexuality-related distress is very common among cancer patients and their partners. Studies have documented that about 1 in 3 cancer survivors report sexuality-related distress, over two-thirds experience sexual dysfunction and pain, 56% endorse lower desire and pleasure, and 40% encounter depression during the cancer experience.[2,3] The physical sequelae of cancer and its treatments affecting sexuality may be temporary such as in the case of loss of hair, asthenia, and loss of body weight or swelling linked to the administration of cortisone during chemotherapy. While at other times, the physical impact is permanent such as the loss of the breast due to mastectomy, and impotence following the resection of abdominal nerves during prostate cancer surgery. In addition, there are relational aspects like conflict within the couple or family that negatively impact cancer survivorship and sexuality outcomes. Many survivors endorse marital discord as a stressor that facilitated their cancer.[4] Problems might also arise in couples who believe that past events might have contributed to causing the cancer, consequently feeling a sense of guilt. This is relevant in the case of cervical, anal and oral cancers due to sexually transmitted human papillomavirus (HPV) infection that resulted in the cancerous cellular changes. Other people might feel that cancer is contagious and therefore engaging in sexual activity may 'spread' the cancer to the partner. Some may feel very unattractive due to the surgical site, and disfigurement due to surgery and/or radiation. Guilt feelings can also arise and interfere with one's state of mind in which an individual is unable to feel free to enjoy fantasies and desires.

Sexuality, gender and cancer: common aspects and cultural variables

Lévi-Strauss defines culture as the expression of thought systems in the world, a means of communication in many ways similar to spoken language.[5] This means that, in an era of globalization, knowing the cultural variables is essential to understanding patients' communication systems and to providing them with the best possible biopsychosocial assistance.

Through its powerful effects on the biological sphere, cancer inevitably produces changes in the equilibrium of marital relationships and in the representation of the Self, both physical and relational. Sexuality is the watershed between the biological and social spheres of individuals. The management of a man–woman relationship represents, at the same time, the invasion of culture in nature and vice versa, insofar as sexual drives are among the instincts that most need to be stimulated by another person, thus configuring a paradigmatic example of social life within nature.

In particular, pathologies like those of the breast, cervix, ovary, prostate and testicles, which are specifically correlated to sexual function, have more evident repercussions on gender identity and sexual health. For a man, infertility and impotence may constitute a blow to his deep sense of manhood. In the same way for women, the loss of their menstrual cycle, hormone alterations and mutilations of their genitalia may alter the way they perceive their femininity, making them feel prematurely elderly, or may create embarrassment during intercourse. After a hysterectomy, for example, some women report concern that their lack of uterus might be experienced or 'felt' during sexual intercourse. Post-operative consequences like the presence of an ostomy in the case of bladder and intestinal cancer, or of a mastectomy following breast cancer, can considerably alter the patients' body image and possibly affect their interest in sexual activity.

The cancer site and the form of the surgical and radiation scars influence a person's appearance, body image, sexual functioning, the partner's attitudes and behaviours regarding intimacy and the marital relationship. Therefore, the impact of cancer on sexuality must be understood in terms of the specificity of the problems associated with the biological and clinical aspects, the physical sequelae, and of the patient and partner's perception that is shaped by his or her culture of reference.

Most of the literature on the medical or psychosocial treatment of cancer is grounded on data collected among the White populations of the United States and the United Kingdom, thus raising the risk that a specific cultural model might be elevated to a normative value of reference. Investigations of the cancer experience that include other countries, ethnic groups and cultures make it possible to understand the global human impact of cancer, thus addressing unmet needs.

Sexuality and prostate cancer

Since the 1990s, there have been an increasing number of studies on the quality of life of patients suffering from prostate cancer, highlighting the emotional scope of this disease. Erectile dysfunction and loss of libido represent the main clinical sequelae of prostate cancer. Pharmacological therapies are not very effective at treating the sexual sequelae and are still quite controversial, to the extent that only 60% of the patients follow these therapies one year after diagnosis. The reasons for this attitude have been singled out in the persisting cultural stereotype that requires men to be sexually virile.[6] Due to the lack of resources and therapies to address sexual dysfunction in male cancer patients and survivors, it is probable that many couples respond with a sense of the inevitability of symptoms that are experienced rather like the unavoidable consequence of age. The difficulty of recognizing the emotional distress that might arise from impotence and the often associated urinary incontinence are reflected in the tendency to underestimate the importance of the loss of sexual function in older age, in general.

Recent studies on the quality of life in the Western world have clearly shown that erectile dysfunction causes distress, marital dissatisfaction and a feeling of loss of status in one's family and social role. The ensuing affective withdrawal also affects the patient's partner who, due to gender roles (e.g. feelings of helplessness and inadequacy at not being able to arouse her partner), appears to be at increased risk for distress.[7] In some cultures, for example the Mediterranean, cultural pressure determines an equation between sexual performance and identity that enhances the need and pursuit of sexual performance, thus establishing a vicious circle that strengthens sexual inhibition.

In the United States, African Americans are considered to be at greatest risk for prostate cancer and have the highest incidence and mortality. *Healthy People 2020*[8] estimates a 34% higher risk, and *Cancer Facts & Figures*[9] reports a 2.4 times greater mortality rate than in European men. This population group also suffer from greater prostate cancer-induced distress.[10] A tendency to equate cancer with a death sentence and the trauma of the loss of their 'manhood' is a further impediment to attending screenings and specialist examinations, even in the presence of symptoms. The patient may adhere to the cultural value of avoiding the 'sick role' perspective, and assuming a stoical attitude, denying symptoms indicative of an illness. Thus they may resort to seeing a physician only once their body is already debilitated, which contributes in turn to the late-stage diagnosis experienced among African Americans.

Health care system challenges create barriers in access to and utilization of care. In addition, diffidence due to medical mistrust and tribal taboos may serve as further obstacles in relating to their medical providers. Given the greater burden of prostate cancer among men of African descent, studies addressing screening efficacy, survivorship, health-related quality of life (HRQOL), and psychosocial including sexual health care are necessary.

Data is still scant on the effect of prostate cancer on HRQOL and sexuality among the Chinese population. However, the response of these patients to erectile dysfunctions, their psychological distress and quality of life appear to match those recorded in the Western world, are shown to be slightly heightened by a traditional culture that emphasizes the manliness-sexual potency equation.[11] In marital relationships, the consequences of prostatectomy (urinary incontinence and impotence) have been found to worsen the quality of life of patients' partners in terms of psychological stress, loss of a sex life and social activities.[12]

A comparative analysis between data on Western (European and American) and Japanese patients reveals significant differences. Japanese men appear to suffer a greater level of impairment of their sexual function but nonetheless seem to be less concerned about the loss of their sexuality,[13] resulting in a lesser impact on their quality of life. Given that there is no apparent biological explanation, the said difference has been attributed to cultural factors. Their prevalently indirect way of communicating, aimed at avoiding situations of conflict, may play an important role in their tendency to not express their needs and/or feelings of loss associated with their sexuality. In Asian cultures, relations are aimed at the pursuit of harmony rather than on building intimate relationships, as is the case in the Western world. The driving principle is to respect the other person's individuality to the point where people refrain from interfering with questions or expressions of dissent or concern that could create conflict and/or disagreement.[14]

Understanding cultural attitudes towards emotional expression is an important parameter for evaluating data on quality of life. A comparative study between American, Asian and Hawaiian men suffering from prostate cancer identifies Filipino men as the group with the greatest difficulties and the lowest scores in quality of life assessments. This datum is interpreted as the expression of a cultural attitude that shows a greater acceptance of the expression of emotions within the Filipino culture compared to other Asian groups.[15]

Sexuality and gynaecological tumours and breast cancer

Tumours of the breast and of the female reproductive system affect women in essential aspects of their gender identity, which in turn determines specific fears about their body image, sexual identity and emotional life. Data found in the literature estimate that, in the Western world, between 50–80% of the women operated for breast cancer report sexual dysfunctions during the first six months after surgery. By the end of the first year, roughly 90% of these women resume a normal sex life although some problems may persist, for example lack of libido (60%), dyspareunia (38%), frigidity (42%), vaginal dryness (30%), vaginismus, and brief intercourse and orgasm disorders.

Chemotherapy and hormone therapy are correlated with the worsening quality of sexual relationships although female sexual dysfunctions are extremely complex to evaluate insofar as they appear to be equally produced by possible relational and affective problems. Among young women especially, a core concern is that changes in their body image might affect their ongoing and future relationship with their partners. The need to address the issue by also involving their partners is highlighted by data that correlate the distress of women with breast cancer to the distress of their partners, and to the communication style within the couple. Cancer patients' partners often represent their principal source of support[16] although the tendency to shoulder caregiver responsibility is an aspect strongly linked to a women's roles. Men may feel insecure and hampered in providing their partner with adequate support. Controlling their emotions, which is an important feature of a man's identity, may be expressed via rejection and avoidance mechanisms that can make the woman feel isolated and misunderstood. This affective rejection may inhibit the couple's intimate relations and the transition from caregiver to sexual partner, both during and after the end of treatment.

The correlation between body image, sex life and concerns about becoming a burden for their partner and family seems to have a transcultural aspect.[4]

A comparative study among Europeans, Chinese and Japanese women on the emotional impact of breast cancer and their perception of the support received from their husbands revealed that, given an equal need of closeness and affective dependence, Japanese and Chinese women expressed more difficulties in the light of a cultural model that requires greater self-sacrifice with respect to one's sexual needs and to the family's need of care.[17] The difficulty faced by Asian women in expressing their needs, which appears to also hinder them from seeking help from support groups, is that speaking in intimate terms, for example about one's sexuality, is considered to be shameful.[18]

Taboos linked to female sexuality are consistently present throughout the Asian world, where a woman's sex life is still primarily for the purpose of reproduction. Thus, information on Asian women's sexuality is scarce. Data collected on women in Malaysia, China, Korea and India highlight that, in most cases, a cancer affecting reproductive organs puts a temporary and sometimes lasting stop to a woman's sex life.[19] The belief still seems to exist that all cancers are contagious, and thus engaging in sexual intercourse with a woman with breast cancer will put her partner at risk for cancer. Cultural prejudices are so deeply rooted that such an occurrence is not manifested as malaise, and a woman's adjustment following cancer is directed at her functional and familial obligations; thus her concerns seem to focus more on how to continue managing her domestic chores. The presence of a female health care professional (doctor or nurse) can be of great help in overcoming embarrassment about discussing issues of sexuality. This consideration is important in outlining strategies aimed at overcoming cultural barriers and facilitating participation in screenings, which is something difficult to achieve among Asian women.

There are contradictory results from the Islamic world: some studies indicate a greater satisfaction among Muslim women than Western women for the support received from their husbands and their family;[20,21] other data suggest concern about undergoing screening tests due to the possible reaction of their husbands following diagnosis of an oncological pathology, and for having violated religious taboos relative to exhibiting their body.[22,23] These studies generally focus on how the concern of Muslim women in coming to terms with the disease is more oriented towards accepting the will of God while the changes in their body are of secondary importance compared to issues of spirituality, including in their love relationships.

However, a qualitative research study on the correlation between cancer and sexuality conducted in Morocco revealed the difficulty of investigating this issue in a conservative social context such as that of the world of Islam.[24] Prudery, shame, personal and religious prejudices on sexuality represent the major hindrances: 'sexuality will stir up the cancer', 'making love would drain my energy', as well as women's concern that gynaecological cancer is a contagious disease. Doctors' scarce attention to the impact of the disease on women's sex lives and emotions has been correlated to concerns about not having the necessary skills and to a persisting prejudice against the importance of sexuality compared to issues of survival. This qualitative study also reports that among the women interviewed, 50% of the cases diagnosed with cancer resulted in separation from their husbands. In some of these cases the separation was initiated by the cancer survivor, because of the couples' inability to accept the physical changes in the woman's body brought about by the disease were experienced as a and the perceived loss of femininity.

Similar results are revealed by a study on breast cancer and sexuality recently conducted in Sudan. Cultural prejudice and embarrassment among both physicians and patients negatively affect the attention focused on sexuality and relative psychosocial needs. Treatment-induced changes in the women's body image negatively affected their perception of being sexually attractive in 55% of cases and their sexual relationships in 58% of cases. Most of the women involved in this study had undergone a mastectomy without reconstruction. Ethnic factors and the patients' cultural level contribute to the difficulties found in addressing sexuality issues. Women with a higher level of education reported more positive sexual satisfaction. Indeed, sexual needs represent an extremely private issue among Sudanese women from regions with a lower level of literacy, making it difficult to tackle it in a straightforward manner, even with their own husbands.[25] Recently married and younger women reported fewer sexual disorders ($P = 0.030$). Their husbands' support was evaluated positively by 79% of the patients, being defined as economic support in 80% of cases, while only 10% reported receiving emotional support.

Women's concerns about undergoing a physical examination of their breast and/or reproductive system represents a sensitive aspect in administering treatment, also for Muslim women living in Western countries. Data collected in the United States highlight a certain reluctance and fear among Muslim women who experience the prescription of Western medicine to undergo routine tests as being intrusive on their rights to privacy and not have their private parts examined.[26]

Ritual and/or religious practices represent a critical factor in the correlation between disease and sexuality in several cultural contexts. For Indian women, their menstrual cycle represents a way of cleansing their body of impurities, and an eventual hysterectomy consequent to a cervical cancer can be rejected insofar as it precludes the possibility of being purified and of maintaining their sexual appeal.[27]

Sexuality and gastrointestinal and bladder cancer: stoma patients

The presence of a stoma following surgery represents a great hurdle in a person's sex life, and is often not mentioned by patients. Specific dysfunctions, stoma care during intercourse and changes in one's body image represent the major problems that these patients face in their intimate relationships and sex life. The location and the type of stoma are another important variable. Compared to patients with an ileostomy, colostomy and urostomy cases appear to have more serious consequences as they are associated with operations in the pelvic area that might damage nerves, thus giving rise to: (1) erectile and/or ejaculatory dysfunctions (i.e. dry orgasm) in men, and (2) vaginal dryness, dyspareunia and perineal numbness in women. Furthermore, the outflow of organic material from an ileostomy is less characterized by faecal odour, making intimate and social relationships easier.

In literature, the incidence of erectile dysfunctions following a colostomy is estimated to be between 43–100% and similar data are reported among patients with urostomy. Problems of retrograde ejaculation (dry orgasm) are detected in approximately 21% of the patients. Fewer research studies have been conducted on the sexual dysfunctions of stomatized women, although dyspareunia was reported in 77% of the cases, especially during the first post-operative year.[28]

In these patients' intimate relationships, they can be particularly sensitive to fear of lack of control over their intestinal or urinary functions and that the odours, sounds or sight of the ostomy might cause disgust in their partner. Stomatized patients are in fact particularly aware of the proximity of the points of excretion to their erogenous areas, this situation adds to sexual discomfort and sexual activity avoidance.

The involvement and support of the partner plays an important role, although this leads us to assume the existence of gender-linked differences. Women appear to more actively pursue social support although, in their love relationships, they are penalized by their partners' greater difficulty in passing from the role of caregiver to that of sexual partner. This gender-linked sensitivity makes women more vulnerable than men in terms of the importance attributed by women to their body image and to physical appeal in their sex life. From the point of view of body image and a personal sense of identity, such a sudden and important change as the one arising from the presence of a stoma is difficult to accept. After surgery, many patients experience a breakdown in their self-esteem and a drop in self-confidence resulting in their perception of no longer being sexually attractive to their partners. For these patients, the possibility of receiving specific psycho-oncological support plays an important role in resuming their normal love lives. Understanding the outcome of surgery in the pre-operative phase is important to maintaining one's body image. Moreover, for some people, body image and self-esteem are closely related and it is important for these aspects be recognized and address in order to avoid provoking phobic attitudes and fears of abandonment and isolation.

The quality of stomatized patients' interpersonal relationships and quality of life has been investigated in a cross-cultural study, which found the geographical origin of the individual to be the principal sensitive factor.[29] The data collected refer to Europe and the Mediterranean Basin. German patients – without revealing significant differences in terms of gender identity or the level of education and social class – achieved higher scores in quality of life assessments. Muslim patients scored the lowest. The reason was identified as lying in the expectations raised by the information received before surgery, the focus on education in stoma care and the acceptance thereof in the social community of reference. The situation in Europe varies widely in terms of the provision of specialized health care and recognition of the psychosocial needs of these patients. The study recorded the tendency to provide fewer health care services in South European countries, especially outside the large hospital facilities. Psycho-educational training on stoma care is of great relevance in the resumption of a patient's sex life and it is important that their partner is also included so that potential fears with respect to damaging the stoma, the possible outflow of faeces or odours and flatulence can be tackled.

Men who have sex with men (MSM), face specific problems that are insufficiently addressed in clinical practice. To date, homosexuality is still perceived as a sensitive issue and may determine the risk of intervening in a way that is inadequate to these patients' specific sexuality problems. Among MSM who practice anal intercourse, the way they express their sexuality can be profoundly modified in case of abdominal-perineal resection of the rectum entailing the closure of the anus and the removal of the rectum. Moreover, in gay cultures, special importance is given to physical appeal as a component of sexual attraction and the presence of a stoma negatively affects patients' relationships and their possibility of making new acquaintances.[30]

Transcultural data on the impact of the presence of a stoma on sexuality are still scarce. In some cultures, such as in Asia, the traditional discretion in addressing issues related to sexuality is magnified and scant data exist on the dimension and the characteristics of the problem. A study on the Chinese population in the United States tracks this difficulty to Chinese men's preoccupation that discussing their weaknesses is tantamount to falling short of their social role ('losing face') and medical examinations are therefore experienced as aggressive and invasive on the part of their interlocutor.[31]

Among Muslim populations, specific problems are linked to the religious factor which entails social isolation, losing one's social role and compromising their personal identity. A large proportion of the literature found that stoma care makes it difficult for Muslim patients to take part in ritual prayer – both in private and in the Mosque – and to practise fasting during Ramadan. The Muslim religion dictates on the purification rituals that are to precede the five daily prayers; these require cleansing rituals that oblige patients to remove the covering of the surgical site often, irritating the surrounding skin. Furthermore, believers might feel that the cleansing practices are insufficient, making them feel impure due to the presence of the stoma or embarrassed by the odours and noises while participating in collective prayers. These complications give rise to renunciation and avoidance behaviours, with a subsequent worsening of general quality of life and interpersonal relations.

Similar difficulties have been recorded among Orthodox Jews who try to comply with the dictates of the Shabbat, which bans the use of running water on Saturdays, and also among some Asian cultures like the Sikh and Hindu, who associate prayer with bodily purification and cleansing rituals. Among Orthodox Jewish women, the presence of a stoma may represent a hindrance to resuming their sex life after the prescribed ritual bath (Mikvah) at the end of their menstrual cycle. This purifying bath must be taken completely naked – precluding a stoma bag – and this creates a situation that is difficult to handle, especially in the presence of an ileostomy or urostomy, which provokes frequent and uncontrollable leakages. In addition, Muslims, Sikhs, Hindus and some Buddhists are conditioned to only use their left hand for *dirty* activities like washing their anal and pubic area, making stoma care impossible as it requires the use of both hands.

Cancer, infertility and sociocultural aspects

Cancer can impact intimacy, sexuality and fertility at some point during the cancer journey. Infertility is the term used when a woman cannot get pregnant. If a woman keeps having miscarriages, this is also called infertility. Infertility may be due to problems in the man or woman. In developed countries and to some degree in developing countries, more women are choosing not to have children, and the way that infertility is perceived and the social pressure for women and men to have children has changed over the years.[32–34] Infertility remains a medical condition that affects 1 in 8 couples of reproductive age in America.[35] Cancer is a major contributor to infertility; and this trend is increasing globally as cancer incidence is growing worldwide. Between 1975 and 2000, cancer increased in incidence for all age groups <45 years. There is evidence that this increase has declined in 15–29 year olds, following a peak in the late 1980s and early 1990s.[36] With the increase in survival, young patients and their partners now face a multitude of overwhelming quality of life and treatment side-effect issues such as infertility or impaired fecundity.[37] The human impact of cancer often includes some physical and psychological distress that diminishes over time; however, this distress can be even more devastating and traumatic among young cancer survivors and families, and among some cultural groups.

Health disparities in infertility and cancer: a global perspective

By 2030, the global cancer burden is expected to nearly double, growing to 21.4 million cases and 13.2 million deaths.[38] The WHO publication, *Global Burden of Disease 2000*, reported that 18% of five-year female survivors who had reproductive cancer, which includes cervix, uterus and ovary cancers, may suffer infertility, and 20% of five-year male survivors who had genitourinary cancer, which includes prostate and bladder cancers, may suffer impotence and incontinence.[39]

Annually more than 130 000 cancer patients are diagnosed in their reproductive years (up to age 45) in the United States,[40] various cancer treatments – including surgery, chemotherapy and radiation therapy – can cause infertility under certain circumstances.[41] Currently, besides a national registry to which the majority of infertility clinics contribute on a voluntary basis,[42] there is no national data on the statistics of infertility or impaired fecundity after cancer treatment, or of infertility in general amongst multiethnic groups except White, Black and Hispanics.[35]

One of the goals of *Healthy People 2020* is to improve sexual health.[8] A recent report suggested African Americans had twofold increased odds (95% confidence interval (CI)) of infertility compared with Whites after adjustment for socioeconomic position (education and ability to pay for basics), correlates of pregnancy intent (marital status and hormonal contraceptive use), and risk factors for infertility (age, smoking, fibroid presence and ovarian volume). The corresponding odds ratio among all women was 1.5 (95% CI, 1.0–2.2). Difficulty paying for basic gynaecological medical care and ovarian volume were associated with infertility among Black but not White women.[43] The report corresponded to the 2002 CDC NSFA data that infertile couples are more likely to be Black (11.5%) than Hispanic (7.7%) or White (7.0%). Therefore, in the United States, Hispanics (57.8%) and European-Americans (57.9%) compared to Black (44.3%) are less likely to have fecundity issues. Most infertility services were used by older childless women (e.g. 29% aged 40–44 years), married childless women (24%), non-Hispanic white women, and women with higher levels of education and income.[35]

What are the causes of infertility in cancer patients?

Figure 4.1 outlines the major physical, social and other determinants of infertility, and the percentage distribution of incidence in males and females.[37] The review of the literature by Huddleston *et al.* suggested that the clinical significance of these differences and the biological versus social

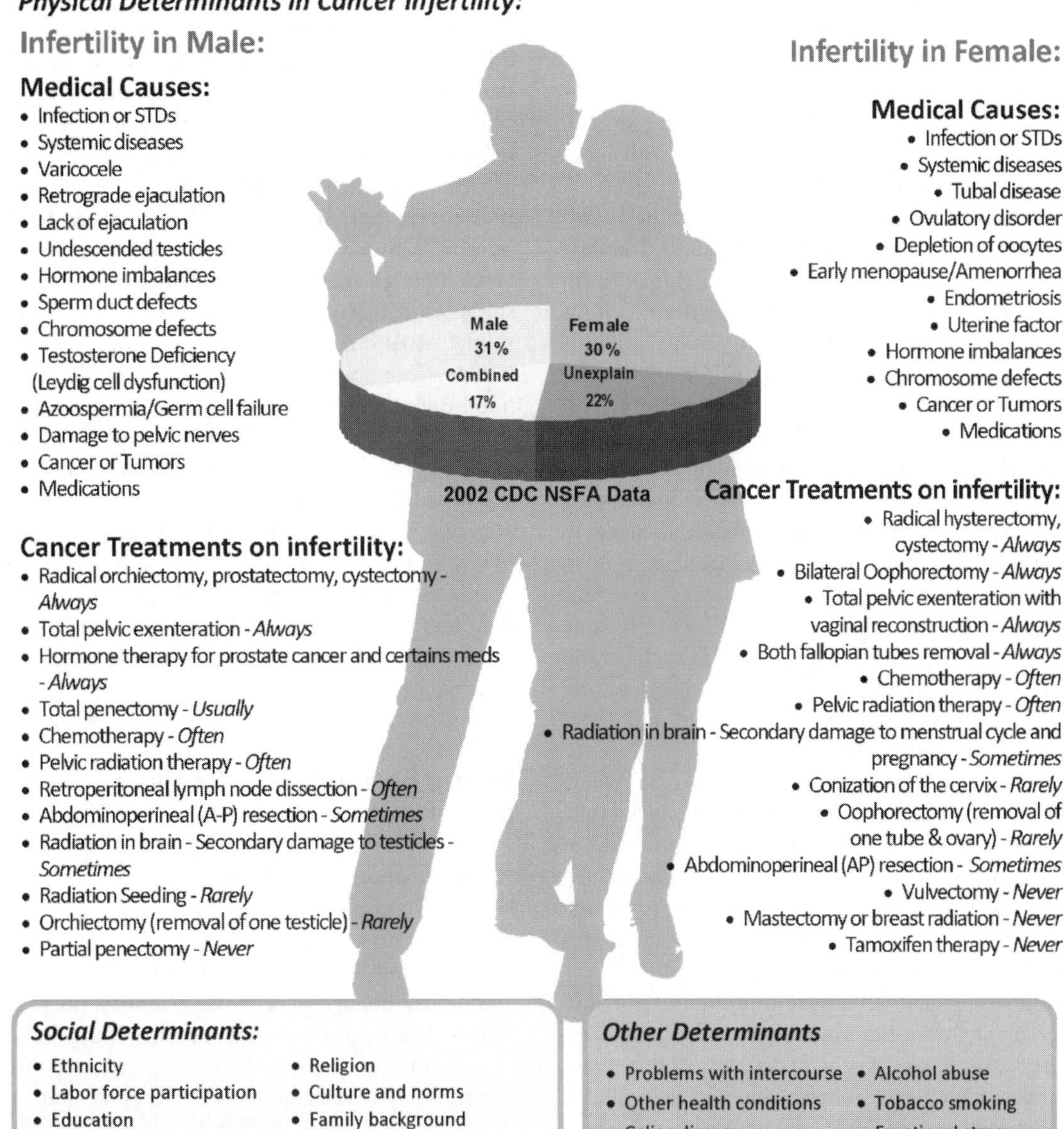

Figure 4.1 Factors affecting fertility[47] was informed by the American Cancer Society (2010)[66,67] and Chandra *et al.* (2006).[68]

underpinnings remain to be determined; further research is needed to fill the gaps in understanding of these racial and ethnic disparities and their origins.[44] Cancer patients may face different fertility issues including difficult fertilization after cancer, infertility, or impaired fecundity along with compounded psychosocial distresses.

Different types of cancers, tumours and cancer treatments (i.e. surgery, radiation therapy, chemotherapy and certain medications) may result in infertility among cancer patients. Various aggressive cancer treatments in female patients which may affect fertility and/or cause infertility include radical cystectomy, hysterectomy, bilateral oophorectomy and fallopian tube removal, chemotherapy, radiation of genitalia, radiation of brain and medication therapy. Cancer treatments in female patients may cause direct damage to ovaries, tubes and uterus, including depletion in number of oocytes and hormonal imbalance resulting in early menopause, germ cell failure leading to premature ovarian failure (POF), uterine and tube fibrosis, uterine vascular insufficiency, and secondary damage to menstrual cycle and pregnancy from brain radiation.[40]

Many aggressive cancer treatments for male patients affect fertility; these treatments include radical orchiectomy, chemotherapy, radiation of genitalia, radiation of brain and medication therapy. Potential impacts of cancer treatments include germ cell failure, azoospermia, damage to sperm duct, damage to pelvic nerves or blood vessels, secondary damage to testicle from brain radiation, which may result in gonadal dysfunction and infertility.[45] Testicular cancer patients are often diagnosed at a young age; potential long-term sequelae after testicular malignancy treatments may include the above negative effects as well as Leydig cell dysfunction and testosterone deficiency.[46]

What are the options?

People from different cultures, religions, family backgrounds and generations, with different education, acculturation level and knowledge, resources, information access and individual values may find different solutions and decisions when facing infertility. This can be more complicated and difficult among cancer patients, survivors and families. Some negative solutions may include abandonment, divorce and remarriage or even polygyny.[48] For a male who wants to become a father, parenthood options may include natural conception, sperm banking, testicular tissue freezing, assisted reproduction technology (ART), instillation of methylene blue dye to open the sperm duct, testicular sperm extraction (TESE), sperm donation, adoption and fostering. For the female who wants to become a mother, parenthood options may include natural conception, *in vitro* fertilization (IVF),[49] embryo, egg or ovarian tissue freezing, *in vitro* maturation, ovarian transposition, radical trachelectomy, using GnRH analogue and oral contraceptives to reduce activity in the ovary and save eggs during chemotherapy, eggs or embryos donation, gestational surrogacy, adoption, and fostering. There is also increasing use of complementary and alternative medicine (CAM) in treating infertility.

Tissue banking and fertility preservation

Women are born with a fixed number of eggs; studies show that the quality of a woman's eggs begins to decline after the age of 32. In the mid thirties, the rate of follicle loss accelerates, resulting in fewer and poorer quality eggs, making conception more challenging. Ultimately, the diminishing number of eggs in the ovaries will result in menopause. Men's sperm parameters peak between ages 30–35 years; and fertility diminishes to some extent after age 40–50. Nowadays, tissue banking and fertility preservation are strategies for women or men who wish to pursue their family at a later age. For some cancer patients and survivors, especially young survivors, sperm, ova, embryo, ovarian and testicular tissue banking can be helpful to achieve fertilization in the event of ovarian or testicular failure. Tissue banking and fertility preservation are suitable for populations who are anatomically able to conceive.

Improved IVF technology as a therapy for infertility among cancer patients

Techniques to successfully harvest and store reproductive cells have vastly improved over the past two decades. Fertility preservation is still an emerging discipline, but advances in medical procedures and technology in the last several years are providing new options for patients. However, *in vitro* fertilization (IVF) pregnancy rates are influenced by multiple factors including genotypes with predisposition toward autoimmune disease and ethnic group membership. One study conducted in the United States revealed that African women experience lower IVF pregnancy rates than Caucasians and Asians.[50] A large-scale study of 25 843 European-Americans and 1429 Asian patients from the national registry found that poorer outcomes among Asian women persisted with decreased IVF success;[44] Asian women undergoing their first IVF treatment attempt did not achieve the same live-birth rates seen in European-American women. This investigation revealed disparities in assisted reproductive technologies (ART) outcomes between Asian- and European-American women with infertility in the United States. The decreased pregnancy rates following ART may indicate fundamental biological or genetic differences between the ethnicities. Although IVF technology has improved over the years, the disparities have actually increased among different ethnicities.

Alternative fertility treatment

There is increasing use of complementary and alternative medicine (CAM) to treat a variety of gynaecological and infertility-related disorders including ovarian and testicular malfunction due to cancer treatments, erectile dysfunction, polycystic ovarian syndrome (PCOS), endometriosis and idiopathic infertility. Acupuncture is the most common form of CAM used for patients under going IVF, and acupuncture and herbal supplements are the most commonly used CAM therapies for male factor infertility.

Summary

The LIVESTRONG Cancer Policy Platform Federal Priority Report (2011)[64] suggests that adolescent and young adult cancer survivors face additional issues, including fertility, education and career challenges. Further research, policy changes and resources are needed to spur developments in medical and psychological interventions to improve overall quality of life and in particular sexual health and fertility outcomes. Appropriate health care provider sensitivity and sexual health training are essential to help couples to understand and prioritize treatment options, identify resources and suitable solutions for making appropriate fertility decisions. Additionally, psychological interventions must focus on helping couples to rebuild perceived control, meaning and purpose, a sense of well-being, and to explore the new relationship and roles beyond parenthood, and sexuality, including exploring new intimate behaviours through comprehensive cancer supportive services and/or self-help strategies.

Pregnancy and cancer

Although cancer patients and survivors may suffer chronic physical conditions caused by cancer treatments, age and overall physical health, research suggests that pregnancy after cancer does not trigger recurrence, even after breast cancer; nor does cancer and its treatments result in increased risk for the offspring of cancer patients.[51,52] However, appropriate medical care is advised for pregnant cancer survivors. One study reported that children of female cancer survivors treated with radiation to the pelvis are more likely to be born pre-term and have a low birth-weight in comparison to those children from sibling controls.[53] People of high paternal age may be susceptible to environmental chemicals and infection in general. Advanced age pregnancy may result in complications such as miscarriage, chromosomal anomalies, pre-eclampsia, caesarean delivery, gestational trophoblast diseases, placenta praevia and placental abruption during pregnancy, and pre-term birth.

Infertility and the impact on patient and family quality of life

In the United States, there is no data available on the effect of infertility on divorce rates. However, the inability to have a family has been known to cause a division in a marriage, and it can lead to divorce, grief and loss of status.[48,54,55] Reproduction and fertility have different meanings in Western and non-Western countries. Couples who are more educated, acculturated or reside in developed countries are more likely to view reproduction as a self-chosen goal or personal choice made by an individual or couple. Because of the advances of feminism and individualism, many women also have a sense of ownership of their own bodies. Immigrant couples from developing countries, peoples from intact indigenous cultures or traditional value systems, the less educated or less Western-acculturated are more likely to be influenced by social normative practice and pressure to bear children. In non-Western societies, having children is also a social obligation, a performance that is due to the family (-in-law) and the community.[34] Some cultures tend to blame women for being unable to bear children; women in these cultures may carry an internalized stigma and experience feelings of shame and guilt at not being able to continue the family name, or extend the family and lineage. This is often true for uneducated women whose only identity comes from being mothers, or for women who live in a submissive culture or relationship. An article in *Newsweek* in 2008 documented that infertility in developing countries is seen as a personal failing, or even a curse for women.[56] The consequences of infertility can include ostracism, physical abuse and even suicide. Stigma and infertility is not limited to women; some men who suffer infertility issues may also lose self-esteem since they are expected to be virile and sexually powerful. Cancer patients already distressed by the journey of cancer may be further scarred by feelings of guilt, blame, remorse, anger, hopelessness or regret at the loss of their ability to have children and reproduce.[2,3,57]

Suggestions for clinicians in addressing sexuality and fertility concerns

Traditionally, the primary concern of physicians is to save patients' lives rather than their quality of life. However, discussions about sexual health and fertility preservation among cancer patients are most effective when they occur before initiation of treatment.[58] In a study published in the *Journal of Clinical Oncology*, a team of University of New South Wales researchers reported that women with breast cancer are often not well informed on fertility issues.[51] According to Schover, 51% of men with cancer report wanting children in the future, and 91% of oncologists agree sperm banking should be offered to eligible men; however, only 10% offer sperm banking routinely.[37] With the increase in survival rate and young cancer survivors, cancer treatment should focus on a comprehensive approach to improve outcomes and quality of life. *Healthy People 2020* suggested employing a 'life course' perspective to health promotion and disease prevention in fertility issues so as to examine the quality of life.[8] Oncology organizations and advocates recommend sexual health intervention and fertility preservation in cancer patients. Lee suggested that as part of informed consent prior to therapy, oncologists should address HRQOL issues with patients, including the possibility of infertility, as early in treatment planning as possible.[59] A multidisciplinary team approach including oncologists, nurses in the specialties of oncology and infertility, a psycho-oncologist, reproductive endocrinology and infertility specialists, andrologists and embryologists is effective in communicating and intervening in the fertility issue.[60] Mick *et al.* suggested clinicians should use a BETTER model approach when communicating with patients about sexual health issues (see Box 4.1).[61] The IOM report *Cancer Care for the Whole Patient* underscores the importance of psychosocial care.[62] Therefore, it is crucial that patients and their partners be provided with the appropriate psychological, counselling and support care needed to address the distress associated with sexual health challenges and infertility.

Box 4.1 BETTER model

where

- B = **Bring** up the topic – start with clinical questions first, then move to relationship and fertility concerns.
- E = **Explain** that sexuality and fertility is an important part of quality of life for many.
- T = **Tell** patients about resources to address their concerns.
- T = **Timing** to discuss sexuality and fertility issues might seem inappropriate now, but questions may come later; encourage questions at any time. Some patients and families who are concerned about fertility may consider options of fertility preservation.
- E = **Educate** patients about side effects of their cancer treatments and changes in sexuality and fertility.
- R = **Record** discussions, assessments, interventions and outcomes.

Cultural beliefs and practices may also pose as barriers to communicating about fertility issues.[63] For example, Asian women do not feel comfortable discussing psychosexual issues with their spouse or doctors but would appreciate if these issues were addressed discreetly on a routine basis in clinical consultations.[19]

Although no national race and ethnicity data exists in the United States about the rates of infertility and the use of infertility services amongst cancer patients or survivors, the 2002 CDC NSFA data revealed that infertile couples are more likely to be Black (11.5%) than Hispanic (7.7%) or White (7.0%); and non-Hispanic white women, and women with higher levels of education and income will be more likely to utilize infertility services.[35] This gives a clue that fertility is also a social disparity issue which can be reduced by education, income and improvements in other social determinants. Many of the aspects such as knowledge deficit, cultural stigma, obesity, substance abuse, healthy lifestyles, emotions, coping and stress relief can be directly or indirectly improved by increasing awareness, resources and services of sexual health counselling and family planning, health education, affordable genetic counselling, health screening, health care, physical activities and healthy food advice, smoking cessation, behavioural and mental health support as well as better environmental zoning.

Conclusion and future directions

Addressing the sexual health of cancer patients is a necessary component of comprehensive cancer treatment and cancer care of the whole person. While there is increasing attention to this HRQOL dimension in survivorship research, practices and policy in developed countries, there is a serious dearth of HRQOL and sexual health data and information among persons from developing nations, immigrant and indigenous/native peoples. Complex and over-burdened health care systems create barriers to access and utilization of medical care. In addition, medical mistrust and tribal taboos may present further obstacles to the receipt of medical care and medical adherence. Given the greater burden of cancer among underserved populations, studies and interventions addressing the continuum of cancer care including sexual health assessments, fertility screenings and sexual health interventions are urgent and compelling.

A 'one-size-fits-all' approach to cancer care does not adequately address the needs of diverse populations. Continued support for programmes to improve access to health care, education and care delivery, especially in a humane, culturally sensitive and competent manner, will maximize our capacity to serve our most vulnerable populations.[64] At the 44th session of the Commission on Population and Development on the theme 'Fertility, reproductive health and development' in April 2011, the United Nations urged Member States, resorting to the appropriate technical and financial support from development partners when needed, to design and implement national cancer control plans and strategies that encompass prevention, early detection, treatment and palliation of cancers of the male and female reproductive systems, especially prostate, breast and cervical cancers, and to strengthen existing health services and health systems to increase the capacity to detect these cancers at earlier stages and allow prompt access to quality treatment.[65] Improved governmental, non-governmental and health care systems efforts are needed to identify, monitor and address fertility and sexuality concerns among cancer patients and their families. Moreover, the inclusion of sexuality, family building and family quality of life interventions prior to and post-treatment are necessary to attend to the human side of cancer and reduce cancer morbidity by improving sexual health quality of life.

Key points

- Emerging global cancer trends present both challenges and opportunities for sexual and reproductive health. The most relevant trends are increasing earlier age at diagnosis for many cancers (i.e. breast, cervical, ovarian, prostate and genital cancers), and advances in treatment promoting survival and cure.
- New developments in fertility therapy promote both options and success for biological children in cancer patients. Yet, disparities in access and utilization of sexual and reproductive health counselling and therapeutics exist and persist. Unfortunately, these disparities are primarily based on patient characteristics (e.g. education, income and health care system factors, such as health care coverage, and overly complex procedures).
- The challenge for psycho-oncologists and partners in the cancer health care team is to: (1) educate our medical colleagues on the significance of sexual and reproductive health as key indicators of cancer outcomes; (2) integrate sexual and reproductive health counselling into our clinical skills and practices; and (3) advocate for patients' access into fertility treatments to provide hope and enhance health-related quality of life among cancer survivors.

References

1. World Health Organization (WHO) (2006) Defining sexual health. Report of a technical consultation on sexual health, 28–31 January 2002, Geneva, WHO, Geneva; http://www.who.int/reproductivehealth/publications/sexual_health/defining_sexual_health.pdf (last accessed January 2012).
2. Carter J., Chi D.S., Brown C.L. *et al.* (2010) Cancer-related infertility in survivorship. *International Journal of Gynecological Cancer*, 20, 2–8.
3. Carter J., Raviv L., Sonoda Y. *et al.* (2011) Recovery issues of fertility-preserving surgery in patients with early-stage cervical cancer and a model for survivorship: The physician checklist. *International Journal of Gynecological Cancer*, 21, 106–116.
4. Ashing-Giwa K., Padilla G., Tejero J. *et al.* (2004) Understanding the breast cancer experience of women: A qualitative study of African American, Asian American, Latina and Caucasian cancer survivors. *Psycho-Oncology*, 13, 408–428.
5. Lévi-Strauss C. (1974) *Anthropologie structurale*, Vol LXXIV, Annuaire du Collège de France, pp. 303–309.
6. Wall D., Kristjanson L. (2005) Men, culture and hegemonic masculinity: Understanding the experience of prostate cancer. *Nursing Inquiry*, 12, 87–97.
7. Street A., Couper J., Love A. *et al.* (2010) Psychosocial adaptation in female partners of men with prostate cancer. *European Journal of Cancer Care*, 19, 234–242.
8. U.S. Department of Health and Human Services (2010) *Healthy People 2020: Maternal, Infant, and Child Health*; http://www.healthypeople.gov/2020/topics objectives2020/overview.aspx?topicid = 26 (accessed December 2011).
9. American Cancer Society (2011) *Cancer Facts & Figures for African Americans 2011–2012*; http://www.cancer.org/acs/groups/content/@epidemiologysurveilance/documents/document/acspc-027765.pdf (accessed January 2012).
10. Ellison G., Coker A., Hebert J. *et al.* (2011) Psychosocial stress and prostate cancer: A theoretical model. *Ethnicity & Disease*, 11, 484–495.
11. Lau J., Kim J., Tsui H.-Y. (2005) Prevalence of male and female sexual problems, perceptions related to sex and association with quality of life in a Chinese population: A population-based study. *International Journal of Impotence Research*, 17, 494–450.
12. Shao Q., Song J., Liu Q., Tian Y. (2010) Symptomatic benign prostate hyperplasia affects the quality of life of the patients' wives. *Zhonqhua Nan Ke Xue*, 16, 132–136.
13. Namiki S., Arai Y. (2011) Sexual quality of life for localized prostate cancer: A cross-cultural study between Japanese and American men *Reproductive Medicine and Biology*, 10, 59–68.
14. Namiki S., Ishidoya S., Ito A. *et al.* (2009) Quality of life after radical prostatectomy in Japanese men: A 5-year follow-up study. *International Journal of Urology*, 16, 75–81.
15. Gotay C., Holup J., Pagano I. (2002) Ethnic differences in quality of life. *Psycho-Oncology*, 11, 103–113.

16. Baider L., Cooper C.L., De-Nour A.K. (eds) (1996) *Cancer and the Family*, John Wiley & Sons, Ltd, Chichester.
17. Kagawa-Singer M., Wellish D. (2003) Patients' perceptions of their husband support. *Psycho-Oncology*, 12, 24–37.
18. Fukui S., Kugaya A., Kamiya M. *et al.* (2001) Participation in psychosocial group intervention among Japanese women with primary breast cancer and its associated factors. *Psycho-Oncology*, 10, 419–427.
19. Khoo S.B. (2009) Impact of cancer on psychosexuality: Cultural perspectives of Asian women. *International Journal of Nursing Practice*, 15, 481–488.
20. Taleghani F., Yekta Z., Nasrabadi A. (2005) Coping with breast cancer in newly diagnosed Iranian women. *Journal of Advanced Nursing*, 54, 265–272.
21. Banning M., Hafeez H., Faisal S. *et al.* (2009) The impact of culture and sociological and psychological issues on Muslim patients with breast cancer in Pakistan. *Cancer Nursing*, 32, 317–324.
22. Faisal A., Cohen M. (2008) Between traditional and modern perceptions of breast and cervical cancer screenings: A qualitative study of Arab women in Israel. *Psycho-Oncology*, 17, 34–41.
23. Zahedin F., Larijani B. (2007) Cancer ethics from the Islamic point of view. *Iran Journal of Allergy, Asthma Immunology*, 6(Supp. 5), 17–24.
24. Errihani H., Elghissassi I., Mellas N. (2008) Impact du cancer sur la sexualité: Qu'en est-il du patient marocain? *Sexologies*, 19, 92–98.
25. Abasher S. (2009) Sexual health issues in Sudanese women before and during hormonal treatment for breast cancer. *Psycho-Oncology*, 18, 858–865.
26. Matin M., LeBaron S. (2004) Attitudes toward cervical cancer screening among Muslim women: A pilot study. *Women & Health*, 39, 63–77.
27. Dein S. (2004) Explanatory models of and attitudes towards cancer in different cultures. *The Lancet Oncology*, 5, 119–124.
28. Weerakon P. (2001) Sexuality and the stoma patients. *Sexuality and Disability*, 19, 121–128.
29. Holzer B., Matzel K., Schiedeck T. *et al.* (2005) Do geographic and educational factors influence the quality of life in rectal patients with a permanent colostomy? *Disease of the Colon Rectum*, 48, 2209–2216.
30. Caldwell K. (1995) Homosexuality: A neglected issue in stoma care. *British Journal of Nursing*, 4, 1009–1012.
31. Chia-Chun L. (2009) Sexuality among patients with a colostomy: An exploration of the influences of gender, sexual orientation, and Asian heritage. *Journal of Wound, Ostomy and Continence Nursing*, 36, 288–296.
32. Schmidt L. (2010) Psychosocial consequences of infertility and treatment, in *Reproductive Endocrinology and Infertility* (eds D.T. Carrell, C.M. Peterson), Springer, New York, pp. 93–100.
33. Greil A.L., Shreffler K.M., Schmidt L., McQuillan J. (2011) Variation in distress among women with infertility: Evidence from a population-based sample. *Human Reproduction*, 26, 2101–2112.
34. Pennings G. (2008) Ethical issues of infertility treatment in developing countries. *ESHRE Monographs*, 1, 15–20.
35. Martinez G., Chandra A., Abma J. *et al.* (2006) Fertility, contraception, and fatherhood: Data on men and women from cycle 6 (2002) of the 2002 National Survey of Family Growth. *Vital Health Statistics*, 23, 1–142.
36. Bleyer A., O'Leary M., Barr R., Ries L. (2006) *Cancer Epidemiology in Older Adolescents and Young Adults 15 to 29 Years of Age, including SEER Incidence and survival: 1975–2000*, NIH Pub. No. 06-5767, National Cancer Institute, Bethesda, MD.
37. Schover L. (2007) Reproductive complications and sexual dysfunction in cancer survivors, in *Cancer Survivorship* (ed. P.A. Ganz), Springer, New York, pp. 251–271.
38. Jemal A., Bray F., Center M.M. *et al.* (2011) Global cancer statistics. *CA: A Cancer Journal for Clinicians*, 61, 69–90.
39. Mathers C., Boschi-Pinto C. (2003) Global burden of cancer in the year 2000: Version 1 estimates, in *Global Burden of Disease 2000*, WHO, Geneva.
40. Fertile Hope (2011); http://www.fertilehope.org/
41. Meirow D., Nugent D. (2001) The effects of radiotherapy and chemotherapy on female reproduction. *Human Reproduction Update*, 7, 535–543.
42. The Society for Assisted Reproductive Technology (SART) (2011); www.sart.org
43. Wellons M., Lewis C., Schwartz S. *et al.* (2008) Racial differences in self-reported infertility and risk factors for infertility in a cohort of black and white women: The CARDIA Women's Study. *Fertility and Sterility*, 90, 1640–1648.
44. Huddleston H.G., Cedars M.I., Sohn S.H. *et al.* (2010) Racial and ethnic disparities in reproductive endocrinology and infertility. *American Journal of Obstetrics and Gynecology*, 202, 413–419.
45. Brydøy M., Fosså S.D., Dahl O., Bjøro T. (2007) Gonadal dysfunction and fertility problems in cancer survivors. *Acta Oncologica*, 46, 480–489.

46. Abouassaly R., Fossa S.D., Giwercman A. *et al.* Sequelae of treatment in long-term survivors of testis cancer. *European Urology* (in press).
47. Ashing-Giwa K., Yeung S., Rosales M. Sexuality, fertility and cancer: Exploring contextual and socio-ecological determinants (in press).
48. Rutstein S.O., Shah I.H. (2004) Infecundity, infertility, and childlessness in developing countries, DHS Comparative Reports No. 9, ORC Macro and the World Health Organization, Calverton, MD, USA.
49. Ginsburg E.S., Yanushpolsky E.H., Jackson K.V. (2001) In vitro fertilization for cancer patients and survivors. *Fertility and Sterility,* 75, 705–710.
50. Gleicher N., Weghofer A., Lee I., Barad D. (2011) Association of FMR1 genotypes with in vitro fertilization (IVF) outcomes based on ethnicity/race. *PLoS ONE,* 6, DOI: 18710.11371/journal.pone.0018781.
51. Peate M., Meiser B., Hickey M., Friedlander M. (2009) The fertility-related concerns, needs and preferences of younger women with breast cancer: A systematic review. *Breast Cancer Research and Treatment,* 116, 215–223.
52. Thewes B., Meiser B., Rickard J., Friedlander M. (2003) The fertility- and menopause-related information needs of younger women with a diagnosis of breast cancer: A qualitative study. *Psycho-Oncology,* 12, 500–511.
53. Signorello L.B., Cohen S.S., Bosetti C. *et al.* (2006) Female survivors of childhood cancer: Preterm birth and low birth weight among their children. *Journal of the National Cancer Institute,* 98, 1453–1461.
54. Snyder K., Thazin M., Pearse W., Moinuddin M. (2010 The fertility-related treatment choices of cancer patients: Cancer-related infertility and family dynamics. *Cancer Treatment Research,* 156, 413–428.
55. Matthews M.A., Matthews R. (1986) Beyond the mechanics of infertility: Perspectives on the social psychology of infertility and involuntary childlessness. *Family Relations,* 35, 579–587.
56. Springen K. (2008) What it means to be a woman. *Newsweek,* 15 September.
57. Carter J., Rowland K., Chi D. *et al.* (2005) Gynecologic cancer treatment and the impact of cancer-related infertility. *Gynecologic Oncology,* 97, 90–95.
58. Redig A.J., Brannigan R., Stryker S.J. *et al.* (2011) Incorporating fertility preservation into the care of young oncology patients. *Cancer,* 117, 1–10.
59. Lee S.J., Schover L.R., Partridge A.H. *et al.* (2006) American Society of Clinical Oncology Recommendations on Fertility Preservation in Cancer Patients. *Journal of Clinical Oncology,* 24, 2917–2931.
60. Nagel K., Cassano J., Wizowski L., Neal M.S. (2009) Collaborative multidisciplinary team approach to fertility issues among adolescent and young adult cancer patients. *International Journal of Nursing Practice,* 15, 311–317.
61. Mick J., Hughes M., Cohen M. (2004) Using the BETTER Model to assess sexuality. *Clinical Journal of Oncology Nursing,* 8, 84–86.
62. Institute of Medicine (IOM) (2008) *Cancer Care for the Whole Patient: Meeting Psychosocial Health Needs,* National Academies Press, Washington, DC.
63. Missmer S.A., Seifer D.B., Jain T. (2011) Cultural factors contributing to health care disparities among patients with infertility in Midwestern United States. *Fertility and Sterility,* 95, 1943–1949.
64. LIVESTRONG (2011) *LIVESTRONG Cancer Policy Platform Federal Priority Report.* Available at: http://www.livestrong.org/pdfs/3-0/LIVESTRONG_Policy Platform_2011 (accessed December 2011).
65. America Cancer Society (2011) ACS global blog: The United Nations includes cancer in a landmark resolution, ACS, New York.
66. American Cancer Society (2010) *Sexuality for the Man With Cancer.* http://www.cancer.org/Treatment/TreatmentsandSideEffects/PhysicalSideEffects/Sexual SideEffectsinMen/SexualityfortheMan/sexuality-for-the-man-with-cancer-toc (accessed January 2012).
67. American Cancer Society (2010) *Sexuality for the Woman With Cancer.* http://www.cancer.org/Treatment/TreatmentsandSideEffects/PhysicalSideEffects/Sexual SideEffectsinWomen/SexualityfortheWoman/sexuality-for-the-woman-with- cancer-toc (accessed January 2012).
68. Chandra A., Martinez G.M., Mosher W.D. *et al.* (2006) Fertility, contraception, and fatherhood: Data on men and women from Cycle 6 (2002) of the National Survey of Family Growth. National Center for Health Statistics. *Vital and Health Statistics* 23, 1–160.

CHAPTER 5
Psychosocial and Psychiatric Disorders

Santosh K. Chaturvedi[1] *and Yosuke Uchitomi*[2]

[1]Department of Psychiatry, National Institute of Mental Health and Neurosciences, Bangalore, India
[2]Department of Neuropsychiatry, Okayama University Graduate School of Medicine, Dentistry and Pharmaceutical Sciences, Okayama, Japan

Introduction and background

Psychosocial distress is commonly noted in persons suffering from cancer. A variety of psychiatric and psychosocial disorders are also observed in cancer patients, at different stages of their disease. The psychosocial disorders are related to the diagnosis of cancer, its physical effects, different treatments and interventions, as well as the outcome of the disease. The commonest psychiatric disorders observed in cancer patients are adjustment disorders, depression, anxiety, delirium and specific cancer-related psychosocial disorders. Many times, the psychiatric disorders are mild and/or of short duration, but at times these disorders can seriously impair the functioning, compliance and quality of life of the cancer patients. Earlier, depression was considered as the only emotional response to cancer and a natural reaction to the disease. Most of the early literature on psychiatric morbidity of cancer was drawn from clinical experience or unstructured interviews with patients and was largely anecdotal. There are considerable methodological problems in assessing the psychiatric morbidity, especially depression and anxiety, among cancer patients. A patient with cancer is expected to have a certain level of psychological distress but when this distress becomes a clinical problem, it needs to be addressed.

A majority of the studies have revealed a significant level of psychiatric morbidity among cancer patients. In clinical practice and in epidemiological studies of these patients, psychiatric disorders have been noted in varying prevalence rates. About 50% of patients with advanced cancer meet criteria for a psychiatric disorder, the most common being adjustment disorders (11–35%) and major depression (5–26%).[1] Generally, studies have found adjustment disorder as the most common psychiatric syndrome in cancer patients with major depression, delirium and anxiety disorders as the next common diagnoses. Conditions like personality disorders, psychoses and substance abuse are comparatively less frequent. In this chapter, the common psychosocial disorders related to cancer are discussed.

Common psychiatric disorders

Delirium

Delirium (sometimes called 'acute confusional state' or 'acute brain failure') is a common clinical syndrome characterized by disturbed consciousness, cognitive function or perception, which has an acute onset and fluctuating course. It usually develops over a few hours to days. However, it can be prevented and treated if dealt with urgently.[2]

Delirium is a serious condition that is associated with poor health outcomes (pneumonia, longer hospital stays, death). It is a distressing experience for family and medical ward staff as well as

Clinical Psycho-Oncology: An International Perspective, First Edition. Edited by Luigi Grassi and Michelle Riba.

for patients, caused by delusion, facing memory loss and nearing death. Delirium also interferes with appropriate assessment of physical symptoms, such as pain, and communication with family and friends. Delirious patients sometimes are not competent to consent to medical treatment, and exhibit impulsive behaviours caused by disinhibition, resulting in suicidal behaviours.

Prevalence

The prevalence of delirium in people in the general adult population is 0.7% (95% CI, 0.4–1.1) among those >55 years,[3] and that on medical wards in hospital is about 14–24%.[4] Up to 51% of post-surgical people[4] and up to 88% of people with terminally ill cancer develop delirium.[5]

Although delirium is common and treatable (but mainly irreversible in the last 24–48 hours of life),[6] very few cancer patients receive beneficial pharmacological and non-pharmacological treatments. One of the barriers that interfere with appropriate treatment may be associated with 'hypoactive subtype of delirium', characterized by people who become withdrawn, quiet and sleepy and who do not express discomfort and distress. Patients with hypoactive delirium were definitely as distressed as those with hyperactive delirium.[7] Hyperactive delirium showing restlessness, agitation and aggressiveness can be easily recognized. Moreover, it is often unrecognized in part because of its fluctuating nature, its overlap with dementia, lack of formal cognitive assessment, under-appreciation of its clinical consequences, and failure of health care professionals to be mindful of delirium.[4]

Diagnosis, signs and symptoms, and risk factors

If delirium is suspected, it is essential to carry out a clinical assessment based on the clinical and diagnostic criteria.[8,9] The Short Confusion Assessment Method (CAM) can be useful for rapid assessment and diagnosis. According to CAM the features of delirium are: (1) acute onset and fluctuating course, (2) inattention, (3) disorganized thinking, and (4) altered level of consciousness.

The risk factors for delirium are presented in Table 5.1 and the common causes of delirium in cancer patients in Table 5.2. After diagnosing, an assessment of risk and of cause for delirium should be carried out.

Delirium in the future DSM-V is currently proposed for the diagnostic category termed Neurocognitive Disorders. This category contains diagnoses that were listed in current classifications as Delirium, Dementia, Amnestic, and Other Cognitive Disorders. It is proposed to divide the new category into three broad syndromes: Delirium, Major Neurocognitive Disorders, and Mild Neurocognitive Disorders. The Neurocognitive Disorders Work Group discussed the notion that visuospatial impairment and impairment in executive

Table 5.1 Common risk factors for delirium.

Age 65 years or older
History of delirium, dementia, cognitive impairment
Low performance status, immobility, low level of activity
Visual or hearing impairment
Dehydration, malnutrition
Many psychoactive and non-psychoactive drugs
Alcohol abuse
Advanced illness and coexisting medical conditions

Table 5.2 Common causes of delirium in cancer patients.

Cancer disease-related
Brain tumour and metastasis, paraneoplastic syndrome, ectopic hormone-producing tumour (ACTH, ADH, insulin-like, parathyroid hormone)
Cancer treatment
Chemotherapy, corticosteroids, brain irradiation
Cancer pain drugs
Opioid analgesics, antidepressants, psychostimulants
Drugs
Benzodiazepines, anticholinergic drugs, alcohol
Infection
Metabolic disturbance
Hypoxia, hypercapnia, hypo- or hyperglycaemia, vitamins (B12, folate), electrolyte imbalance (Na, K, Ca), anaemia, dehydration, poor nutritional status, liver or renal dysfunction
Environmental
Admission to hospital, physical restraints, bladder catheter

function are key symptoms of delirium; the Group has also added a clarification that a pre-existing neurocognitive disorder does not account for the cognitive changes. Nothing is mentioned in the current criteria about accompanying symptoms. Though not necessary or sufficient in themselves to make the diagnosis, they should be recognized as frequent symptoms of delirium. Evidence is questionable for a subcategory for chronic delirium. The Group is still discussing whether to add subsyndromal delirium in parallel with minor neurocognitive disorder.[10]

Prevention, management and prognosis

Multicomponent approaches to reduce risk factors for delirium should ideally be provided for all newly admitted elderly patients, which are proven to prevent delirium resulting from orientation and therapeutic interventions for cognitive impairment, minimizing the use of psychoactive drugs, and so on.[9]

When delirium develops, the possible underlying cause or combination of causes should be identified and managed. Ensure effective communication and reorientation (e.g. explaining where the person is, who they are, and what your role is) and provide reassurance for people diagnosed with delirium. Consider involving family, friends and carers to help with this. Provide a suitable and safe care environment. Family members feel more distressed about facing delirious patients, therefore information, education and reassurance about the nature of delirium and its meaning are critically important management as well.[7] Information for patients with delirium and their family is available which: explains that delirium is common and usually temporary; describes people's experience of delirium; encourages people at risk and their families to tell their health care team about any sudden changes or fluctuations in usual behaviour; encourages the person who has had delirium to share their experience of delirium with the health care professional during recovery; and advises the person of any support groups. Ensure information meets cultural, cognitive and language needs.

In terminal delirium, over half of the bereaved families reported experiencing high levels of emotional distress and felt the need for some improvement in the specialized palliative care service. Control of agitation symptoms with careful consideration of ambivalent family wishes, providing information about the pathology of delirium, being present with the family, respecting the patient's subjective world, explaining the expected course with daily changes, and relieving family care burden can be useful care strategies.[11]

If delirium is significantly distressing for the patients, or the person with delirium is considered a risk to themselves or others, consider pharmacological interventions; short-term antipsychotic medication and implement safety precautions and procedures. All four guidelines (Australian, Canadian, UK and USA) recommend low-dose use of haloperidol (0.25–0.5 mg). Start at the lowest clinically appropriate dose and titrate cautiously according to symptoms. Some of the guidelines recommend atypical antipsychotics like olanzapine, risperidone and quetiapine. Open-label prospective studies revealed that aripiprazole,[12] perospirone,[13] mianserin,[14] and trazodone[15] might be effective for delirium, whereas melatonin[16] was effective in a randomized placebo-controlled study. If there is difficulty distinguishing between the diagnoses of delirium, dementia or delirium superimposed on dementia, treat for delirium first.

In conclusion, there is still a need to improve the understanding of pathophysiology of delirium and the efficacy of specific drug and/or non-drug therapy in delirium subtypes and subgroups based on the large, multicentre trials in this field.

Major depressive disorder

Depression has a great impact on the cancer patient's psychological distress, quality of life and increase in the subjective perception of pain, suicidal ideation and attempts, decreased adherence to treatment, prolonged length of hospital stay, increased family distress and worse prognosis.

Prevalence

Depression occurs throughout the course of their illness. Studies on depression in cancer patients have revealed that 4.5–58% of patients experience some form of depression, including major depression, dysthymia and adjustment disorders with depressive mood, and that 1–38% have major depression.[17] Recent meta-analytical pooled prevalence of DSM-defined major depression was 16.5% (95% CI, 13.1–20.3) in palliative care settings, and 16.3% (13.4–19.5) in oncological and haematological settings.[18]

Although depression is common and treatable (but may be irreversible in the last four weeks of life),[19] very few cancer patients receive beneficial psychosocial and psychiatric treatments. The recent systematic review provides evidence that antidepressants are effective in treating depression in palliative care settings as well. Their superiority over placebo is apparent within 4–5 weeks and increases with continued use.[20]

The barriers that interfere with appropriate treatment are: patient's reluctance to talk about psychological issues with medical staff, oncologist's thoughts that depression is an understandable reaction to cancer, lack of oncologist's knowledge and skills about psychological assessment and management skills, lack of psychiatrist's knowledge about oncology, difficulties in distinguishing appropriate sadness to cancer from depressive physical symptoms not attributable to cancer.[21] Also, cultural, organizational and specific issues continue to represent a problem in the delivery of mental health interventions in medical settings.

Diagnosis and severity assessment of depression

If thinking of depression, consider asking cancer patients who may have depression two questions, specifically:

- During the last month, have you often been bothered by feeling down, depressed or hopeless?
- During the last month, have you often been bothered by having little interest or pleasure in doing things?

These are two core symptoms of major depression, namely depressed mood and a marked loss of interest or pleasure. To diagnose as major depression, one or both of the hallmark core symptoms must be present for at least two weeks, along with at least four other symptoms (significant weight loss/gain or decrease/increase in appetite, insomnia or hypersomnia, psychomotor agitation or slowing, fatigue or loss of energy, feelings of worthlessness or excessive guilt, diminished ability to think or concentrate, or indecisiveness, recurrent thoughts of death or suicidal ideation).

Difficulty in diagnosing depression comes from somatic and vegetative symptoms, such as fatigue, appetite disturbance or weight loss, sleep difficulties, and difficulties with memory and concentration, because these symptoms can be attributable to cancer and its treatment. More emphasis may need to be placed on psychological symptoms, such as feelings of worthlessness, excessive guilt, hopelessness and helplessness. Persistent suicidal ideation is strongly associated with major depression.

Non-Western, especially Japanese patients had difficulty with Western biopsychiatric concepts of depression. Sadness, worry and stress, not depression were more commonly used terms, thus mental health providers need more euphemisms: worry, maybe sadness, stress, anxiety. These patients are reluctant to discuss psychological issues, especially emotional disclosure to their physicians. They would like not to view their condition as an individual issue. Focusing on community and contextual factors, such as family, work, financial and housing issues, was seen as more acceptable. The physicians might avoid the term depression during these discussions.[22,23]

Depression in cancer patients should be distinguished from demoralization. The depressed person has lost the ability to experience pleasure generally, whereas a demoralized person may enjoy the present moment, if distracted from demoralizing thoughts. The demoralized person feels inhibited in action by not knowing what to do, feeling helpless and incompetent; the depressed person has lost motivation and drive, and is unable to act even when an appropriate direction of action is known.[24] Diagnosing severity of depression simultaneously would be useful for moderate and severe major depression responding well to antidepressant pharmacotherapy.

The Mood Disorders Work Group for DSM-V is putting forth a proposal for the addition of Mixed Anxiety/Depression as a new diagnosis. The patient has three or four of the symptoms of major depression (which must include depressed mood and/or anhedonia), and they are accompanied by anxious distress. The symptoms must have lasted at least two weeks, no other DSM diagnosis of anxiety or depression must be present, and they are both occurring at the same time. Anxious distress is defined as having two or more of the following symptoms: irrational worry, preoccupation with unpleasant worries, having trouble relaxing, motor tension, fear that something awful may happen. The new Mixed Anxiety/Depression will be a hot area in the field of psycho-oncology.

Assessing risk factors of depression in cancer patients

Comprehensive assessment of risk factors of depression in cancer patients leads to better prevention and early treatment. Table 5.3 describes the common risk factors of depression in cancer patients.

Management and prognosis

Clinical practice guidelines for the psychosocial care of cancer patients are available in some countries. The National Institute for Clinical Evidence (NICE) guidelines for the management of depression in adults with a chronic physical health problem in the United Kingdom propose that screening for depression should be undertaken in primary-care and general hospital settings for high-risk groups, which include those with significant physical illnesses.[25]

Table 5.3 Common risk factors of depression in cancer patients.

- Physical: pain, low performance status
- Metabolic: abnormal electrolytes, vitamin B12, folate, parathyroid and thyroid hormone, ACTH, cortisol, cachexia, paraneoplastic syndrome
- Brain tumour, vascular vulnerability, Parkinsonism, Lewy body disease
- Drugs: corticosteroids, interferon, interleukin-2, vincristine, vinblastine, procarbazine, paclitaxel
- Psychiatric: history of depression and suicide, substance abuse
- Others: recent life events, recent loss of spouse or significant other, younger age, living alone, poor social support, economic difficulties

When beginning treatment with cancer patients with depression and their families, information and support should be provided, a time for appropriate decision and informed consent, support for families and carers, being respectful of, and sensitive to, diverse familial, cultural, ethnic and religious backgrounds, coordination of cancer care and choosing depression treatments.

After carefully assessing symptoms, risk factors and functional impairment, moderate/severe major depression or mild/less major depression (minor depression, adjustment disorders with depressive mood, 'reactive depression') should be evaluated next. For mild/less major depression, in principle, low-intensive psychosocial interventions should be provided, such as a peer support group, supportive psychotherapy, problem-solving technique and/or anxiolytics and hypnotics.

For moderate/severe major depression, intensive-psychosocial interventions should be provided, such as more formal cognitive-behavioural psychotherapy or pharmacotherapy. Before choosing antidepressants, consider administration route of antidepressants (e.g. bowel obstruction, stomatitis), adverse effect profiles (nausea, constipation, erectile dysfunction, urinary retention, etc.), estimated prognosis and time enough for responding to antidepressants (at least four weeks),[19,20] physical status, especially, liver and renal dysfunction, drug interactions and patient's preferences for avoidable adverse effects. Selective serotonin reuptake inhibitors (SSRIs) with safety and less adverse effect profiles, such as citalopram and sertraline, are the starting drugs. The newer agents, such as mirtazapine, duloxetine, venlafaxine, are also considered especially for patients with cancer pain.

Although SSRIs and SNRIs (serotonin–norepinephrine reuptake inhibitors) have been shown to be effective in treating hot flushes in women with a history of breast cancer, paroxetine (an irreversible inhibitor of CYP2D6) use during tamoxifen treatment is recently reported to be associated with an increased risk of death from breast cancer. Caution should be exercised when using SSRIs and SNRIs, which can reduce or abolish the benefit of tamoxifen in women with breast cancer by inhibiting its bioactivation by CYP2D6.[26]

The older agents, such as tricyclic antidepressants, are usually avoided except for patients with neuropathic cancer pain because of the drugs' anticholinergic and anti-alpha-adrenergic properties. Amytriptyline as well as mirtazapine are listed in the essential drugs for palliative care endorsed by the International Associations of Hospice and Palliative Care (IAHPC).Vulnerable and elderly patients should be started at low doses with careful dose escalation and be monitored every1–2 weeks for adverse effects and response. When facing death, antipsychotics rather than antidepressants should be considered for reducing and sedating some of the distressing symptoms caused by terminally ill depression.

In conclusion, a more sensitive, collaborative and comprehensive approach to the diagnosis and treatment of depression, including clinical education, enhanced role of nurses, and integrating oncology and specialty care, is required in the clinical oncology setting.

Anxiety disorders

Anxiety symptoms have often been observed as part of depression in cancer patients. Anxiety can also be a part of the normal stress response, adjustment disorder, depressive disorders and delirium. Generalized anxiety disorder is not as frequent as depressive disorder in these patients. The common anxiety symptoms noted in cancer patients are persistent tension and worrying, panic attacks and palpitations. In addition to the stress of the cancer and its effects, the treatment methods and some of the drugs that are commonly used in cancer patients can also produce anxiety, for example bronchodilators, which are frequently used in lung cancer patients, interferon and steroids.

Cancer patients become anxious when there is uncertainty and communication with the health professional has not been appropriate or satisfactory. Other situations which can make a cancer patient anxious are costs of treatment, future of family members, lack of adequate response to cancer treatment and other unfinished business. Effective communication skills and breaking bad news methods can reduce or minimize this anxiety.

Prevalence

The prevalence of anxiety in patients diagnosed with cancer increases with advancing disease and declines with the patient's physical status. In cancer patients, anxiety is commonly associated with depressive symptoms, which makes the determination of exact prevalence of anxiety symptoms and syndromes a challenging task. Another factor that interferes with the assessment of prevalence of anxiety in cancer patients is the overlap of physical and autonomic symptoms of anxiety in cancer and anxiety disorders, such as in depressive disorders. A recent meta-analysis found prevalence of anxiety disorders to be 9.8% (6.8–13.2) in palliative care settings and 10.3% (5.1–17.0) in oncological and haematological settings.[18] There is a lack of data regarding the influence of cultural factors in the moulding anxiety disorders in cancer.

The anxiety symptoms in relation to cancer often go undetected and under-treated as these are considered as a natural reaction to the cancer diagnosis, the physical effects of the treatment and also the different therapies for the disease. Anxiety increases as the disease progresses and may also be precipitated by the withdrawal of active treatment due to any reason.[27]

Diagnosis of anxiety disorders

The common symptoms of anxiety are given in Table 5.4. The physical or somatic manifestations of anxiety, such as autonomic hyperactivity, insomnia, or dyspnoea, often overshadow the psychological or cognitive ones. Physical symptoms are the most common presenting symptoms of anxiety in patients with advanced illness also.

The assumption that a high level of anxiety is inevitably encountered during the terminal phase of illness is neither helpful nor accurate for diagnostic and therapeutic purposes. Anxiety decreases gradually and sometimes spontaneously, but can be easily reactivated by another development in the course of disease or treatment.

Table 5.4 The common symptoms of anxiety in cancer patients.

Somatic / Physical
- Muscular aches and fatigue
- Restlessness
- Trembling, tremors
- Jumpiness, edgy, jitteriness
- Tension headache
- Autonomic over-activity: palpitations, sweating, dizziness, dry mouth, nausea, diarrhoea, 'lump in throat', cold clammy hands, paresthesias, hot or cold spells
- Inability to relax body

Psychological
- Apprehension about future, death
- Worry about illness, anxiety
- Fears, ruminations
- Dread of misfortune in self or others
- Inability to relax mind
- Irritability
- Difficulty concentrating, distractible
- Difficulty falling sleep, unrefreshing sleep, tired on waking, nightmares
- Misinterpretation of bodily sensations

Risk factors of anxiety in cancer patients can be assessed by evaluating a number of features given in Table 5.5.

Management and prognosis

The patient's subjective level of distress is the primary reason for the initiation of treatment. It is necessary to consider the risks and benefits of treatment. The specific treatment of anxiety in cancer often depends on aetiology, presentation and setting. Other considerations include problematic patient behaviour such as non-adherence due to the anxiety, as well as family and staff reactions to the patient's distress.

The common pharmacological agents that can be used for management of anxiety disorders in cancer patients are low-dose benzodiazepines such as clonazepam, alprazolam, lorazepam, beta-blockers, buspirone and hydroxizine. Low-dose antidepressants can also be used for management of anxiety disorders, such as trazodone or citalopram. Tricyclic antidepressants as well as SSRIs are useful for longer term anxiety disorders in patients with cancer.

Table 5.5 Risk factors of anxiety in cancer patients can be assessed by evaluating the following:

Anxiety as a reaction to:
- Receiving bad news,
- Awareness of terminal condition,
- Fears and uncertainty about, poor relationship with family or staff.

Disease- and treatment-related anxiety:
- Poor pain control,
- Related metabolic disturbances,
- Delirium,
- Discomforts of medical procedures.

Medication-induced anxiety:
- Due to steroids, antiemetics, opioids, bronchodilators including,
- Withdrawal of medications, like opioids, benzodiazepines.

Other risk factors:
- Pre-existing anxiety disorders, independent of the disease
- Past history of mood disorder
- Family history of mood disorder
- History of substance use, alcoholism, drug dependence
- Concurrent life events, social stress
- Lack of social support from families and friends
- Personality traits hindering adjustment, such as rigidity, pessimism, extreme need for independence and control, or anxious avoidant personality

Psychological methods such as psychotherapy and counselling, and behavioural methods such as mindfulness meditation and relaxation exercises can also be useful in managing anxiety disorders, with or without pharmacological therapy.

Adjustment disorders

The diagnostic criteria for adjustment disorders in the DSM and ICD systems are reported to be imprecise and vague. Adjustment disorder refers to someone who is distressed and 'not coping', having recently encountered a disease-related stressor, like a malignant diagnosis, a treatment complication, a non-response to treatment, or the awareness of impending death.[27] In the proposed DSM-V, adjustment disorder will be considered as the development of emotional or behavioural symptoms in response to an identifiable stressor(s) occurring within three months of the onset of the stressor(s). In the case of the subtype 'related to bereavement', 12 months of symptoms are required after the death of a close relative or friend, before the diagnosis may be employed.[10]

Prevalence

These are the most common psychiatric syndromes seen in cancer patients. The majority of patients have adjustment disorder mainly with depressed mood, anxious mood and mixed emotional disturbances. Prevalence of adjustment disorder alone was 15.4% (10.1–21.6) in palliative care settings and 19.4% (14.5–24.8), in oncological and haematological settings in a recent meta-analysis.[18]

Diagnosis, risk factors and severity assessment of adjustment disorders

A diagnosis of adjustment disorder should be considered when an acute stress response persists in a stereotyped fashion and interferes significantly with functioning. Adjustment disorder is classified according to subtype, which corresponds with the presenting symptoms. The subtypes of adjustment disorder include those with depressed mood, anxiety, mixed anxiety and depressed mood, disturbance of conduct, mixed disturbance of emotions and conduct, and unspecified.

Risk factors identified for development of adjustment disorders are: low ego strength, passive or avoidant coping style, inadequate or inappropriate information, poor social support, communication problems, treatment-related stressors, number of unresolved concerns and level of partner's distress.[28] Lack of coping flexibility may also predispose a person dealing with the stress of a malignant disease.

Management and prognosis

Management of adjustment disorders can be done effectively with supportive methods and counselling. Behavioural and cognitive behavioural approaches are also worth trying. The pharmacological treatment is symptomatic. Low-dose antidepressant medications or benzodiazepines for a short period of time may be useful.

Adjustment disorders are likely to recur with repeated stressful situations during the course and progression of the disease. Cancer patients with adjustment disorders can respond to psychiatric treatment, but some patients go on to develop major depressive disorders. Those suffering from pain, which can be managed or controlled, significantly predicted a good treatment response, whereas a worse performance status predicted a poor treatment response.[29]

Somatization and abnormal illness behaviour in cancer patients

There is a common belief among health professionals that physical or somatic symptoms occur only in medical, physical or 'organic' disorders, and that psychiatric disorders present mainly with emotional, psychological or cognitive symptoms. Similarly, when physical or somatic symptoms occur in a person with a diagnosed medical disease, these symptoms are suspected or believed to be due to the underlying medical disease, its complication or its treatment. Somatic symptoms and somatization in depressive disorders and anxiety disorders are common clinical and research observations. Thus, it is likely that the depressive, anxiety or other psychiatric disorders in cancer may manifest with physical or somatic symptoms. Psychological factors affecting medical conditions in a category in DSM-V, could be useful in documenting illness behaviours in cancer patients as the factors that influence the course of the malignancy, as shown by a close temporal association between the psychological factors and the development or exacerbation of, or delayed recovery from, the malignancy (e.g. poor adherence), interfere with the treatment of the malignancy. These factors constitute additional well-established health risks for the individual and influence the underlying pathophysiology to precipitate or exacerbate symptoms or to necessitate medical attention.[10]

Prevalence

Residual or persistent fatigue in survivors of childhood cancer, survivors of Hodgkin's disease and cancer patients referred for psychiatric consultation have been noticed.[30,31] In a prospective study of patients with Hodgkin's disease and non-Hodgkin's lymphoma nearly a fifth of patients, who were disease-free and off treatment, continued to exhibit illness behaviour such as complaints of feeling tired, poor concentration and irritability, probably due to psychological factors. Somatization is common in patients referred for psychiatric consultation with about 28% demonstrating prominent somatic presentation with multiple somatic symptoms. There is an association between somatization, depression and cancer.[30] Common somatic complaints observed in cancer patients are pain, fatigue, sensory symptoms, anorexia, weight loss, tiredness, exhaustion, weakness, reduced energy, tremors, lethargy and mixed symptoms. A study reported high prevalence of psychological distress in cancer patients (37%) and among patients with psychological distress somatization was more frequent followed by depression and anxiety.[32]

An important issue related to somatic symptoms in cancer is the difficulty in deciding whether certain physical symptoms are due to cancer, treatment by cytotoxic drugs, radiotherapy, psychiatric disorder, or a combination of these, because somatic symptoms of depression overlap those of cancer. However, they present a challenge since the management of cancer pain and fatigue due to chemotherapy would be managed differently from pain and fatigue as somatoform symptoms.

The somatic symptoms in cancer are not life-threatening, rather these fluctuate during the course of the disease. They have important implications in the management and prognosis of cancer due to the associated disability and poor outcome with reduced quality of life. Somatic symptoms magnify disability resulting from cancer, interfere with treatment adherence and decisions, cause delay in recovery, result in poor outcome and recurrence, reduce overall well-being and quality of life.

Diagnosis of somatization

Cancer-related somatic symptoms have cognitive, psychological and physiological causes each of which is amenable to treatment. The occurrence of somatoform disorders in cancer patients is likely to complicate the treatment and outcome of cancer. In advanced cancer, depression and somatic symptoms have been known to be due to endocrine and metabolic brain syndromes, cerebral metastasis, neurological infections, nutrition deficits and anti-tumour therapies. Breathlessness, muscle pain, dizziness and palpitation are common symptoms of anxiety and panic attack, which have been noted in cancer patients.

Somatization in disease-free cancer patients is perhaps related to anxiety and depression. Cancer patients with somatization also have excessive somatic concern and preoccupation, but whether this is the cause or effect of suffering from persistent somatic symptoms is difficult to conclude. It could be the effect of persistent somatization since most subjects had no previous evidence of somatization. Depressive symptoms and depressive disorders were encountered commonly in these patients, and this association between depression and somatization is similar to that documented in psychiatric populations.

Assessment of somatic symptoms and differentiating their aetiology needs careful evaluation of association with stress and psychological factors. When somatic symptoms arise or are aggravated after stress, psychological or emotional factors, they are likely to be psychological somatic symptoms. Those related to progression of disease or treatments are probably more physical. Some somatic symptoms may have both physical and psychological factors implicated. Lastly, there may be somatic symptoms which may not be clearly physical or psychological in origin and may be idiopathic.[31]

Diagnosis of abnormal illness behaviour in cancer patients

The occurrence of unexplained somatic symptoms, persistent fatigue and tiredness in disease-free cancer patients has raised doubts of the occurrence of abnormal illness behaviour in cancer patients. The study by Grassi and Rosti[33] confirmed the association between psychological disorders and abnormal illness behaviour in cancer and pointed out a role for personality variables (external locus of control) and low social support in favouring maladaptive responses to cancer. In another study by Grassi and colleagues,[34] different forms of abnormal illness behaviours such as denial, irritability, dysphoria, measured using the Illness Behaviour Questionnaire, were noted in cancer patients in association with depression.

Management and prognosis

The management of somatization would include a combination of psychosocial and pharmacological methods. Psychotherapy, counselling, reassurance and reattribution of the somatic symptoms can be useful. Low-dose antidepressants, both tricyclics and SSRIs can also be effective, though one needs to be cautious of drug side-effects which may be further misinterpreted as worsening of the disease or new somatic symptoms.[35] Fatigue in terminally ill cancer patients is determined by both physical and psychological factors; hence it may be important to include psychological intervention in the multidimensional management of fatigue in addition to physical and nursing interventions.[36]

Other psychiatric disorders

Other psychosocial disorders encountered in cancer patients are sleep disorders, psychosis, psychosexual dysfunctions, anticipatory nausea and vomiting, alcoholism and substance use disorders.

Sleep disorders

Sleep disturbances are common in cancer patients, but there are few specific data on their prevalence. Sleep problems may be a symptom of cancer itself, part of the stress reaction to having cancer, as sequelae to some other cancer symptom such as pain, or a side-effect of cancer treatment. Insomnia is the more common sleep problem, although hypersomnia also occurs. Most insomnias are related either to pain or to psychophysiological factors. For management of insomnia in cancer, evidence supports cognitive-behavioural therapy in cancer; no sleep agents have superior effectiveness.[37]

Psychosis

Schizophrenia and other functional psychoses are comparatively less frequent than the other above-mentioned disorders but contrary to the earlier beliefs cancer is not rare in patients with schizophrenia as compared to the general population. Recently the impact of cancer in patients with severe mental illness has been the object of discussion among mental health professionals. The different organization in mental health care systems in different countries is making an attempt to understand if and how people with severe psychiatric disorders are in fact looked after in terms of screening of cancer, prevention and treatment. Problems can emerge in using drugs that could worse psychotic symptoms. Vinca alkaloids can produce hallucinations. Opioid treatment also could create problems in psychiatrically ill patients who develop cancer. It has been reported that severe mental illness is associated with behaviours that predispose an individual to an increased risk of some cancers, including lung and breast cancer, although lower rates of other cancers are reported in this population. Severe mental illness is also associated with disparities in screening for cancer and with higher case-fatality rates. This higher rate is partly due to the specific challenges of treating these patients, including medical comorbidity, drug interactions, lack of capacity and difficulties in coping with the treatment regimen as a result of psychiatric symptoms. To ensure that patients with severe mental illness receive effective treatment, inequalities in care need to be addressed by all health care professionals involved, including those from mental health services and the surgical and oncology teams.[38]

The management is the same as in schizophrenia with any medical disorder, with caution over drug interactions between anticancer treatment and antipsychotics.

Psychosexual dysfunctions

Psychosexual dysfunctions can occur in patients who have a malignancy of sexual organs or related body parts like testis, prostate, cervical cancers, uterus, ovary or breast. The dysfunction could be due to direct effect of the disease, hormonal derangements, chemotherapy, radiation treatment or hormonal treatment.

Sexuality and intimacy are altered following mastectomy. Besides the woman affected by breast cancer or mastectomy, some researchers have found that approximately 36% of husbands reported that mastectomy had a 'bad' or 'somewhat bad' influence on their sexual relationships, and moderate to severe sexual difficulties even a year after mastectomy.

A review of sexual functioning morbidity estimates for major organ sites, indicates that a large number of cancer patients have problems in sexual functioning. The highest rates are in those patients where the cancer is at a sexual or reproductive body site. The exact prevalence of psychosexual problems is not known among cancer patients, but it is thought to be much more common than expected. Cancer survivors experience rates of sexual dysfunction ranging up to 90%; actual rates may be even higher than reported rates due to widespread reluctance of patients to discuss sexual problems with staff.

Sexual problems among cancer patients usually start acutely, after diagnosis, or treatment. In some cases, such as in prostate cancer or cervical cancers, sexual problems may be the earliest sign of disease. Problems in sexual excitement and arousal are common, orgasmic problems are also quite frequent while in some there may be pain during intercourse. Sexual activity and satisfaction is affected by the malignancy, its effect on the health, changes in body image, foul smelling or blood-stained discharges from the tumour site, chemotherapy, radiotherapy or surgery. Loss of libido could be due to the above factors, but it could at times be a manifestation of depression associated with cancer. General weakness and cachexia could also contribute to the sexual weakness and disinclination. Fatigue after the treatment can be very severe and interfere with sexual activity.

The management would include sexual and marital counselling besides any medications for underlying medical or psychiatric causes of the dysfunction or difficulty. Also regarding this important area, cultural implications are important, given the role of social habits, religious and traditions in modulating the expression of sexuality and sexual disorders secondary to cancer.

A recent review[39] noted moderate support for the effectiveness and feasibility of psychological interventions targeting sexual dysfunction following cancer but attrition rates were high, placebo response was notable, and there were often barriers impeding survivors from seeking out psychological interventions for sexual concerns. Despite the prevalence of sexual difficulties following cancer treatment, psychological interventions are a viable, but not often sought after option to help improve sexual functioning, intimacy and quality of life for cancer survivors and their partners.

Anticipatory nausea and vomiting (ANV) (conditioned response to chemotherapy)

The conditioned side-effects are thought to develop through a classical conditioning. These conditioned responses can occur before, during or after chemotherapy. The anticipatory nausea and vomiting are found to be associated with a higher anxiety level, post-chemotherapy nausea and vomiting are also reliable predictors of anticipatory side-effect.

The management of the anticipatory nausea and vomiting is gradual desensitization, counselling or low-dose benzodiazepines.

Non-pharmacological approaches, which include behavioural interventions, may offer the greatest promise in relieving symptoms. Little evidence supports the use of complementary and alternative methods, such as acupuncture and acupressure, in relieving ANV. Behavioural interventions, especially progressive muscle relaxation training and systematic desensitization, should be considered important methods for preventing and treating ANV.[40]

Alcoholism and substance use disorders

Alcoholism may coexist in many cancer patients, as a risk factor for many malignancies especially involving the gastrointestinal system, head and neck, and hepatic systems. Similarly, nicotine use, both smoke and smokeless is associated with pulmonary and head and neck cancers. Patients with dependence on alcohol, nicotine or other substances may need additional help to manage these drug dependencies.

Similarly, there can be evidence of cannabis and opiate abuse or dependence, which would need appropriate management. One has to be cautious not to under-medicate for cancer pain in a patient who has a substance use disorder. Misconceptions that treatment of cancer pain with morphine would necessarily lead to addiction also need to be dispelled.

Psychiatric emergencies

Psychiatric emergencies warrant immediate attention similar to other oncological emergencies (Table 5.6). Early diagnosis and treatment can result in effective management of these psychiatric emergencies.[41,42] The most common psychiatric emergencies are delirium, depression, suicidal behaviours and severe anxiety in cancer patients. There are, however, some difficulties in carrying out a psychiatric and psychosocial assessment of cancer patients without a history of psychiatric disorders encountered in the emergent setting. When the patients are agitated, confused, self-harmful and leave the hospital against medical advice, these disorders require the same urgent and aggressive attention as do other distressing physical symptoms.

When emergent, carry out the assessment of risk and cause for agitated and suicidal behaviours (Table 5.6). Suicidal statements are commonly thought, and when asked, expressed by cancer patients, often resulting from their frustration or wish to share or end their distressed situation. However, it could be dangerous when they have actual plans with suicidal attempts, especially if juxtaposed with delirium, depression, or substance abuse. So, it is important to ask if they have a suicidal plan as well as psychiatric and psychosocial disorders.

Table 5.6 Psychiatric emergencies: assessment of agitated, confused, suicidal, or treatment refusal in cancer patients.

1. Oncological emergencies (spinal cord compression, superior vena cava syndrome, hypocalcaemia, acute dyspnoea, seizures, acute urinary and bowel obstructions, massive haemorrhage, cardiac tamponade and acute embolic phenomenon)
2. Excited, agitated, restlessness, anxious
   - Major depression, adjustment disorders with anxious mood
   - Acute exacerbation of major psychosis, alcohol and substance abuser, dementia and other organic brain disorders, panic disorder, generalized anxiety disorder, personality disorders
   - Uncontrolled pain, anticipated painful images of medical procedures, surgery, or advanced illness
   - Akathisia due to dopamine-2 receptor antagonist; prochlorperazine, metoclopramide, haloperidol, chlorpromazine
   - Steroid psychosis
   - Grief reaction
3. Confused, somnolent
   - Delirium
   - Encephalitis, brain tumour, brain haemorrhage, hepatic encephalopathy, dementia with delirium, alcohol and substance withdrawal, epileptic seizure and other organic brain disorders
   - Drug intoxication
4. Suicidal
   - Depression, adjustment disorders with anxious mood
   - Delirium, drug intoxication
5. Refusal against medical advice
   - Cognitive impairment, dementia, delirium
   - Major depression, adjustment disorders with anxious mood

Role of cultural factors and cultural implications

As discussed throughout the chapter, sociocultural and traditional factors have an important role in the etiopathogenesis, manifestation, presentation and management of psychosocial disorders related to cancer. The implications of the cultural aspects are important in view of current globalization and immigration. It is crucial for health care providers to recognize the influence of cultural factors and be able to provide culturally sensitive care for their patients. The knowledge about a person's cultural background can improve psychosocial care. Hence, there is a need for cultural sensitivity and respect for cultural norms, preferences, taboos and traditions of the patient. Promoting cultural awareness and cultural competence among health care professionals should improve their confidence and skills in providing comprehensive care for cancer patients and families from different backgrounds. Cultural competence is effective when based on knowledge of a culture, on appreciation of cultural differences, on awareness of biases and prejudices, and on attitudes of humility, empathy, curiosity, respect and sensitivity.

A recent meta-analysis on prevalence of depression, anxiety and adjustment disorder in oncological, haematological and palliative care settings evaluated 24 studies of individuals across 7 countries in palliative care settings, and 70 studies across 14 countries in oncological and haematological settings, and reported comparable rates using the ICD and DSM systems, indicating little cross-national variations.[18]

Key points

- Psychosocial and psychiatric disorders are common in cancer patients at different stages of the disease, and may be related to the cancer treatments as well. Identification and appropriate management of these disorders is important for the holistic care of cancer patients.
- Adjustment disorders are common; however, there can be varied manifestations of depression, anxiety, panic, somatoform and illness behaviour disorders, or specific sleep, psychosexual or substance use disorders.
- Combination diagnoses are common; all types of depression and mood disorder are noted. The presence of psychosocial disorders may interfere with the patient's adherence to cancer treatment, and also aggravate their quality of life.
- A recent meta-analysis concluded that depression and anxiety is less common in patients with cancer than previously thought, although some combination of mood disorders occurs in 30–40% of patients in hospital settings without a significant difference between palliative care and non-palliative care settings.[18]
- Clinicians should be cautious and vigilant for different mood complications, not just depression. Psychiatric emergencies occurring in cancer patients need prompt intervention. The role of psychological treatments in the management of psychological problems is well acknowledged by physicians and other clinicians caring for patients in oncology.

References

1. Miovic M., Block S. (2007) Psychiatric disorders in advanced cancer. *Cancer*, 15, 1665–76.
2. Caraceni A., Grassi L. (2011) *Delirium: Acute Confusional States in Palliative Medicine*, 2nd edn, Oxford University Press, New York.
3. Folstein M.F., Bassett S.S., Romanoski A.J., Nestadt G. (1991) The epidemiology of delirium in the community: The Eastern Baltimore Mental Health Survey. *International Psychogeriatrics*, 3, 169–76.
4. Inouye S.K. (2006) Delirium in older persons. *New England Journal of Medicine*, 354, 1157–1165.
5. Lawlor P.G., Gagnon B., Mancini I.L. *et al.* (2000). Clinical utility, factor analysis, and further validation of the memorial delirium assessment scale in patients with advanced cancer: Assessing delirium in advanced cancer. *Cancer*, 88, 2859–67.
6. Breitbart W., Cohen K.R. (1998) Delirium, in *Psycho-Oncology* (ed. J.C. Holland), Oxford University Press, New York, pp. 564–575.
7. Breitbart W., Gibson C., Tremblay A. (2002) The delirium experience: Delirium recall and delirium-related distress in hospitalized patients with cancer, their spouses/caregivers, and their nurses. *Psychosomatics*, 43, 183–94.
8. American Psychiatric Association (APA) (1999) Practice guidelines for the treatment of patients with delirium. *American Journal of Psychiatry*, 156S, 1–20.
9. National Collaborating Centre for Mental Health, Commissioned by the National Institute for Health and Clinical Excellence (NICE) (2010) *Delirium: Diagnosis, prevention, and management.* (Clinical guideline CG103.); www.nice.org.uk/CG103 (accessed December 2011).
10. http://www.dsm5.org/ProposedRevision/Pages/proposedrevision.aspx?rid=32# (accessed December 2011).
11. Morita T., Akechi T., Ikenaga M. *et al.* (2007) Terminal delirium: Recommendations from bereaved families' experiences. *Journal of Pain Symptom Management*, 34, 579–89.
12. Boettger S., Friedlander M., Breitbart W., Passik S. (2011) Aripiprazole and haloperidol in the treatment of delirium. *Australia and New Zealand Journal of Psychiatry*, 45, 477–82.
13. Takeuchi T., Furuta K., Hirasawa T. *et al.* (2007) Perospirone in the treatment of patients with delirium. *Psychiatry and Clinical Neurosciences*, 61, 67–70.

14. Uchiyama M., Tanaka K., Isse K., Toru M. (1996) Efficacy of mianserin on symptoms of delirium in the aged: An open trial study. *Progress in Neuropsychopharmacology & Biological Psychiatry*, 20, 651–6.
15. Okamoto Y., Matsuoka Y., Sasaki T. *et al.* (1999) Trazodone in the treatment of delirium. *Journal of Clinical Psychopharmacology*, 19, 280–2.
16. Al-Aama T., Brymer C., Gutmanis I. *et al.* (2011) Melatonin decreases delirium in elderly patients: A randomized, placebo-controlled trial. *International Journal of Geriatric Psychiatry*, 26, 687–94.
17. Massie M.J. (2004) Prevalence of depression in patients with cancer. *Journal of the National Cancer Institute Monographs*, 32, 57–71.
18. Mitchell A.J., Chan M., Bhatti H. *et al.* (2011) Prevalence of depression, anxiety, and adjustment disorder in oncological, haematological, and palliative-care settings: A meta-analysis of 94 interview-based studies. *The Lancet Oncology*, 12, 160–74.
19. Shimizu K., Akechi T., Shimamoto M. *et al.* (2007) Can psychiatric intervention improve major depression in very near end-of-life cancer patients? *Palliative and Supportive Care*, 5, 3–9.
20. Rayner L., Price A., Evans A. *et al.* (2011) Antidepressants for the treatment of depression in palliative care: Systematic review and meta-analysis. *Palliative Medicine*, 25, 36–51.
21. Grassi L., Nanni M.G., Uchitomi Y., Riba M. (2010) Pharmacotherapy of depression in people with cancer, in *Depression and Cancer* (eds D. Kissane, M. Maj, N. Sartorius), John Wiley & Sons, Ltd, Chichester, pp. 151–176.
22. Okuyama T., Endo C., Seto T. *et al.* (2009) Cancer patients' reluctance to discuss psychological distress with their physicians was not associated with underrecognition of depression by physicians: A preliminary study. *Palliative and Supportive Care*, 7, 229–33.
23. Furler J., Kokanovic R., Dowrick C. *et al.* (2010). Managing depression among ethnic communities: A qualitative study. *Annals of Family Medicine*, 8, 231–6.
24. Massie M.J., Lloyd-Williams M., Irving G., Miller K. (2010) The prevalence of depression in people with cancer, in *Depression and Cancer* (eds D. Kissane, M. Maj, N. Sartorius), John Wiley & Sons, Ltd., Chichester, pp 1–36.
25. National Collaborating Centre for Mental Health, Commissioned by the National Institute for Health and Clinical Excellence (NICE) (2009) *Depression in adults with a chronic physical health problem: Treatment and management*. (Clinical guideline CG91); www.nice.org.uk/CG91 (accessed December 2011).
26. Kelly C.M., Juurlink D.N., Gomes T. *et al.* (2010) Selective serotonin reuptake inhibitors and breast cancer mortality in women receiving tamoxifen: A population-based cohort study. *British Medical Journal*, 340, c693.
27. Macleod A.D. (2007) *The Psychiatry of Palliative Medicine. The Dying Mind*, Radcliff Publishing, New York, pp. 5–18.
28. Walker L., Walker M., Sharp D. (2003) Current provision of psychosocial care within palliative care. In *Psychosocial Issues in Palliative Care* (ed. M. Lloyd Williams), Oxford University Press, Oxford, pp. 49–65.
29. Shimizu K., Akizuki N., Nakaya N. *et al.* (2011) Treatment response to psychiatric intervention and predictors of response among cancer patients with adjustment disorders. *Journal of Pain Symptom Management*, 41, 684–91.
30. Chaturvedi SK, Hopwood P, Maguire, P. (1993). Non organic somatic symptoms in Cancer. *European Journal of Cancer*, 29A, 1006–1008.
31. Chaturvedi S.K., Maguire P. (1998) Persistent somatization in cancer: A follow up study. *Journal of Psychosomatic Research*, 45, 249–256.
32. Carlson L.E., Angen M., Cullum J. (2004) High level of untreated distress and fatigue in cancer patients. *British Journal of Cancer*, 90, 2297–2304.
33. Grassi L., Rosti G. (1996) Psychiatric and psychosocial concomitants of abnormal illness behaviour in patients with cancer. *Psychotherapy and Psychosomatics*, 65, 246–52.
34. Grassi L., Rosti G., Albieri G., Marangolo M. (1989) Depression and abnormal illness behavior in cancer patients. *General Hospital Psychiatry*, 11, 404–11.
35. Chaturvedi SK, Maguire P, Somashekhar BS (2006). Somatization in cancer. *International Review of Psychiatry*, 18, 49–54.
36. Okuyama T., Akechi T., Shima Y. *et al.* (2008) Factors correlated with fatigue in terminally ill cancer patients: A longitudinal study. *Journal of Pain Symptom Management*, 35, 515–23.
37. Dy S.M., Apostol C.C. (2010) Evidence-based approaches to other symptoms in advanced cancer. *Cancer Journal*, 16, 507–13.
38. Howard L.M., Barley E.A., Davies E. *et al.* (2010) Cancer diagnosis in people with severe mental illness: Practical and ethical issues. *The Lancet Oncology*, 11, 797–804

39. Brotto L.A., Yule M., Breckon E. (2010) Psychological interventions for the sexual sequelae of cancer: A review of the literature. *Journal of Cancer Survivorship*, 4, 346–60.
40. Figueroa-Moseley C., Jean-Pierre P., Roscoe J.A. *et al.* (2007) Behavioral interventions in treating anticipatory nausea and vomiting. *Journal of the National Comprehensive Cancer Network*, 5, 44–50.
41. Roth A.J., Breitbart W. (1996) Psychiatric emergencies in terminally ill cancer patients. *Hematology Oncology Clinics of North America*, 10, 235–59.
42. Roth A.J., Levenson J.A. (2006) Psychiatric emergencies, in *Quick Reference for Oncology Clinicians: The Psychiatric and Psychological Dimensions of Cancer Symptom Management*, IPOS Press, pp. 19–25.

CHAPTER 6

Neurocognitive Effects of Anticancer Treatments

Tim Ahles[1], *Sanne Schagen*[2] *and Janette Vardy*[3]

[1]Neurocognitive Research Laboratory, Department of Psychiatry and Behavioral Sciences, Memorial Sloan-Kettering Cancer Center, New York, NY, USA

[2]Department of Psychosocial Research and Epidemiology, Netherlands Cancer Institute, Antoni van Leeuwenhoek Hospital, Amsterdam, the Netherlands

[3]Sydney Cancer Centre, University of Sydney, Concord Repatriation General Hospital, Concord, NSW, Australia

Introduction

Cognitive changes associated with central nervous system (CNS) cancers (e.g. brain tumours, CNS lymphoma) and treatment for these malignancies (e.g. cranial surgery and radiation) have long been recognized.[1] Additionally, the advent of cures for paediatric cancers and the associated emergence of cognitive changes, and learning/developmental disabilities has been studied since the 1980s.[2] However, over the last 15–20 years, increasing evidence suggests that treatments for non-CNS tumours can have both acute and long-term effects on cognitive functioning that can range from subtle changes to problems which affect the attainment of educational and occupational goals, and quality of life. Understanding these cognitive changes and the impact on survivors' functioning is critical since hundreds of thousands of patients are treated worldwide each year for these cancers (e.g. breast, colon, prostate) and the number of long-term survivors who may have to cope with these cognitive changes is growing dramatically. This chapter will focus on treatment-related cognitive changes associated with adjuvant treatment for breast cancer as an example of the emerging findings in this field (see Box 6.1).

Box 6.1 Major findings.

- Multiple aspects of cancer and cancer treatments are likely related to post-treatment cognitive change.
- Risk for post-treatment cognitive problems is likely the interaction of vulnerability factors (including age, cognitive reserve, genetics, lifestyle and environmental exposures) and specific cancer treatments.
- Emerging data from imaging and animal studies suggest that chemotherapy can affect brain structure and function.
- Treatment trials evaluating the efficacy of medications and cognitive rehabilitation approaches are being conducted, but additional research is required to define optimal treatment approaches.
- Lack of studies examining racial/ethnic variation or low socioeconomic status and post-treatment cognitive problems.

Background

Although references to cognitive changes associated with chemotherapy can be found dating back to the 1970s, serious scientific attention was not paid to the topic until the mid 1990s.[1] Cancer survivors report changes in attention, concentration,

Clinical Psycho-Oncology: An International Perspective, First Edition. Edited by Luigi Grassi and Michelle Riba.

working memory and executive function (i.e. ability to multitask) (see clinical case study below). A series of cross-sectional studies of breast cancer survivors reported that 17–75% of women experienced cognitive deficits in these domains from 6 months to 10 years post-exposure to chemotherapy. The lack of pre-chemotherapy assessment of cognitive performance limited the conclusions that could be drawn from these studies since some survivors may have had cognitive deficits pre-treatment that did not change over time or others may have had high normal performance on neuropsychological testing pre-treatment but mid-range normal performance post-treatment. Consequently, a number of investigators began longitudinal studies that included pre-treatment (post-surgery, but prior to adjuvant treatment) neuropsychological assessments of various domains of cognitive function. Consistent with the cross-sectional studies, the results of the longitudinal studies suggest that only a subgroup of patients experience post-treatment cognitive problems. Estimates of the frequency of post-treatment cognitive change vary among studies, likely due to differences in patient populations, assessment instruments used, criteria for defining change, and other aspects of study methods. Many investigators believe that the incidence of post-treatment cognitive problems is in the range of 15–25%, although percentages as high as 61% have been reported.[3] However, the longitudinal studies have found a less consistent pattern of post-treatment cognitive decline (some finding no evidence of cognitive change) and have challenged some basic assumptions made by many researchers in the field.

Clinical case study

Ms A is a 45-year-old woman diagnosed with stage II breast cancer. Her treatment consisted of mastectomy followed by chemotherapy (AC-T), and radiation therapy. She is currently taking tamoxifen. She is married and the mother of three children (ages 7, 10 and 14) and works as a partner in a corporate law firm. She took a medical leave of absence during her treatment, but is now trying to return to work on a full-time basis. Ms A reported that she experienced multiple symptoms during treatment including nausea, fatigue and problems with attention, concentration and short-term memory. After the end of radiation therapy, she reported that her symptoms began to improve over a 12-month period. However, in terms of her cognitive symptoms, she feels that she has recovered only to 75% of her previous capacity and she reports that the persistence of her cognitive problems only became obvious when she returned to work. Her current cognitive symptoms include problems with attention, short-term memory, word-finding and multitasking. She admits to becoming fatigued more easily and that her sleep quality is not as good as before her diagnosis; however, she denies major symptoms of anxiety or depression. The cognitive assessment revealed significant attentional difficulties. On a continuous performance task, Ms A had problems quickly and efficiently processing stimuli and her responses were less consistent as the test progressed. Ms A had an impaired learning slope on a verbal list learning task. Her ability to retain what she had learned was Average but this is likely lower than expected for her given her pre-morbid academic and occupational functioning. Also she made many false positive errors on a recognition task (Impaired). Her attentional difficulties impact her retrieval of information. The results of the evaluation are consistent with Ms A's report of shortened attention span, forgetfulness and difficulty with word-finding and multitasking.

Normal pre-treatment cognitive function

Many investigators assumed that breast cancer patients would have normal cognitive function at pre-treatment. However, several studies have found that 20–30% of breast cancer patients have lower than expected cognitive performance based on age and education at the pre-treatment assessment (in all cases assessments occurred between surgery and the onset of adjuvant treatment). Interestingly, lower than expected level of performance does not appear to be related to psychological factors (depression or anxiety), fatigue, or surgical factors (e.g. type and length of general anaesthesia).[4] No explanation for this phenomenon currently exists; however, two non-mutually exclusive hypotheses have been proposed.[5] First, there may be some aspect of the biology of cancer (e.g. an inflammatory response triggering neurotoxic cytokines) that may contribute to lower than expected cognitive performance. Second, there may be common risk factors for the development of breast cancer and the development of mild cognitive changes over years (e.g. poor DNA repair mechanisms have been linked both to increased risk of cancer and of neurodegenerative disorders such as Alzheimer's disease).

Chemotherapy is the major cause of cognitive change

As the colloquial term 'chemobrain' implies, most investigators initially assumed that cognitive changes were associated primarily with exposure to chemotherapy. However, longitudinal studies that included cancer patients not exposed to chemotherapy and healthy controls revealed that the no chemotherapy cancer group sometimes performed as poorly as the chemotherapy group or at an intermediate level between the chemotherapy exposed group and the healthy controls. This pattern of results also raised the question of whether endocrine therapy could impact cognitive functioning. Initial examination of this issue produced mixed results, but most studies were not powered to adequately examine the independent effects of endocrine therapy. However, a recent longitudinal study examining patients not treated with chemotherapy who were randomized to tamoxifen or exemestane revealed that patients treated with tamoxifen, but not exemestane experienced cognitive problems compared to healthy controls.[6] Even though investigators assumed that they were studying the effects of chemotherapy, in reality, most breast cancer patients receive multimodality treatment including surgery with exposure to general anaesthesia, radiation therapy and endocrine therapy in addition to chemotherapy. This in combination with the evidence for pre-treatment cognitive issues lead Hurria and colleagues to propose the phrase cancer and cancer treatment associated cognitive change as a more accurate descriptor of the phenomenon.[7]

Pattern of cognitive change

Longitudinal studies and clinical description have suggested that the majority of patients experience cognitive changes during active treatment with chemotherapy, likely due to multiple factors including anaemia, nausea, fatigue/disrupted sleep, distress and sedating medication. Recovery post-chemotherapy occurs over 6–12 months for many patients. However, a subgroup report 'hitting a plateau at 70–80% of pre-treatment functioning' and then no further improvement. This lower level of cognitive functioning was then thought to remain stable over time. This assumption has been challenged by data from a study by Wefel *et al.* which suggests that some patients continue to deteriorate over time and others show no deficits immediately post-chemotherapy, but then develop declines in cognitive functioning after 12 months post-treatment.[3] Clinically, the first author has seen women in their 60s who report a gradual worsening of their cognitive symptoms as if the cancer treatment has accelerated the normal process of cognitive ageing.

Cognitive changes are subtle

Cognitive changes associated with adjuvant treatment are frequently described as relatively subtle changes. In contrast to disorders like Alzheimer's disease or major head trauma, this may be an accurate description. However, this description may be misleading on at least two levels. First, most longitudinal studies have a long list of exclusion criteria, which frequently include a history of learning disability, head trauma, neurological disorders and major psychiatric disorders, all of which may be risk factors for post-treatment cognitive decline. Therefore, the current research may be underestimating the impact of treatment-related cognitive changes because the people who are most vulnerable may be excluded from the studies.

Second, even subtle changes in cognitive functioning may be problematic for someone who has a lifestyle with high cognitive demands. Even within the same profession, the demands on working memory and multitasking capacity may vary considerable. For example, the first author has seen several nurses clinically who experienced significant problems post-cancer treatment when returning to work in high-stress environments like emergency rooms and intensive care units but who were able to function well in slower paced outpatient clinics. Additionally, survivors have reported being able to return to work, but feeling like they have been passed over for promotions or other opportunities for advancement. Further research examining this interface of cognitive change and environmental demand is clearly needed.

Psychological factors do not impact cognitive decline

Most studies of cancer treatment-related cognitive change have found no association between cognitive decline and factors like depression, anxiety and fatigue. However, this may be, in part, related to the fact that patients with clinical levels of psychiatric problems have been excluded, thereby weakening the chance of finding associations between cognitive functioning and psychological factors. As noted below, in the clinical setting, the evaluation of depression and anxiety are critical when assessing a cancer survivor who reports cognitive issues.

Interestingly, Schagen and colleagues[8] have demonstrated that cancer survivors who were given information about the association between cognitive problems and chemotherapy and who had a history of treatment with chemotherapy reported higher levels of cognitive problems and performed less well on a word-learning test compared to survivors not provided with this information. The investigators hypothesize that the provision of information connecting chemotherapy and cognitive problems induces a stereotype threat that affects both self-report of cognitive problems and neuropsychological test performance. These intriguing findings suggest that psychological factors may play a more significant role in cancer treatment-related cognitive changes than previously assumed. Additional factors that have not been adequately studied are the psychological and physiological impact of stress and trauma history and their relationship to cognitive changes associated with cancer treatments.

Risk factors for post-treatment cognitive decline

Since there is an emerging consensus that only a subgroup of patients treated with similar regimens experience persistent post-treatment cognitive decline, a next logical step is to examine risk factors that increase vulnerability to cognitive change. Age is a well-established risk factor for cognitive decline in other disorders, and researchers have speculated that older adults may be more vulnerable to cognitive side-effects of cancer treatments. Lower than expected cognitive performance at pre-treatment may also be a risk factor for post-treatment cognitive changes if it is an indication of low cognitive reserve. Cognitive reserve represents innate and developed cognitive capacity which is influenced by various factors including genetics, education, occupational attainment and lifestyle. Research has demonstrated that people with low cognitive reserve are more vulnerable to the development of neurocognitive disorders (Alzheimer's disease) and to cognitive decline following a variety of insults to the brain. Further, research has demonstrated poorer cognitive outcomes secondary to neurotoxic exposures (e.g. lead) in people with low cognitive reserve. Based on the theory of cognitive reserve, one would predict that patients with lower than expected cognitive performance at pre-treatment who are exposed to chemotherapy would demonstrate poorer cognitive performance post-treatment. Ahles and colleagues found support for an interaction of age, cognitive reserve and exposure to chemotherapy as risk factors for cognitive decline. In the context of a longitudinal study they demonstrated that older patients who had lower levels of pre-treatment who were exposed to chemotherapy demonstrated significantly reduced performance on post-treatment measures of processing speed (see Figure 6.1).[9]

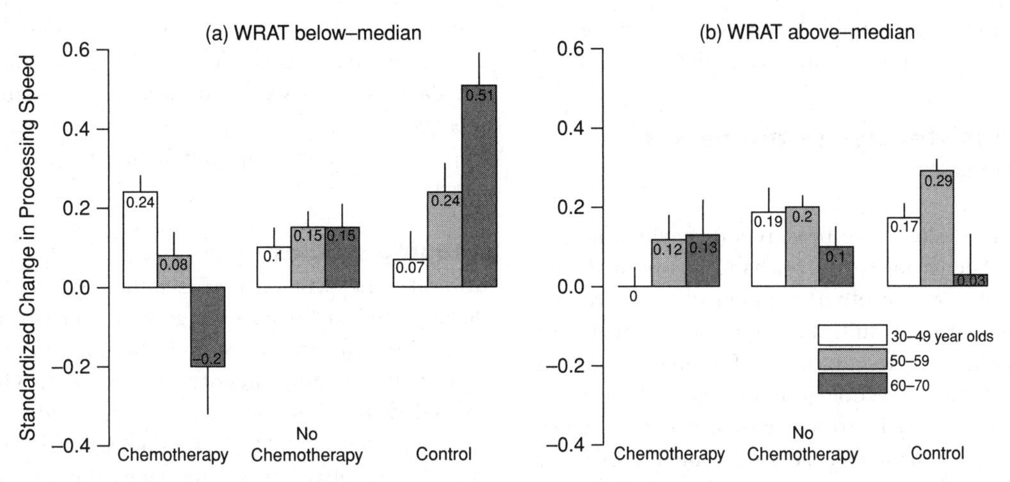

Figure 6.1 Pre- to post-treatment change in processing speed by treatment, age groups, and level of cognitive reserve. Reprinted with permission. © 2008 American Society of Clinical Oncology. All rights reserved. Ahles, Tim A. *et al.* Journal of Clinical Oncology, Issue 28, 2010: 4434–4440.

Genetic factors have also been examined as potential risk factors for cognitive decline. Apolipoprotein E (ApoE) is a complex glycolipoprotein that facilitates the uptake, transport and distribution of lipids. It appears to play an important role in neuronal repair and plasticity after injury. A four-exon gene codes for ApoE on chromosome 19 in humans. There are three major alleles: E2, E3 and E4. These alleles differ in amino acids at positions 112 and 158: E2 (cysteine/cysteine), E3 (cysteine/arginine), and E4 (arginine/arginine). Animal models suggest a link between the E4 allele and increased mortality, extent of damage and poor repair following trauma.[10] The human E4 allele has been associated with a variety of disorders with prominent cognitive dysfunction including healthy individuals with memory complaints, Alzheimer's disease, and poor outcomes in stroke and traumatic brain injury. The Dartmouth group evaluated the relationship of the ApoE genotype to neuropsychological performance in long-term cancer survivors treated with standard dose chemotherapy. The results demonstrated that survivors with at least one E4 allele scored significantly lower in the visual memory and spatial ability domains, with a trend to score lower in the psychomotor domain, as compared to survivors who did not carry an E4 allele.[11]

Small *et al.*[12] studied catechol-o-methyl transferase (COMT), which influences the metabolic breakdown of catecholamines through the methylation of dopamine (DA). The valine version (val allele) is almost four times as active as the methionine version of the gene (met allele). Thus individuals homozygous for the val allele presumably metabolize DA much more rapidly than those with the met allele. COMT becomes a major modulator of dopaminergic tone in the frontal cortex, accounting for ~60% of the metabolic degradation of DA. These researchers found that breast cancer patients who had the COMT-val allele and were treated with chemotherapy performed less well on tests of attention, verbal fluency and motor speed as compared to COMT-met homozygotes.

Other genetic factors that have been suggested as potential candidates for increasing risk for chemotherapy-induced cognitive change include genes that regulate DNA repair (e.g. X-ray repair cross-complementing protein 1, (XRCC1); Meiotic recombination 11 homolog A, (MRE11A)), cytokine regulation (e.g. Interleukin 1, IL1; IL6; tumour necrosis factor alpha TNF-alpha), neurotransmitter activity (e.g. BDNF), and blood–brain barrier efficiency (e.g. multidrug resistance 1, (MDR1); organic anion transporting polypeptide, (OATP)). However, no studies have directly examined the relationship between these genes and chemotherapy-induced cognitive function.[5]

Inconsistencies in the pattern of results

Several studies have been reported which do not find evidence for cognitive changes associated with chemotherapy or other treatments.[1] This inconsistent pattern of results may be related to high variability in study design, choice of comparison groups and the neuropsychological tests used (these issues will be discussed further below). However, given the discussion of risk factors outlined above, the pattern of post-treatment cognitive deficits may be influenced by sample characteristics like age and education (typically reported) and genetic variability (typically not measured). Therefore, if a study population consists of young, highly educated (one proxy for cognitive reserve) patients, then one might expect less evidence of post-treatment cognitive deficits as compared to a study that includes older, less-educated individuals. Generally, the studies which do not find evidence for chemotherapy-induced cognitive decline included younger patients with high levels of education. Further, many of these studies covaried out the effects of age and education or other proxies of premorbid IQ rather than examining these variables as risk factors; therefore, the investigators may have inadvertently covaried out the very effect that they were studying. Finally, within a relatively small study, the proportion of patients with adverse genetic alleles (e.g. ApoE) may vary significantly and affect the pattern of results depending on whether the proportion of ApoE 4-positive patients is high or low. Although these causes for variation in the pattern of results cannot be sorted out completely based on the current literature, they suggest specific hypotheses for future research.

Impact of chemotherapy on brain structure and function

Because of the relatively subtle nature of post-treatment effects and the inconsistent results, some investigators have questioned whether cancer treatments actually alter brain function. Emerging data from imaging and animal model studies increasingly provide important evidence for the impact of chemotherapy on brain structure and function.

Imaging studies

Several cross-sectional, post-treatment studies have documented reductions in grey matter, primarily in frontal structures and the hippocampus, and white matter integrity in cancer survivors treated with chemotherapy.[13,14] McDonald *et al.*[13] have reported the first longitudinal study of breast cancer patients exposed to chemotherapy who were evaluated with neuropsychological testing and structural and functional magnetic resonance imaging (MRI) at pre-treatment and 1 and 12 months post-treatment. Patients not exposed to chemotherapy and healthy controls were evaluated at similar intervals. Voxel-based morphometry was used to evaluate grey matter density between groups and over time. The analysis revealed that patients treated with chemotherapy had decreased grey matter density in bilateral frontal, temporal (including hippocampus), and cerebellar regions and right thalamus. Recovery was seen in some regions at the year-one assessment, but persistent decreases were seen in bilateral cerebellum, right thalamus, medial temporal lobe, left middle gyrus and right precentral medial frontal, and superior frontal gyri. No significant changes in grey matter over time were seen in the no chemotherapy cancer group or the healthy controls.

Cross-sectional studies of cancer survivors utilizing functional imaging techniques including functional magnetic resonance imaging (fMRI),[15] functional positron emission tomography (fPET),[16] and electroencephalographic evaluation (EEG)[17] have demonstrated both areas of decreased and increased activation during performance of a cognitive task in survivors exposed to chemotherapy as compared to controls. The interpretation of an increase in brain activation is a matter of debate, but many investigators believe that this represents compensatory activation of alternate brain structures in an attempt to maintain task performance.

If this interpretation is correct, it may provide a partial explanation for the lack of correlation between survivors' self-report of cognitive problems and performance on neuropsychological tests. In the context of a standard neuropsychological assessment with a supportive tester and one task to focus on at a time, the person may be able to activate alternate brain structures in order to perform successfully on the test. However, in their home or work environment, the cognitive demands may exceed the capacity of compensatory activation, causing a decline in cognitive functioning. Therefore, the person may accurately perceive cognitive problems that are not adequately captured in a typical neuropsychological evaluation. Clearly, this is an area that requires further investigation. McDonald *et al.* are currently analysing the data from the fMRI component of their longitudinal study.

Animal studies

Seigers and Fardell[18] recently reviewed the literature examining animal studies of chemotherapy-induced cognitive impairment. Several studies that have utilized a variety of common chemotherapeutic agents have demonstrated changes in memory and learning which parallel the deficits seen in cancer survivors. Further, the animal studies have demonstrated evidence for a variety of potential mechanisms for the effect of chemotherapy on the brain including: (1) inhibition of hippocampal neurogenesis; (2) oxidative damage; (3) white matter damage; (4) decreased hypothalamic-pituitary-adrenal axis activity; and (5) reduced brain vascularization and blood flow.

In addition to these general findings, several specific findings help to increase our understanding of the results from the clinical studies. First, there has been an assumption that most chemotherapy agents cannot affect cognition because they do not cross the blood–brain barrier in significant concentrations. However, Deitrich *et al.*[19] have demonstrated that concentrations of carmustine, cisplatin and cytarabine that are ineffective in killing tumour cells did increase cell death and decrease cell division in the subventricular zone, in the dentate gyrus of the hippocampus and in the corpus callosum. Therefore, even very small amounts of chemotherapy in the brain may have toxic effects. Second, studies of 5-fluorouracil (5-FU) have demonstrated both acute and progressive changes in white matter which is consistent with the Wefel *et al.*[3] study which demonstrated both acute and delayed post-treatment cognitive changes in breast cancer patients treated with chemotherapy regimens that included 5-FU. Finally, emerging evidence supports the efficacy of antioxidants in blocking the behavioural and physiological (e.g. decreased hippocampal neurogenesis) effects when coadministered with chemotherapy. Although this is a very interesting proof of principle, this is not an intervention that can be taken immediately to the clinic because of concerns that antioxidants may decrease the therapeutic efficacy of chemotherapy. However, understanding the mechanism(s) of treatment-related cognitive change will allow for a rational approach to drug development with the goal of designing drugs that protect the brain but do not interfere with the efficacy of cancer treatments.

Taken together, data from imaging and animal studies support the hypothesis that chemotherapy effects brain structure and function and begin to provide evidence for candidate mechanisms of chemotherapy-induced cognitive change. Similar studies examining other aspects of cancer treatments such as endocrine therapy for breast cancer and hormone ablation therapy for prostate cancer are clearly needed.

Interventions

Despite the increasing concern regarding cognitive changes associated with chemotherapy, few studies designed to evaluate interventions to treat cognitive changes have been conducted. When evaluating a cancer survivor clinically, it is important to evaluate fatigue/sleep disorders (insomnia, sleep apnoea), anxiety and depression, pain and pain medications which may alter cognitive functioning. Additionally, since the majority of cancer patients are diagnosed over the age of 65, comorbidities (e.g. diabetes and hypertension) and polypharmacy will be common. Common medical problems of the elderly and medications used to manage these problems can impact cognitive functioning as well. A thorough clinical assessment is critical since the appropriate treatment of problems such as sleep disorders or depression can result in both the resolution of that problem and improvement in cognitive functioning.

In terms of medication management of cognitive deficits, two studies have found support for the efficacy of modafinil, a psychostimulant, in improving memory and attention, and reducing fatigue.[20] Studies examining the use of medications utilized for the treatment of Alzheimer's disease (cholinesterase inhibitors) and herbs (Ginkgo biloba) are currently in process. Although these medication approaches make sense empirically, they do not represent targeted approaches based on known mechanisms of chemotherapy-induced cognitive change. The animal studies described provide a model for defining the mechanisms of cognitive change associated with cancer treatments and testing interventions for preventing these changes.

Cognitive rehabilitation approaches are emerging as a treatment option for cancer survivors experiencing cognitive problems. Ferguson and colleagues have developed an intervention termed Memory and Attention Training (MAAT) that includes several components including education regarding cognitive problems, compensatory strategies (e.g. memory aids), problem-solving to define goals so that strategies for goal attainment can be designed, and arousal reduction (e.g. relaxation training). A preliminary single-arm study and a small randomized study have provided preliminary support for the efficacy of the MAAT intervention.[21] Studies examining the efficacy of computer-based and group-based cognitive rehabilitation interventions are currently underway. One debate in the rehabilitation area is whether these interventions restore cognitive functioning, presumably through enhanced neuroplasticity, or whether the effects are primarily compensatory in nature. These are not mutually exclusive hypotheses and elements of both processes may be at work. Studies that include pre- and post-treatment assessments utilizing structural and functional neuroimaging techniques may help to shed light on the neuroplasticity hypothesis.

The International Cancer and Cognition Task Force

In 2003, approximately 30 researchers from around the world convened a workshop in Banff, Canada prior to the International Psycho-Oncology Society (IPOS) meetings to discuss the state of the science in the area of chemotherapy-induced cognitive change.[22] From this initial meeting, the International Cancer and Cognition Task Force (ICCTF) was formed at the 8th IPOS World Congress of Psycho-Oncology in Venice, Italy in 2006.[23] Below is the mission statement of the ICCTF (www.icctf.com/):

> The mission of the ICCTF is to advance our understanding of the impact of cancer and cancer-related treatment on cognitive and behavioral functioning in adults with non-central nervous system cancers. Members of the ICCTF conduct local, national and international research to help elucidate the nature of the cognitive and neurobehavioral sequelae associated with cancer and cancer therapies, the mechanisms that underlie these changes in function, and interventions to prevent or manage these undesired symptoms and/or their side effects.

A critical outcome from the Venice Conference was the setting up of working groups which were charged with the development of guidelines for salient issues related to the study of cognition and behaviour in cancer patients. Six working groups were planned focusing on issues relevant to: (1) neuropsychological assessment; (2) trial design; (3) prevention, management and intervention for cognitive dysfunction; (4) clinical epidemiology and translational guidelines; (5) imaging; and (6) animal studies. The recommendations of the first two working groups were reported at the 2006 meeting in Amsterdam and were summarized in a recent publication.[24] The Neuropsychological Assessment Working Group recommended the inclusion of three

Box 6.2 ICCTF recommended neuropsychological tests for inclusion in test batteries.

Hopkins Verbal Learning Test-Revised
- Assesses short- and long-term memory
- Adequate psychometric properties and six alternate forms
- Is available in multiple languages (English, Dutch, French, German, Italian and Spanish).

Trail-Making Test
- Assesses psychomotor speed and executive function
- Adequate psychometric properties
- Although the test is not language-dependent, the instructions have been translated into multiple languages.

Controlled Oral Word Association Test
- Assesses speeded lexical fluency and aspects of executive function
- Adequate psychometric properties
- Available for use in multiple languages.

neuropsychological measures (Hopkins Verbal Learning Test-Revised, Trail Making Test, and the Controlled Oral Word Association Test of the Multilingual Aphasia Examination) in test batteries to allow for the potential of comparing data across studies and/or for combining data (see Box 6.2). The Trial Design Working Group offered suggestions on a variety of topics including the use of longitudinal versus cross-sectional designs, the importance of pre-treatment cognitive assessments, and the selection of appropriate control groups (see Box 6.3). Overall, the goal of the working groups is to make recommendations that harmonize studies of cognitive function in cancer patients in order to move the field forward by increasing the comparability of results across international studies.

Box 6.3 ICCTF methodological recommendations.

- Preferred design is a longitudinal study which includes pre-treatment assessment.
- Cross-sectional designs with appropriate control groups may be useful for proof-of-concept trials.
- Comparison groups would ideally include disease-specific controls (e.g. cancer patients not exposed to chemotherapy) and healthy controls, matched on age and education.
- Inclusion and exclusion criteria need to be appropriate for the study question, but cannot be so restrictive as to reduce the generalizability of the results (e.g. excluding patients on SSRIs for the treatment of depression or hot flushes could significantly reduce patient eligibility).

Another major goal of the ICCTF is to explore opportunities to conduct coordinated, international studies. To date, published studies in this area have been conducted in Australia, Belgium, Canada, Denmark, France, Germany, Japan, the Netherlands, the United Kingdom and the United States. Although there are difficulties comparing the results of these studies, there do not appear to be major differences in the general pattern of results across countries. However, no studies have directly addressed the issue of differences in the incidence, severity, etc. of cognitive problems across populations from different countries. The ICCTF network could potentially design such a study. Of particular interest would be the examination of populations with expected genetic variation based on racial and ethnic background.

To date, most of the studies reported have had small to modest sample sizes, which has limited investigators' ability to obtain precise estimates of the prevalence of cognitive problems and to conduct subgroup analyses to examine risk factors etc. In order for the field of cognition and cancer to move forward, a critical next step is conducting large-scale studies that would allow for the more accurate identification of the incidence of cognitive side-effects of cancer treatments, factors that confer vulnerability to cognitive side-effects, including genetic polymorphisms that are associated with change in performance on neuropsychological testing and in brain structure and function based on imaging. There are many challenges to conducting collaborative research across institutions including standardization of testing and imaging protocols. However, the Alzheimer's Disease Neuroimaging Initiative (ADNI) serves as a model for such a study (http://adni.loni.ucla.edu/). The goal of ADNI is to understand the rate of progression of mild cognitive impairment and Alzheimer's disease. Patients diagnosed with mild cognitive impairment and Alzheimer's disease, as well as healthy, elderly controls from over 50 sites in the United States and internationally are evaluated with a comprehensive assessment that includes neuropsychological testing, imaging, biomarkers and genetics. ADNI investigators have developed protocols for collecting reliable and valid data across institutions and imaging scanner platforms. Additionally, data from ADNI is uploaded to the Internet so that data can be accessed by researchers around the world. Very similar methods and protocols could be adapted for a study of cognitive changes associated with cancer treatments.

Cultural implications

A limitation of all of the research conducted thus far is that studies have been primarily conducted in large cancer centres and the patients have tended to have high education and socioeconomic status. No studies have focused on patients from underserved populations who may have lower education levels and live in poverty. One could predict that patients from underserved populations may be more vulnerable to cognitive changes associated with cancer and cancer treatments for a variety of reasons including lower education/cognitive reserve, poorer diet and health care and high exposure to environmental toxins. Further, genetic variation based on race and ethnicity may influence the incidence and severity of post-treatment cognitive changes. For example, research has suggested variability in the incidence of the ApoE 4 polymorphism across racial/ethnic populations; therefore, groups that have higher incidence of the ApoE 4 polymorphism and other genetic vulnerability factors may have a higher incidence of cancer treatment-related cognitive changes in those populations. Further, the association between ApoE 4 and Alzheimer's disease has been shown to differ across racial/ethnic groups; therefore, the same genetic polymorphism may confer a different level of risk for post-treatment cognitive decline based on race and ethnicity.[25] Finally, extrapolating from the work of Schagen *et al.*[8] discussed above, certain racial/ethnic groups may be more vulnerable to the induction of stereotype threat which may translate into higher levels of self-reported cognitive problems and poorer performance on neuropsychological tests.

There are various challenges to conducting research on cognitive changes associated with cancer treatments across racial, ethnic and low socioeconomic status groups. Many of the traditional neuropsychological tests have been developed and norms obtained on Western, English-speaking populations. Therefore, not all tests have been appropriately translated and normative data obtained for particular groups of interest. Additionally, even when translated, the test may not be culturally relevant which makes comparisons across cultural groups challenging. Finally, the quality of educational systems vary greatly across socioeconomic strata; therefore, years of education are likely not equivalent across groups (e.g. in areas of the United States, a significant proportion of high school graduates are functionally illiterate). Tests of premorbid IQ and/or reading ability can help to control for this variation.

Conclusions

Increasing evidence has suggested that various aspects of breast cancer and breast cancer treatment can have a long-term effect on cognitive functioning in a subgroup of patients. Data from imaging studies in patients and animal model studies are providing clues regarding the impact of cancer treatments on brain structure and function that can lead to the definition of mechanisms for post-treatment cognitive change. However, a critical next step in moving the field forward is large-scale, multi-institutional studies designed to provide an accurate estimate of the incidence and course of post-treatment cognitive decline, the relative cognitive effects of various chemotherapy regimens and endocrine therapies, risk factors for cognitive decline, mechanisms (biological and psychological) underlying cognitive changes, the effect of cognitive changes on a survivor's daily life and ability to function, and interventions designed to prevent or reduce the negative cognitive impact of cancer treatments. Further, similarities and differences between breast cancer and other types of cancer and cancer treatment clearly need additional investigation. A major gap in the field is the lack of studies examining the cognitive impact of cancer treatments across racial and ethnic groups and across lower levels of socioeconomic status. Data collected on highly educated, affluent Caucasian patients may not generalize to other populations given known genetic variation across racial and ethnic groups, and the deleterious effects of poverty, including poor nutrition and health care, impoverished environments which translate into lower cognitive reserve, and higher levels of toxic environmental exposures.

Key points

- Emerging data from studies examining cognition and cancer have led to new insights and challenged various assumptions.
- Pre-treatment cognitive problems suggest that some aspect of the biology of cancer may affect cognitive function or that there may be common risk factors for the development of cancer and mild cognitive change over time. These data, along with the results of studies examining the cognitive effects of endocrine therapy suggest that chemotherapy is not the only aspect of cancer treatment that influences cognitive functioning.
- Factors including age, cognitive reserve and genetic factors (ApoE and COMT) are being identified as increasing risk for post-treatment cognitive decline and imaging studies and animal model studies are beginning to define the impact of cancer treatments on brain structure and function.
- Studies examining the efficacy of medication and cognitive rehabilitation interventions are underway, but are hampered by the lack of understanding of the mechanism(s) for cancer treatment-related cognitive change. The ICCTF has brought together researchers from around the world who are studying cognition and cancer with the goals of providing a forum for exchange of emerging results and to provide recommendations for study design, assessment, etc. However, although research in this area is being conducted in many countries, most studies have focused on relatively homogenous populations from a racial/ethnic perspective and most study populations have consisted of high education and income patients.
- Therefore, a major gap in the field is examining differences based on race and ethnicity and socioeconomic status.

References

1. Ahles T.A., Correa D.D. (2010) Neuropsychological impact of cancer and cancer treatments, in *Psycho-Oncology*, 2nd edn, (ed. J.C. Holland), Oxford University Press, New York, pp. 251–257.
2. Anderson F.S., Kunin-Bastan A.S. (2009) Neurocognitive late effects of chemotherapy in children: The past 10 years of research on brain structure and function. *Pediatric Blood and Cancer*, 52, 159–164.
3. Wefel J.S., Saleeba A.K., Buzdar A.U. *et al.* (2010) Acute and late onset cognitive dysfunction associated with chemotherapy in women with breast cancer. *Cancer*, 116, 3348–3356.
4. Ahles T.A., Saykin A.J., McDonald B.C. *et al.* (2008) Cognitive function in breast cancer patients prior to adjuvant treatment. *Breast Cancer Research and Treatment*, 110, 143–152.
5. Ahles T.A., Saykin A.J. (2007) Candidate mechanisms for chemotherapy-induced cognitive changes. *Nature Reviews Cancer*, 7, 192–201.
6. Schilder C., Seynaeve C., Beex L.V. *et al.* (2010) Effects of tamoxifen and exemestane on cognitive function of postmenopausal patients with breast cancer: Results from the neuropsychological side study of the Tamoxifen and Exemestane Adjuvant Multinational Trial. *Journal of Clinical Oncology*, 28, 1294–1300.
7. Hurria A., Somlo G., Ahles T. (2007) Renaming "chemobrain". *Cancer Investigation*, 25, 373– 377.
8. Schagen S.B., Das E., Vermeulen I. (2011) Information about chemotherapy-associated problems contributes to cognitive problems in cancer patients. *Psycho-Oncology*, (e-pub ahead of print).
9. Ahles T.A., Saykin A.J., McDonald B.C. *et al.* (2010) Longitudinal assessment of cognitive changes associated with adjuvant treatment for breast cancer: The

impact of age and cognitive reserve. *Journal of Clinical Oncology*, 28, 4434–4440.

10. Bookheimer S., Burggren A. (2009) APOE-4 genotype and neurophysiological vulnerability to Alzheimer's disease and cognitive aging. *Annual Review of Clinical Psychology*, 5, 343–362.
11. Ahles T.A., Saykin A.J., Noll W.W. *et al.* (2003) The relationship of APOE genotype to neuropsychological performance in long-term cancer survivors treated with standard dose chemotherapy. *Psycho-Oncology*, 12, 612–619.
12. Small B.J., Sharp Rowson K., Walsh E. *et al.* (2011) Catechol-o-methyltransferase genotype modulates cancer treatment-related cognitive deficits in breast cancer survivors. *Cancer*, 117, 1369–1376.
13. McDonald B.C., Conroy S.K., Ahles T.A. *et al.* (2010) Gray matter reduction associated with systemic chemotherapy for breast cancer: A prospective MRI study. *Breast Cancer Research and Treatment*, 123, 819–828.
14. Deprez S., Amant F., Yigit R. *et al.* (2011) Chemotherapy-induced structural changes in cerebral white matter and its correlation with impaired functioning in breast cancer patients. *Human Brain Mapping*, 32, 480–493.
15. de Ruiter M.D., Reneman L., Boogerd W. *et al.* (2011) Cerebral hyperresponsiveness and cognitive impairment 10 years after chemotherapy for breast cancer. *Human Brain Mapping*, 38, 1206–1219.
16. Silverman D.H., Dy C.J., Castellon S.A. *et al.* (2007) Altered frontocortical, cerebellar, and basal ganglia activity in adjuvant-treated breast cancer survivors 5–10 years after chemotherapy. *Breast Cancer Research and Treatment*, 103, 303–311.
17. Kreukels B.P.C., van Dam S.A.M., Ridderinkhof K.R. *et al.* (2008). Persistent neurocognitive problems after adjuvant chemotherapy for breast cancer. *Clinical Breast Cancer*, 8, 80–87.
18. Seigers R., Fardell J.E. (2011) Neurobiological basis of chemotherapy-induced cognitive impairment: A review of rodent research. *Neuroscience and Biobehavioral Reviews*, 35, 729–741.
19. Dietrich J., Han R., Yang Y. *et al.* (2006) CNS progenitor cells and oligodendrocytes are targets of chemotherapeutic agents in vitro and in vivo. *Journal of Biology*, 5, 1–23.
20. Joly F., Rigal O., Noal S., Giffard B. (2011) Cognitive dysfunction and cancer: Which consequences in terms of disease management? *Psycho-Oncology*, 20, 1251–1258.
21. Ferguson J.R., McDonald B.C., Rocque M.A. *et al.* (2012) Development of CBT for chemotherapy-related cognitive change: Results of a waitlist control trial. *Psycho-Oncology*, 21, 176–186.
22. Tannock I.F., Ahles T.A., Ganz P.A., van Dam F.S. (2004) Cognitive impairment associated with chemotherapy for cancer: Report of a workshop. *Journal of Clinical Oncology*, 22, 2233–2239.
23. Vardy J., Wefel J.S., Ahles T.A. *et al.* (2008). Cancer and cancer-therapy related cognitive dysfunction: An international perspective from the Venice Cognitive Workshop. *Annals of Oncology*, 19, 623–629.
24. Wefel J.S., Vardy J., Ahles T.A., Schagen S. (2011) International Cognition and Cancer Task Force recommendations to harmonise studies of cognitive function in cancer patients. *The Lancet Oncology*, 12, 703–708.
25. Venketasubramanian N., Sahadevan S., Kua E.H. *et al.* (2010) Interethnic differences in dementia epidemiology: Global and Asia-Pacific perspectives. *Dementia and Geriatric Cognitive Disorders*, 30, 492–498.

CHAPTER 7

Screening for Distress, the 6th Vital Sign, as the Connective Tissue of Health Care Systems: A Roadmap to Integrated Interdisciplinary Person-centred Care

Barry D. Bultz[1], *Matthew J. Loscalzo*[2] *and Karen L. Clark*[2]
[1]Department of Psychosocial Resources, Tom Baker Cancer Centre, and Division of Psychosocial Oncology, Faculty of Medicine, University of Calgary, Calgary, Alberta, Canada
[2]Sheri & Les Biller Patient and Family Resource Center; Department of Supportive Care Medicine and Department of Population Sciences, City of Hope, Duarte, CA, USA

Introduction: Integrated interdisciplinary patient-centred care

Interdisciplinary teams

Interdisciplinary teamwork has long been heralded as the pathway to excellence in patient care. No health care professional would ever admit that they possess the knowledge or skillset to attend to all of their patient's needs. Despite consensual agreement to this viewpoint, health care systems have been slow to commit to an interdisciplinary model of patient care. Rather, health care and the contributing professions seem content to focus on doing what they have been trained to do, remaining in their own discipline silo and to a large extent to ignore or minimize patient concerns outside of their scope of practice.[1] Lack of interdisciplinary integration and coordination can have a negative impact on the cancer experience, especially for those patients most at psychosocial risk. There is also the stress on physicians and nurses who will be caring for patients with complex needs especially when there is no systematic approach to symptom identification or management in place.

Cancer care for the whole person

The Institute of Medicine's (IOM) 2008 report, *Cancer Care for the Whole Patient: Meeting Psychosocial Health Needs* documented the substantial scientific evidence that supportive care can yield significant benefits for cancer patients and survivors.[2] These benefits are robust and extend to the patient, their families, health care providers, institutions where they are treated and local communities. Comprehensive cancer care programmes have emerged because of dramatic advances in early detection, disease-directed treatments and the recognition that the needs of the 'whole' patient must be addressed as an essential part of cancer care. Patient-centred also referred to as whole-patient-centred care requires programmes to be relevant to

Clinical Psycho-Oncology: An International Perspective, First Edition. Edited by Luigi Grassi and Michelle Riba.

what patients and their families experience as they move along the cancer continuum.

In this chapter, we will describe some of the challenges patients experience and the current practices employed by the health care team to address these challenges. We will also describe how Screening for Distress can become the connective tissue of cancer care and how screening has challenged professionals to think beyond mere collaboration to a model of integration that truly puts the patient at the centre of care. To illustrate how Screening for Distress has begun changing clinic culture, the authors will present two models of care, from two very different social contexts, Canada and the United States, where the evolution from profession-centric to person-centred care has been shown to be feasible although still quite provocative.

Background

Current cancer care

With dramatic advances in laboratory and clinical research, cancer care has moved from an acute illness model to one that is, for the most part, chronic and outpatient-oriented. Clinics function in such a way that patients initially see their family physician with a health concern that is followed up with further assessments and referral to other specialized health professionals for a complete assessment. If there is a confirmed cancer diagnosis, referral to an appropriate physician or tertiary cancer clinic usually follows.

Once diagnosed, cancer care focuses on eradication of the malignancy via surgery, chemotherapy, and/or radiation, leaving emotional support for the patient and attention to psychosocial concerns as an afterthought, if considered at all. In smaller oncology practices, psychosocial services may be non-existent. Because of this void in many health care programmes, patients and advocacy groups increasingly have vocalized their concern about the limited psychosocial resources available to help patients and families cope with the complex and multiple challenges often associated with their cancer experience.

Concerns about the specific psychosocial needs of cancer patients in the professional literature go back to the beginning of the twentieth century.[3] Although patient concerns have not changed much since that time, the health care environment certainly has. The time of a generalist physician working in a rural setting, close to the populations they served but isolated from large institutions has given way to highly qualified subspecialists working in highly technologically advanced institutions. In the past, it was physical space and lack of technology that created lack of coordination, but today it may be the highly specialized and technological skills that are barriers to coordination and timely communication among patients, families and multispecialists. But within the supportive care oncology community, there is also a challenge of how best to provide whole-person-centred cancer care. Fortunately, screening patients and families has provided the information on how best to address patient needs. This data has been quite clear and consistent around the world.[4–6]

Major issues

Moving beyond pain as the 5th Vital Sign to distress as the 6th Vital Sign

Given the high prevalence rates of reported symptoms and patient problems, like pain being branded the 5th Vital Sign, it was proposed that a similar approach be used for distress. Distress was eventually endorsed as the 6th Vital Sign in Canada[7] and then supported as a new standard by national and international societies[8] and accreditation organizations.[9] In 2010, the Union for International Cancer Control (UICC) endorsed the value of branding distress as the 6th Vital Sign stating that 'We expect that recognizing distress as the 6th Vital Sign will improve the treatment of cancer patients, improve outcomes for cancer patients, and improve the effectiveness of cancer care systems around the world' (E. Cazap).[10]

Moving beyond psychiatric labelling, cancer-related symptoms became broadly seen as distress[11] and research using this broad definition embraced the full range of patient symptoms likely to be experienced across the cancer journey from time of diagnosis through to end-of-life care and beyond to survivorship. In taking the broad view on distress, the National Comprehensive Cancer Network (NCCN) has defined distress as: *a multifactorial unpleasant emotional experience of a psychological (cognitive, behavioral, emotional), social, and/or spiritual nature that may interfere with the ability to cope effectively with cancer, its physical symptoms and its treatment. Distress extends along a continuum, ranging from common normal feelings of vulnerability, sadness, and fears to problems that can become disabling, such as depression, anxiety, panic, social isolation, and existential and spiritual crisis.*[11] With this definition in mind, research has broadened the definition of distress beyond anxiety and depression to include a complete range of symptoms from fatigue, sleeplessness, nutritional issues, quality of life, to practical and financial pressures to social and family concerns to religious and existential concerns.

Not surprisingly, confronting one's mortality in the face of cancer for many is highly stressful with untreated distress often the most relevant predictor of subsequent psychological distress.[12] When problems such as fatigue, pain, weakness and other physical symptoms are added, the distress of cancer patients is increased. Distress is a normal part of life for a cancer patient and is therefore less stigmatizing than psychiatric labels. The early identification of patient biopsychosocial problems (practical, physical, psychological, social and spiritual) is essential to relieve distress, prevent crises and minimize system disruption. Because psychological and social problems are complex and possess the added barriers of stigma, there is the belief that patients with these concerns take up valuable clinic time, and professional avoidance of emotional content relegates these concerns to a lower value when compared to physical care. The problem-based approach embraced by Screening for Distress and distress being branded the 6th Vital Sign in large part de-stigmatizes the history-taking process by helping patients perceive distress areas as problems rather than personal weaknesses, both in the phrasing of questions and by intermixing items dealing with physical, emotional, social, spiritual and practical issues.[13] Supported in the literature[14,15] NCCN recommends Screening for Distress for all cancer patients to identify and address problems before a crisis develops, and necessitates higher levels of intervention.

Cella (1998),[16] Zabora *et al.* (2003),[17] Carlson *et al.* (2004)[18] and Loscalzo and Clark (2007)[19] have conducted large studies that illustrate that patient needs are complex and variable based on tumour site, stage of disease, gender and socioeconomic background. Though each of these studies has used different tools to identify patient concerns, there is a commonality of identified issues. One of the earliest prevalence studies reporting patient concerns was carried out by Cella.[16] Cella reported that concerns go beyond anxiety and depression, and documented the highest of distressing symptoms to be *fatigue* and *pain* (Figure 7.1), suggesting that at least in oncology settings distress is complex and physical symptoms are likely to play a significant role and are very likely to contribute to the patient's overall distress profile. Subsequently targeting one symptom alone and not the array of concerns is likely to have limited benefit. Zabora has published extensively on distress and reports on anxiety and depression as well, adding the dimensions of common cancer-related problems (Figure 7.2).[17] Consistent with the Cella and Zabora seminal studies, Carlson *et al.* (2004) reported a cross-sectional study of 3000 patients with different cancers and stages attending a tertiary centre; a full range of physical, psychosocial and practical concerns exist in 35–45% of all patients (Figure 7.3).[18]

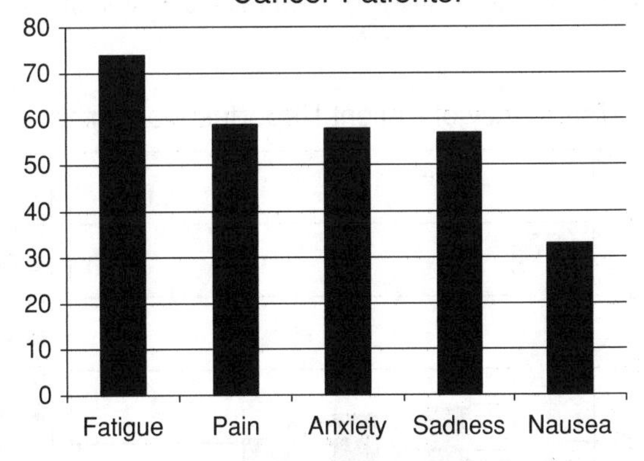

Figure 7.1 Cella (1998) Factors influencing quality of life in cancer patients: anemia and fatigue. This article was published in Seminar of Oncology, Vol 25 (Supl. 7), Cella *et al.*, Factors influencing quality of life in cancer patients: anemia and fatigue, pp. 43–46, Copyright Elsevier (1998).

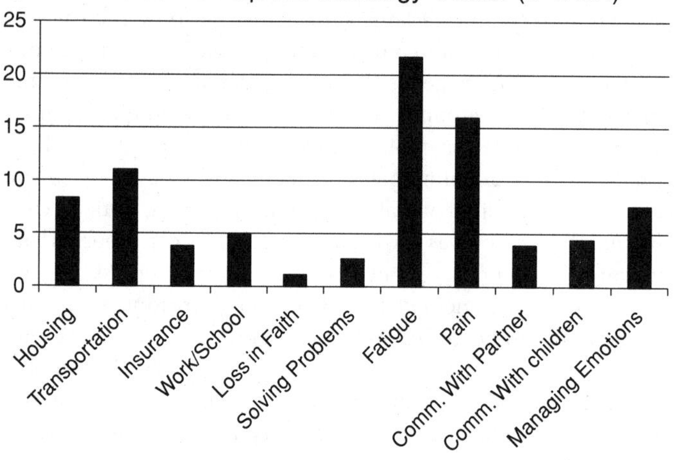

Figure 7.2 Zabora *et al.* (2003) Managing complications in cancer: identifying and responding to the patient's perspective. Reprinted from Seminars in Oncology Nursing, Vol 19, James R Zabora, Matthew J Loscalzo, Jason Weber; Managing complications in cancer: identifying and responding to the patient's perspective, Page 124. Copyright (2003), with permission from Elsevier.

Again, these three figures highlight that cancer patients' concerns can be multiple in number and likely to exist in clusters. While focusing on one symptom may facilitate a deeper understanding of the patient experience, this approach from a clinical perspective is too simplistic given what we are learning about how patients are facing their cancer. Loscalzo *et al.* (2007) implemented the use of an innovative screening of cancer patients at first visit to assist them with distress due to cancer-related problems.[19] Based on 15 years of experience with Screening for Distress, his team developed a 36-question screening instrument that addressed physical, practical, social, psychological and spiritual problems. Patients rated the severity of the problem on a scale of 1 to 5, and indicated if they wanted staff assistance (Table 7.1). Data from the first 2071 patients to complete this screening was analysed to identify common patient problems, demographics and trends. The five most common causes of problem-related distress were: *fatigue, sleeping, finances, pain* and *controlling my fear and worry about the future*. The five most common problems for which patients circled 'Yes' to ask for assistance were: *understanding my treatment options, fatigue, sleeping, pain* and *finances*. Compared to the entire

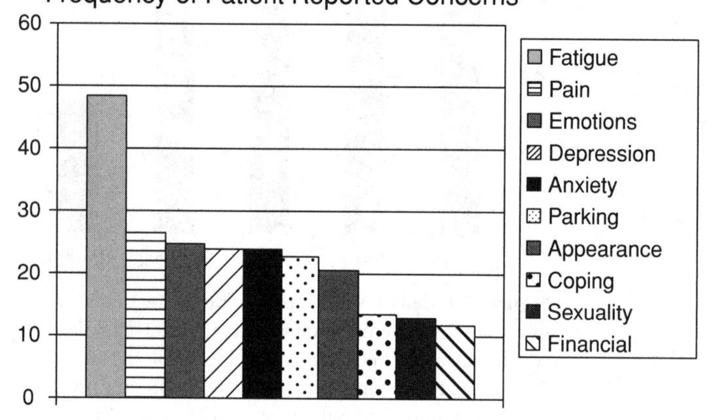

Figure 7.3 Carlson *et al.* (2004) High levels of untreated distress and fatigue in cancer patients. Reprinted by permission from Macmillan Publishers Ltd on behalf of Cancer Research UK: British Journal of Cancer, Vol 19, Issue 12, High levels of untreated distress and fatigue in cancer patients, Carlos *et al.*, copyright (2004).

Table 7.1 Loscalzo and Clark (2007) Problem-related distress in cancer patients drives requests for help: A prospective study. Loscalzo MJ, Clark KL. (2007) Problem-Related Distress in Cancer Patients Drives Requests for Help: A Prospective Study. Oncology 21, 1133–1138. Reproduced with permission.

How Can We Help You and Your Family? Problems and Rankings

Biopsychosocial problems	%≥3	%Yes
Fatigue (feeling tired)	41.9	9.6
Sleeping	32.5	8.1
Finances	31.1	7.8
Pain	29.4	7.9
Controlling my fear and worry about the future	28.2	6.0
Me being dependent on others	27.5	3.5
Being an anxious or nervous person	27.4	5.4
Feeling down depressed or blue	27.4	5.4
Understanding my treatment options	23.1	15.0
Managing my emotions	22.9	4.4
Questions and concerns about the end of life	20.8	4.1
Solving problems due to my illness	20.3	5.3
Managing work, school, home life	20.0	3.3
Losing control of things that matter to me	19.6	2.7
Finding community resources near where I live	19.4	6.3
Sexual function	16.7	2.9
Thinking clearly	16.6	2.6
Needing someone to help coordinate my medical care	14.0	6.3
My ability to cope	13.9	1.8
Recent weight change	13.5	3.5
Transportation	12.9	5.2
Talking with the health care team	12.5	5.6
Someone else totally dependent on me for their care	12.3	1.6
Controlling my anger	12.1	2.0
Writing down my choices about medical care for the medical team and my family if I ever become too ill to speak for myself	11.6	5.3
Talking with the doctor	11.4	5.4
Having people nearby to help me or needing more practical help at home	11.0	2.7
Nausea and vomiting	11.0	3.3
Getting medicines	9.9	3.1
Ability to have children	9.1	2.1
Talking with family, children, friends	7.7	1.5
Substance abuse (drugs, alcohol, nicotine, other)	5.1	1.3
Thoughts of ending my own life	4.8	0.4
Any other problems you would like to tell us about	4.6	4.2
Abandonment by my family	4.5	0.7
Spiritual concerns	4.4	0.8

Note: All 36 of the questions from the screening instrument *How Can We Help You and Your Family* are listed in descending order based on the percentage of patients who marked each problem ≥3. The percentages of patients who marked the problem ≥3 and the percentage who circled 'Yes' are listed in separate columns. The top 5 percentages in each column are shaded in grey.

population, patients who circled 'Yes' on a particular problem demonstrated a robust increase in problem-related distress.

These studies highlight that the cancer patient's challenges are complex with a strong interplay existing between physical, psychosocial and practical concerns. But most significantly within the context of this chapter, for the treating team, these concerns serve as a roadmap to guide clinicians on how to approach and support patients while working with other specialists to adequately address the complexities of cancer and to maximize support and evidence-based care. At a minimum, Screening for Distress can serve as an aid to the health care team by clearly defining patient concerns, facilitating a conversation between the patient and usually the primary nurse or physician. These challenging but essential conversations are critical for careful coordination leading to higher levels of efficiency, quality and safety with the appropriate referral in a timely way.

Operationalizing Screening for Distress: the connective tissue in interdisciplinary patient care

In the United States despite endorsements by NCCN and more recently by the American Society of Clinical Oncology and the American College of Surgeons only 30% of NCCN organizations (all NCI Designated Comprehensive Cancer Centers) routinely screen for distress.[20] In the United Kingdom, Mitchell (2010) reports that few clinicians outside of palliative care teams screen for distress using standardized measures.[21] Much debate is also continuing about the benefit of screening for depression and anxiety and whether screening with the use of ultra-short tools is more beneficial than longer questionnaires.[22] Carlson *et al.* (2011) in a recent RCT demonstrated that screening leading to referral and education improved patient outcomes.[23] There is clearly increasing international momentum to introduce screening as the standard of clinical care in larger institutions. This greater acceptance to screen for emotional concerns and psychosocial problems is based on consumer demand, increased awareness of the importance of psychosocial perspective by physicians, availability of psychosocial experts, expanding research and emerging technology.

Technology has demonstrated the ability to bring people closer together and to make meaningful connections that previously have not been possible. The speed of technological advances is only expected to increase, but, ultimately, caring for and healing patients will always be about trusting and respectful relationships. The authors and others[24–26] have shown that automation can decrease resource intensity while creating systems that provide enhanced interdisciplinary timely communication, tailored interventions, clinical summaries, and real-time triage. In the longer term, automation can also create a database that is immediately updated and available for research and programme development.

Model programmes: clinical cases

With global attention being given to Screening for Distress, the 6th Vital Sign[27] going beyond screening for research purposes alone, it seems appropriate to focus our attention on implementation of screening tools into standardized cancer care. However, screening alone, without attention to clinical concerns, provides some but not full advantage to the patient,[23] family and staff. It is our belief that Screening for Distress can create an opportunity for the health care team to have a conversation with the patient followed by assessment and a referral to the appropriate professional in a timely way. Ultimately, screening has the capacity to transform health care systems to encourage new partnerships that maximize interdisciplinary care.

We will now share two model programmes that demonstrate the integration of screening as the core and connective tissue of their integrated multidisciplinary programmes.

Tom Baker Cancer Centre, Calgary, Canada, with support from the Canadian Partnership Against Cancer, the Cancer Journey Portfolio, and the Screening for Distress Toolkit Working Group, chose a Minimum Data Set comprised of the Edmonton Symptom Assessment Survey and a Problem Checklist as a screening tool (Figure 7.4).[28]

Alberta Health Services
Tom Baker Cancer Centre

Personal Well-being Checklist

Completed by:
- ❒ **Patient**
- ❒ **Family**
- ❒ **Health Professional**
- ❒ **Assisted by family or health professional**

Patient Label

1. EDMONTON SYMPTOM ASSESSMENT SYSTEM (ESAS):

Date: ____________________

Please circle the number that best describes:

No Pain	0	1	2	3	4	5	6	7	8	9	10	Worst possible pain
Not Tired	0	1	2	3	4	5	6	7	8	9	10	Worst possible tiredness
Not nauseated	0	1	2	3	4	5	6	7	8	9	10	Worst possible nausea
Not depressed	0	1	2	3	4	5	6	7	8	9	10	Worst possible depression
Not anxious	0	1	2	3	4	5	6	7	8	9	10	Worst possible anxiety
Not drowsy	0	1	2	3	4	5	6	7	8	9	10	Worst possible drowsiness
Best appetite	0	1	2	3	4	5	6	7	8	9	10	Worst possible appetite
Best feeling of wellbeing	0	1	2	3	4	5	6	7	8	9	10	Worst possible feeling of wellbeing
No shortness of breath	0	1	2	3	4	5	6	7	8	9	10	Worst possible shortness of breath
Other problem	0	1	2	3	4	5	6	7	8	9	10	

STAFF TO COMPLETE SHADED SECTION

Action Taken			Referred to:	Notes
Directly managed	Managed by other care team member	Referral required		
			❒ Pain	
			❒ Fatigue Class	
			❒ Fatigue Coordinator	
			❒ Physical Activity/ ENHANCE Program	
			❒ Counselling Referral	
			❒ Spiritual/Pastoral Care	
			❒ Resource Class	
			❒ Resource Counselling	
			❒ Rehabilitation	
			❒ Living Well With Cancer Class	
			❒ Optimal Nutrition Class	
			❒ Nutrition	
			❒ Speech and Language	
			❒ Patient Advocate	
			❒ Home Care	
			❒ Other:	

2. CANADIAN PROBLEM CHECKLIST

Please check all of the following items that have been a concern or problem for you in the past week including today:

Emotional:
- ❒ Fears/Worries
- ❒ Sadness
- ❒ Frustration/Anger
- ❒ Changes in appearance
- ❒ Intimacy/Sexuality
- ❒ Change in who I am

Practical:
- ❒ Work/School
- ❒ Finances
- ❒ Getting to and from appointments
- ❒ Accommodation
- ❒ Quitting Smoking

Informational:
- ❒ Understanding my illness and/or treatment
- ❒ Talking with the health care team
- ❒ Making treatment decisions
- ❒ Knowing about available resources
- ❒ Taking medications as prescribed

Spiritual:
- ❒ Meaning/Purpose of life
- ❒ Faith

Social/Family:
- ❒ Feeling a burden to others
- ❒ Worry about family/friends
- ❒ Feeling alone

Physical:
- ❒ Concentration/Memory
- ❒ Sleep
- ❒ Weight
- ❒ Mobility
- ❒ Physical Activity

Date: RN Signature:

*Integrated Symptom Relief Service-Screening for Distress - Version 3.2 *Questionnaire adapted from the Cancer Journey Action Group, Canadian Partnership Against Cancer's minimum data set*

Figure 7.4 Personal Well-being Checklist.

Room on the screening form was later created for documentation, so that appropriate referrals could be initiated by the attending nurse or physician. From the outset, it was understood that Screening for Distress was to be followed by assessment and intervention.

At the Tom Baker Cancer Centre in Calgary, two clinics (Neuro-Oncology and Head and Neck Tumor Groups) were selected to model an *Integrated Symptom Relief Service*. Operationally, the *Integrated Symptom Relief Service* seeks to establish a cancer care system which effectively integrates resources to ensure patients' concerns are managed by the right professionals in a timely and coordinated manner. The ultimate goal is to move toward a vision of person-centred care, where care focuses on what has been identified as being important to the patient and ultimately addresses a full range of needs. The key driver of the *Integrated Symptom Relief Service* is the implementation of Screening for Distress which uses standardized measures to rapidly screen patients for psychosocial, practical and physical concerns. Screening for Distress allows concerns to be speedily identified and shared with the health care team. With experience, training and clinical skill, health care providers should, using the screening tool as a guide, be able to open up a directed conversation with the patient to efficiently address patient concerns and refer as required.

Here is how it works: patients attending either of these clinics complete the screening tool (the Minimum Data Set) (Figure 7.4), the nurse coordinator in these clinics reviews the findings from the screening tool, opens a conversation with the patients, determines the nature and types of concerns and refers to the appropriate health care provider as necessary. Actions are reported on the completed form and inserted in the patient chart. To help guide the team, a simple guide has been developed using cut scores as illustrated in the referral pathway guide (Figure 7.5). What is important to keep in mind is that Screening for Distress needs to use a standardized questionnaire that rapidly and simply identifies frequently raised patient concerns so that the guesswork around symptom management can be easily addressed, without stigmatizing patient concerns, and thus referral to appropriate professionals can be initiated in a timely and appropriate way.

City of Hope, California, USA developed a touch screen automated program called *SupportScreen*, based on more than 15 years of screening experience in academic cancer centres and a small community hospital. *SupportScreen* is a patient-friendly data entry system that identifies physical problems, psychosocial concerns, alerts the health care team to risk factors and barriers to care, triages to multispecialists, refers to community resources and provides personalized educational information based on the specific needs of the patient and family member – all in real time (Figure 7.6). *SupportScreen* builds new partnerships by facilitating patient, family, physician and multispecialist communication and is used to maximize the effectiveness of clinical encounters as well as overall cancer care. *SupportScreen* has been successfully implemented at City of Hope and licensed to other medical centres to create a systematic bridge to new levels of communication, trust and partnership, which is essential to managing the financial and resource challenges that are undermining the solvency of the present health care system.

Both the Canadian and American Screening for Distress programmes are driving the health care system to integrate multidisciplinary teams into standardized clinical practice. The problems manifested by patients and their families and the support that the disease-directed teams require in managing the patient are often complex and simply cannot be addressed within the profession-centric care model. Person-centred care cannot exist by professionals remaining in their professional silos but must seek a model of care that encourages respect for what each profession can do to enhance cancer care for the whole person.

Interdisciplinary whole-person-centred care

What we have learned from psychosocial research prevalence studies has confirmed that patients may suffer from a full range of physical, practical and psychosocial concerns. While extension of life is seen as the primary objective for patients

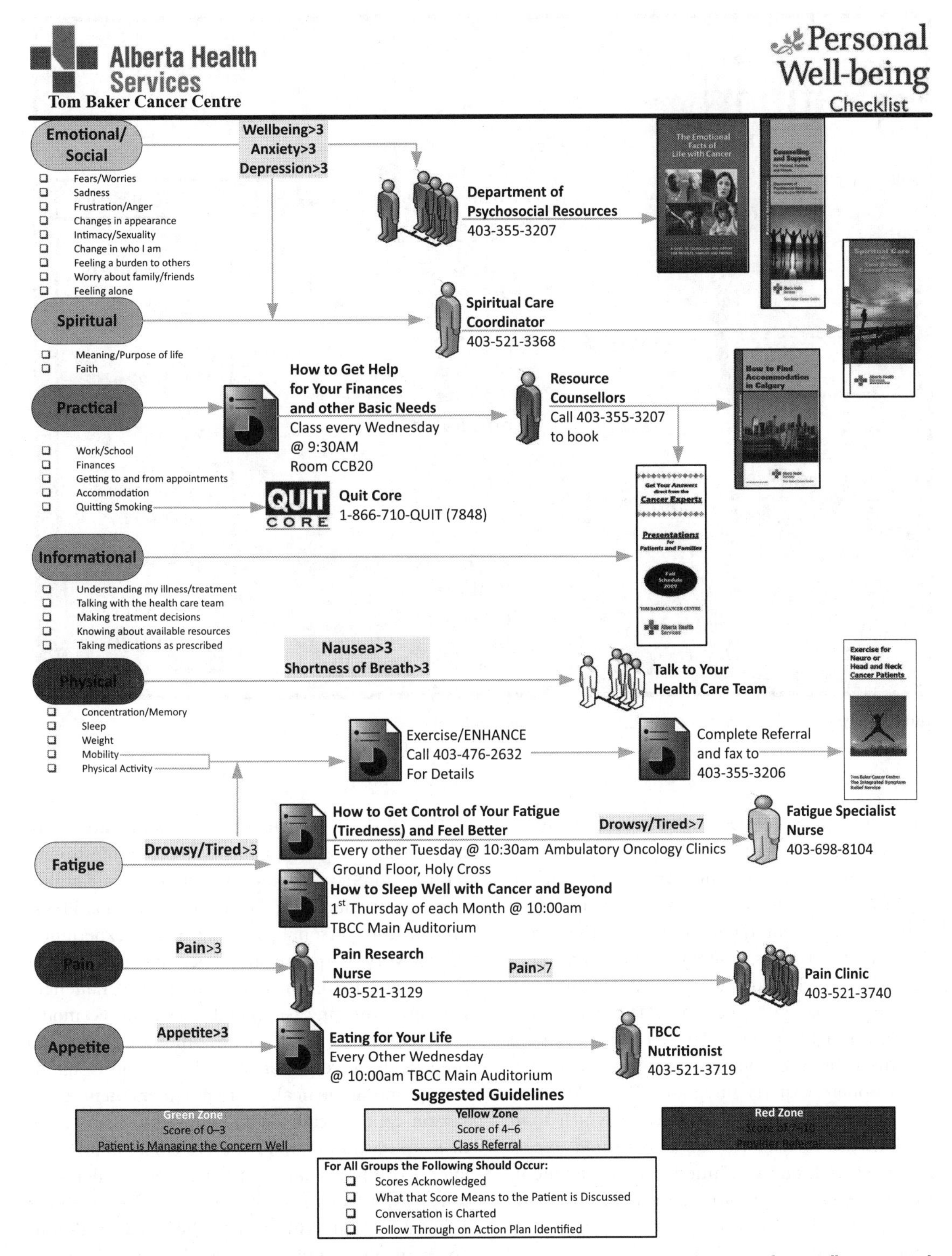

Figure 7.5 Integrated Symptom Relief Service Referral Pathways, Tom Baker Cancer Centre, Calgary, Alberta, Canada.

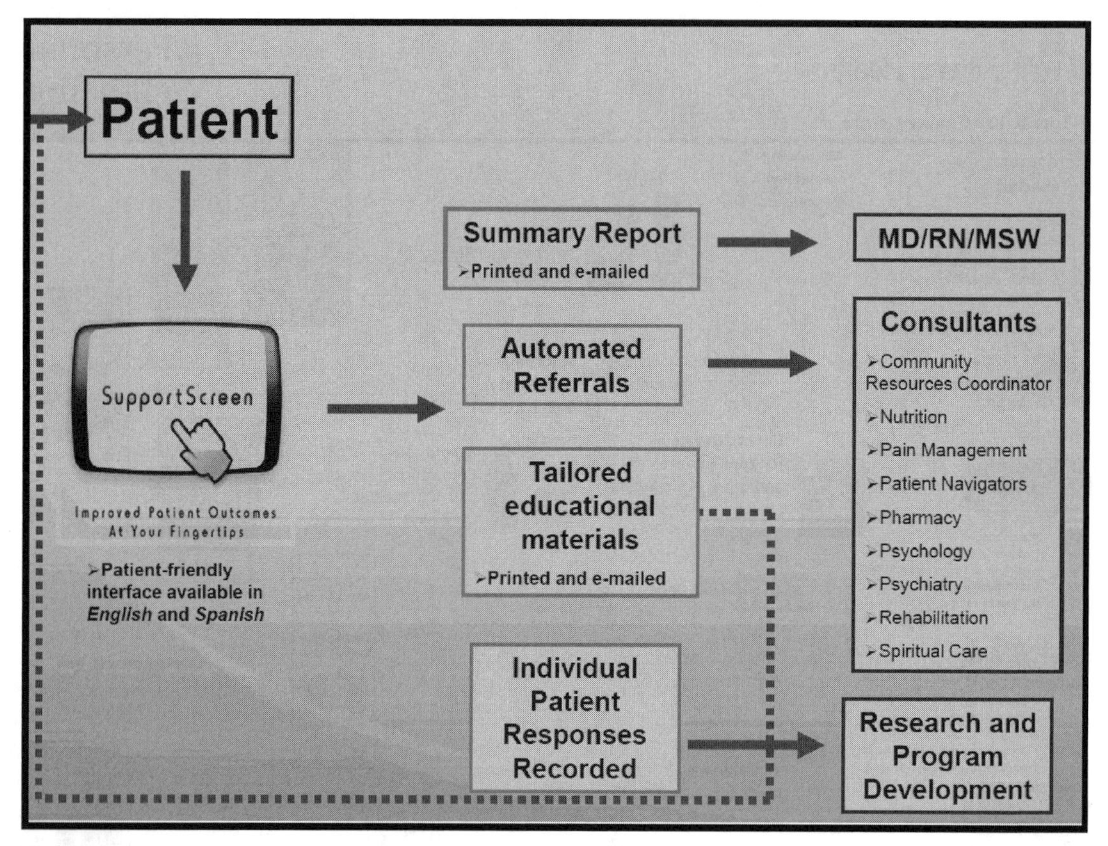

Figure 7.6 *SupportScreen* real-time outputs, City of Hope, California.

and their families, disease progression, symptom management and quality of life are also emerging as central concerns for patients and health care institutions and patient advocates. The data, knowledge and paradigm shifts resulting from Screening for Distress highlight the importance of utilizing simple tools to better understand and improve the patient experience. These tools are providing insights into just how complex patient concerns really are and how important it is that compassionate experts integrate effort. As there is no 'gold standard' with respect to which tool/questionnaire to use, we can and should expect further research and continued tool development. However, what we are learning today is that symptom management is too complex to be ignored or managed by any single professional.

The goal of excellence in patient care is to unite and integrate compassionate professionals with comprehensive skills to help patients, families and staff manage the challenges of serious illness and to find personal meaning in the experience. By its very structure and open commitment to *person-centred* over *profession-centric* care challenges the silo-protecting 'supposed' collaborative model and invites new partnerships among patients and their health care providers and even more significantly among the health care providers themselves. Person-centred care drives the health care team to *integrate* (rather than merely collaborate) their effort, compassionate expertise and to define a transparent way to work together and to celebrate a bigger vision. This is not the traditional top-down medical model and has the potential to be

You are not a serious cancer program, unless you are screening for distress.

Colum J. Smith, MD
Vice President and Chief Medical Officer
Saskatchewan Cancer Agency, Canada

What we measure is what we act upon.

Robert McMurty, MD
Chief Medical Advisor on the Future of Health Care in Canada

I love the program, it helps to identify patient needs and concerns and puts their mind at ease while going through treatment.

Christina Eckhart, Patient

My patients are complex on multiple levels. The automated screening and triage, real-time communication and the provision of tailored educational materials, allows me to be the doctor. The clinic visit is focused and incredibly efficient – no need to fish for potentially sensitive but essential information, it is all there already.

Robert J. Morgan, Jr, MD, FACP
Professor of Medical Oncology
Associate Director for Medical Education, Medical Oncology & Therapeutics Research
City of Hope Comprehensive Cancer Center, Duarte, CA, USA

By having this information in real-time, my initial encounter with the patient is more effective and efficient. Often problems are identified by *SupportScreen* that the patient has not volunteered to the health care team.

Arti Hurria, MD
Director, Cancer and Aging Research Program
City of Hope Comprehensive Cancer Center, Duarte, CA, USA

[Screening for Distress] gives us a good tool to really evaluate where the patient is, in relation to us and the services we have to offer him, and eventually personalize more what we have to offer.

Health Administrator, Quebec, Canada[a]

Having the tool has certainly brought out conversations that I feel confident wouldn't have happened otherwise. So, I find it very useful.

Cancer Patient Navigator, Nova Scotia, Canada[a]

One of the first people that I did [screened] was someone who I had known for several months and I had several connections with. Our interaction was: "Is everything going OK?", "Yes everything's fine". They looked fine and were coming for their treatments. He was one of the first people I administered the tool to and he scored high. It gave him the opportunity to really focus on the issues that were causing him distress rather than the general comment about "is everything OK". We could actually go through the list of everything and he was able to pick out the things that were causing him distress. So, after that, I felt that there were probably many more patients . . . I was just taking it for granted that things are OK because they tell me without really getting into it too deeply.

Cancer Patient Navigator, Nova Scotia, Canada[a]

Figure 7.7 Quotes supporting Screening for Distress.
[a]*Source:* Fillion L., Cook S., Blais M-C. *et al.* (2011) Implementation of Screening for Distress with professional cancer navigators. *Oncologie*, 13, 277–289.

profoundly transformative. In fact, in the two models above, it already has.

It is hard to appreciate the full impact of designing a supportive care programme based on person-centred care. When it comes to thinking about health care, the focus has generally been on thinking in silos. As part of a new model of health service delivery, as well as excellent academic medicine, all clinical care services must think of the patient as the unit of care and not the parts. This means comprehensive integrated interdisciplinary patient care. This is a courageous undertaking and because we are so routed in traditional biomedical care the path ahead will likely be challenged. But changes to culture take time and the impetus for change has never been greater.

Person-centred care must be built into the system at many levels. While Screening for Distress is able to identify problems and to link patients to the support and education they need on an individual level, screening is not about psychosocial issues alone. Based on our research, it is about the multiple symptoms patients are likely to experience. Because cancer care is highly specialized and patient needs complex, an integrated model of service delivery could help reduce the suffering and burden of cancer for the patient and health care system. Given what we are learning from the Canadian model of Screening for Distress and the American model of the *SupportScreen* program it is rapidly becoming apparent that Screening for Distress is emerging as the connective tissue of integrated interdisciplinary patient care. Screening has engaged patients, families and the health care teams in clearly defined efforts to use data to focus professional effort, to apply evidence-based interventions and to begin to transform the way health care is provided (see Figure 7.7 for specific examples).

Summary and conclusion

This is a unique time; health care internationally is being challenged to be more efficient and to become more person-centred. The profession-centric view has been challenged on multiple levels. There have been major lessons learned from how patients, families and communities are actively engaged and becoming partners in their own health caring.

Screening has been widely supported and there have been major advances because of it. The 6th Vital Sign has been a major accomplishment and the data has led us inexorably to the reality that we must all be person-centred. This reality is necessary not only based on the Hippocratic Oath and the values of all the world's great religions and democratic societies but also because it is the most efficient and realistic way for health care to be able to address the many and complex needs of varying populations. Screening for Distress can be metaphorically seen as the connective tissue of the health care system and the data confirms the potential benefits gleaned from Screening for Distress in oncology practice.

Person-centred care ultimately drives the challenge to professionals, health care leaders, social planners to integrate and synergize resources to maximize quality with efficiency, create true working partnerships and to advance a true science of caring.

Key points

- Interdisciplinary teamwork has long been heralded as the pathway to excellence in patient care.
- Screening for Distress data is providing information about how best to address patients' and families' concerns.
- Distress has been endorsed as the 6th Vital Sign internationally.
- Screening for Distress can be a roadmap for health care providers to do the hard work of clearly defining patient problems and referring patients to the right professional in a timely way.
- Both the Canadian and American Screening for Distress programmes are driving the health care system to integrate multidisciplinary teams into standardized clinical care.
- Patients may suffer from a full range of physical, practical and psychosocial concerns.
- Symptom management is too complex to be ignored or managed by any single professional.
- Clinical care must think of the patient as the unit of care.
- Screening for Distress is emerging as the connective tissue of integrated interdisciplinary patient care.

Acknowledgements

We would like to acknowledge the work of Ms Shannon Groff, Ms Andrea Williams and the Screening for Distress Coordinating Team under the Cancer Journey Portfolio, Canadian Partnership Against Cancer, Amy Waller, Paula Jones as well as all the staff at the Tom Baker Cancer Centre involved in the Integrated Symptom Relief Service.

Suggested further reading

Fillion L., Cook S., Blais M-C. *et al.* (2011) Implementation of Screening for Distress with professional cancer navigators. *Oncologie*, 13, 277–289.

Bultz B.D., Groff S.L., Fitch M. *et al.* (2011) Implementing Screening for Distress, the 6th Vital Sign: A Canadian strategy for changing practice. *Psycho-Oncology*, 20, 463–469.

Loscalzo M., von Gunten C.F. (2009) Interdisciplinary teamwork in palliative care: Compassionate expertise for serious complex illness, in *Handbook of Psychiatry in Palliative Medicine*, 2nd edn (eds H.M. Chochinov, W.S. Breitbart) Oxford University Press, New York.

Loscalzo M.J., Bultz B.D., Jacobsen P.B. (2010) Building psychosocial programs: A roadmap to excellence, in *Psycho-Oncology*, 2nd edn (eds J.C. Holland, W.S. Breitbart, P.B. Jacobsen *et al.*), Oxford University Press, New York, pp. 569–574.

Simone J.V. (2002) Understanding cancer centers. *Journal of Clinical Oncology*, 20, 4503–4507.

Holland J. (1998) Establishing a Psycho-oncology Unit in a Cancer Center, in *Psycho-Oncology* (ed. J. Holland), Oxford University Press, New York, pp. 1049–1054.

Jacobsen P.B. (2010) Translating psychosocial oncology research to clinical practice, in *Psycho-Oncology*, 2nd edn (eds J.C. Holland, W.S. Breitbart, P.B. Jacobsen *et al.*), Oxford University Press, New York, pp. 642–647.

Bultz B.D., Jacobsen P.B., Loscalzo M. (2009) Psychosocial programme development, in *Handbook of Communication in Oncology and Palliative Care* (eds D. Kissane, B. Bultz, P. Butow), Oxford University Press, New York, pp. 521–529.

Loscalzo M., Clark K., Holland J. (2011) Successful strategies for implementing biopsychosocial screening. *Psycho-Oncology*, **20**, 455–462. Published online at: http://onlinelibrary.wiley.com/, DOI: 10.1002/pon.1930.

Bultz B.D., Johansen C. (eds) (2011) Special Issue: Screening for Distress, the 6th Vital Sign. *Psycho-Oncology*, 20, 569–674.

References

1. Schofield P., Carey M., Bonevski B., Sanson-Fisher R. (2006) Barriers to the provision of evidence-based psychosocial care in oncology. *Psycho-Oncology*, 15, 863–872.
2. Institute of Medicine (IOM) (2008) *Cancer Care for the Whole Patient: Meeting Psychosocial Health Needs*, National Academies Press, Washington, DC.
3. Peabody F.W. (1927) The care of the patient. *Journal of the American Medical Association*, 88, 877–882.
4. Carter G., Lewin T., Gianacas L. *et al.* (2011) Caregiver satisfaction with out-patient oncology services: Utility of the FAMCARE instrument and development of the FAMCARE-6. *Supportive Care in Cancer*, 19, 565–572.
5. Velikova G. (2010) Patient benefits from psychosocial care: Screening for distress and models of care. *Journal of Clinical Oncology*. Published online before print Oct 12, DOI: 10.1200/JCO.2010.31.0136.
6. van Scheppingen C., Schroevers M., Smink A. *et al.* (2011) Does screening for distress efficiently uncover meetable unmet needs in cancer patients? *Psycho-Oncology*, 20, 1099–1611.
7. Canadian Association of Psychosocial Oncology Conference Statement of Endorsement: Screening for Distress as the 6th Vital Sign, April 2009, Vancouver, BC.
8. IPOS 11th World Congress of Psycho-Oncology Statement of Endorsement: Screening for Distress as the 6th Vital Sign in Oncology, June 2009, Vienna, Austria.
9. Accreditation Canada (2008) Cancer care and oncology services standards. Available at: www.accreditation.ca/accreditation-programs/qmentum/standards/cancercare/ (accessed December 2011).
10. Union for International Cancer Control (2010) Distress the 6th Vital Sign in cancer care. Available at: www.uicc.org (accessed December 2011).
11. National Comprehensive Cancer Network (2009) NCCN Clinical Practice Guidelines in Oncology (NCCN Guidelines®). Distress Management. Version 1.2009. Available at: http://www.nccn.org/professionals/physician_gls/f_guidelines.asp (accessed December 2011).
12. Ashbury F.D., Findlay H., Reynolds B., McKerracher K. (1998) A Canadian survey of cancer patients' experiences: Are their needs being met? *Journal of Pain Symptom Management*, 16, 298–306.
13. Bultz B.D., Berman N.J. (2010) Branding distress as the 6th Vital Sign: Policy implications, in *Psycho-Oncology*, 2nd edn (eds J. Holland, W.S. Breitbart P.B. Jacobsen *et al.*) Oxford University Press, New York, pp. 663–666.
14. Sellick S.M., Edwardson A.D. (2007) Screening new cancer patients for psychological distress using the hospital anxiety and depression scale. *Psycho-Oncology*, 16, 534–542.

15. Zabora J., BrintzenhofeSzoc K., Jacobsen P. *et al.* (2001) A new psychosocial screening instrument for use with cancer patients. *Psychosomatics*, 42, 241–246.
16. Cella D. (1998) Factors influencing quality of life in cancer patients: Anemia and fatigue. *Seminars in Oncology*, 25(suppl 7), 43–46.
17. Zabora J.R., Loscalzo M.J., Weber J. (2003) Managing complications in cancer: Identifying and responding to the patient's perspective. *Seminars in Oncology Nursing*, 19, 1–9.
18. Carlson L.E., Angen M., Cullum J. *et al.* (2004) High levels of untreated distress and fatigue in cancer patients. *British Journal of Cancer*, 90, 2297–2304.
19. Loscalzo M.J., Clark K.L. (2007) Problem-related distress in cancer patients drives requests for help: A prospective study. *Oncology*, 21, 1133–1138.
20. Jacobsen P.B., Ransom S. (2007) Implementation of NCCN distress management guidelines by member institutions. *Journal of National Comprehensive Cancer Network*, 5, 99–103.
21. Mitchell A.J. (2010) Short screening tools for cancer-related distress: A review and diagnostic validity meta-analysis. *Journal of National Comprehensive Center Network*, 8, 487–494.
22. Palmer S.C., Coyne J.C. (2003) Screening for depressions in medical care: Pitfalls, alternatives, and revised priorities. *Journal of Psychosomatic Research*, 54, 279–287.
23. Carlson L.E., Groff S.L., Maciejewski O., Bultz B.D. (2011) Screening for Distress in lung and breast cancer outpatients: A randomized controlled trial. *Journal of Clinical Oncology*, 28, 4884–4891.
24. Clark K.L., Bardwell W.A., Arsenault T. *et al.* (2009) Implementing touch screen technology to enhance recognition of distress. *Psycho-Oncology*, 18, 822–830.
25. Loscalzo M., Clark K., Dillehunt J. *et al.* (2010) SupportScreen: A model for improving patient outcomes at your fingertips. *Journal of National Comprehensive Center Network*, 8, 496–504.
26. Velikova G., Wright E.P., Smith A.B. *et al.* (1999) Automated collection of quality of life data: A comparison of paper and computer touch screen questionnaires. *Journal of Clinical Oncology*, 17, 998–1007.
27. Bultz B., Johansen C. (2011) Screening for Distress, the 6th Vital Sign: Where are we, and where are we going? *Psycho-Oncology*, 20, 569–571.
28. Bultz B.D., Groff S.L., Fitch M. and Screening for Distress Toolkit Working Group (2009) Guide to Implementing Screening for Distress, the 6th Vital Sign, Part A: Background, Recommendations, and Implementation; http://www.partnershipagainstcancer.ca/wp-content/uploads/2.4.0.1.4.5-Guide_CJAG.pdf (accessed December 2011).

CHAPTER 8
Psychological Intervention

Maggie Watson
Psychology Research Group, Institute of Cancer Research, Royal Marsden Hospital, and Research Department of Clinical, Health and Educational Psychology, University College London, UK

Introduction

In psycho-oncology there has been accumulating evidence over the last three decades confirming the value of psychological intervention. This has contributed to specific discussion about how the psychological and emotional needs of cancer patients, their partners, families and those close to them might best be met (see Watson and Kissane (2011) in the recommended further reading for a more detailed exposition of psychotherapy models). The development and delivery of psychological intervention has now become a detailed, skilled and organized activity guided by evidence. Linked to this has been the publication of guidelines from academic organizations, health care providers and governmental sources that aim to rationalize and improve psychological care within oncology practice (see details of guidelines in the recommended further reading).

Background

The need for effective psychological care for people with cancer stems, to some extent, from evidence indicating that substantial levels of distress and difficulties are experienced by patients and those close to them.[1,2] Also cancer treatments are acknowledged as being extremely challenging. Supporting patients through these challenges and difficulties is part of a holistic approach to cancer care that sees the patients as the focus of treatment and not the tumour. One of the most mature and frequently cited studies documenting level of psychological difficulties[3] showed that 47% of cancer patients had symptoms of psychiatric disorder according to the DSM-III classification system; the majority being adjustment disorders with accompanying anxiety and depression. While this study helped put patients' psychological needs on the map it also, by using a psychiatric nosology, set the area back. Patients with cancer might now have diagnosed psychiatric disorders where in reality their reactions, those primarily of ordinary people in extra-ordinary situations, might have been better conceptualized in psychological terms. While the data overwhelmingly confirm that going through cancer is distressing, difficult, challenging and for some, seemingly insurmountable, the figures on levels of psychological problems and distress vary depending on what is being measured and how it is measured.[4] Generally assessment of need focuses on trying to evaluate how much worry or anxiety, general distress or depression someone experiences. Occasionally needs are assessed more broadly to ascertain whether there are relationship problems, communication issues, psychosexual and/or body image issues, financial problems, serious physical and/or treatment problems, or spiritual and/or existential concerns. Issues about what to assess, how needs are defined and how to identify or screen for those in need, have been dealt with comprehensively elsewhere.[5]

Clinical Psycho-Oncology: An International Perspective, First Edition. Edited by Luigi Grassi and Michelle Riba.

Many people cope using their personal resources and adapt to the new situation given time. Some do not, and it is these who may need access to formal specialist services. As a proviso, it is important to acknowledge that all patients need good communication and information provision, they need to feel cared about by cancer professionals, and need to feel able to voice their concerns to those health professionals they meet as part of their routine cancer treatment. This has been one of the motivators behind training to improve communication skills in cancer professionals and, in itself, represents a type of psychological intervention. However, the aim here is to discuss formal psychological intervention as something that is broader and more complex, and practised by professionals who have had training in specific psychological care skills.

It is important that those dealing with patients on an everyday basis in their clinical practice have enough skill to offer some level of psychological care and feel knowledgeable about when to refer on to others with a higher level of skill. Routine provision of psychological care by oncology professionals sends a message to the patient that this is not only an accepted part of oncology care, but confirms the legitimacy of patients voicing psychological problems to oncology staff. In this respect there is a need to integrate training in managing psychological problems into cancer care. It should also be expected that those who provide a formal 'psychological intervention' will have satisfied certain standards for training regardless of whether they need to provide basic level or advanced level care.

What is psychological intervention?

How should psychological intervention be defined and why does it matter? Hodges and colleagues[6] focusing on the lack of definition in the literature, emphasize the importance of defining terms because this helps to clarify what treatments are included under the term 'psychological intervention' and this, in turn, helps achieve a clearer evaluation of the evidence on therapy and what professional training might be offered. They could find no explicit definition in their review of 66 relevant studies and little consistency between reviewers in how they manage this issue, and they proposed that a checklist be used to bring some consistency in study reporting. The importance of defining formal 'psychological intervention' is not only to allow a clearer analysis of the evidence on efficacy but also to inform what will be done in clinical practice. Manne and Andrykowski[7] use the definition described by Strupp[8] where a psychological intervention is: '. . . an interpersonal process designed to bring about modification of feelings, cognitions, attitudes and behaviour'. However, this may be too broad as it could equally apply to innumerable direct or indirect interactions. Hodges and colleagues[6] propose that, rather than use a global term of psychological intervention, the value of outcome data could be more clearly ascertained if researchers described what they did on a number of domains including 'content, proposed mechanism, target outcome and methods of delivery'.

A more specific definition of formal psychological intervention is proposed here and includes four characteristics:

(i) *A direct intervention by a recognized trained professional;*

(ii) *The intervention follows an evidence-based method;*

(iii) *The intervention method and therapy outcome is clearly described and defined making it possible for others to know how to use the intervention, and assess its' effects and efficacy;*

(iv) *The primary focus of the intervention is to work with people to increase their personal resources in dealing with aspects of cancer that cause undue stress/distress and in this respect, targets for change will be behavioural, emotional, cognitive and relational/interpersonal.*

Who should provide psychological intervention?

In the UK, the National Institute for Health and Clinical Excellence (NICE)[9] has operationalized psychological care within a four-tier stepped care model (see Box 8.1). This has the effect of defining 'intervention' according to level of skill required by the professional working with the patient. At the most basic level (level 1) it is a requirement that all oncology staff have some skills that will help provide good emotional support and information to patients. The training in these skills should be integrated into the routine training of each profession. As problems and emotions become more difficult and patients are seen to struggle to cope, so too the type of psychological care offered becomes more complex, detailed and specific, and the level of professional skill needed to provide the care is increased. While mental health professionals are described within this model as being the most skilled (level 4), staff functioning at levels two and three may also provide formal psychological intervention that requires a level of skill over and above what is currently normally achieved within usual training for that profession. Oncology staff providing psychological care at levels two and three are expected to have additional training (often from mental health professionals) so they have the knowledge needed to provide care which is 'psychological', that is, to a professional standard over and above basic skills. This training should be available regardless of type of oncology professional involved and according to the NICE level at which they aim to function.

Box 8.1 Derived from the UK National Institute for Health and Clinical Excellence stepped care four-tier model of psychological support.

LEVEL 1

All health professionals:

Effective information giving, compassionate communication and general psychological support.

LEVEL 2

Health professionals with additional expertise:

Psychological interventions such as anxiety management and problem solving.

LEVEL 3

Trained and accredited professionals:

Counselling and specific psychological therapies according to an explicit theoretical framework.

LEVEL 4

Mental health specialists:

Specialist psychological and psychiatric interventions.

The NICE model does not proscribe in detail a psychological intervention type but acknowledges that there is variation in patient need and a hierarchy of professional skills is required. All levels of the stepped care model are considered important, and access by patients to all these levels of professional skill according to need, is recommended. The NICE guidelines should not be seen to discount the many informal support programmes, informational and social support agencies/networks developed for cancer patients, many of which have their advent in the charitable sector and likely provide important support. However, all good psychological care should be evidence-based no matter what type is provided and by whom.

Although there is evidence that non-psychologist-led interventions show lower effect sizes[10] it is not clear what improvements could be achieved in non-psychologist therapists' skills if they are given adequate training. This issue would benefit from further research. A few studies have shown that non-psychologists can be trained to use specific formal psychological therapies, for example CBT;[11,12] however, the evidence for impact on depression is less clear.[11] Access to mental health professionals is likely to continue to be limited and passing skills down is an important role they have in training others and improving patient access to good psychological care. The integration of mental health professionals into training of oncology staff remains underdeveloped, with the consequence that opportunities are being missed for the passing down of psychological skills.

Recent evidence on the nature of psychosocial care delivered by oncologists indicates that less than half (47%) initiate a referral to psychosocial support services and 48% report starting patients on psychiatric medication, mainly selective serotonin reuptake inhibitors (SSRIs) and benzodiazepines;[13] a questionable quick fix. Ironically, the majority of patients want to discuss psychological concerns with cancer doctors but only a minority of patients are willing to mention them.[14] The burden of time is often perceived by oncologists as a barrier to them asking about concerns but evidence shows that responding to patients' emotional needs may shorten consultation times.[15] Up-skilling cancer professionals should increase confidence in managing many of the patients' psychological concerns observed in routine practice.

Does intervention work: What is the evidence?

The amount of evidence on efficacy of psychological intervention for adult patients is substantial. There are a number of meta-analyses and supra-meta-analyses.[16–20] One review included '673 reports comprising 488 unique projects conducted over a 25-year time'.[21] These authors concluded that it was important to ascertain whether intervention 'should be targeted to individuals experiencing specific difficulties or if, based on their potentially preventive value, most cancer patients could be helped by them'. Despite the number of studies they report accessing they overlooked one of the largest randomized controlled trials[22] perhaps due to the limited bibliographic database they used. In particular it is possible to challenge these authors when they claim that 'just a single non-profit organization among the dozens that exist, ... provided free counselling, support groups, referral, and financial assistance ...' when by doing so they exclude those studies provided from within a free-to-all national health service such as in the UK and other European countries.[23,24] Therefore the conclusions of this review need to be approached with some caution. The UK NICE guidelines[9] help to clarify the issue raised by Moyer and colleagues[21] by describing a stepped care model which advocates providing different types and levels of psychological care according to patient need rather than trying to decide whether either a targeted programme or blanket preventative approach is needed.

Moyer and colleagues acknowledge that evidence for benefit to patients exists but argue that it 'stands in contrast to the services available to, and being used by, cancer patients'. This is an important issue also taken up Manne and Andrykowski[7] who make the point that efficacy and effectiveness evidence do not always provide clear guidelines on what psychological intervention will work with patients in routine clinical practice. This is not a problem unique to psycho-oncology but applies to many areas of psychology and medicine where what works in the context of randomized controlled designs, may not be what happens in routine practice. However, the main aim is to provide sufficient robust data to conclude there is an empirically supported treatment and then effectiveness data can be subsequently collected, for example through clinical audit, to ascertain how well the treatment can be used in the specific context of everyday clinical care.

Newell and colleagues[18] provided one of the better reviews and concluded that group therapy, education, counselling and cognitive behaviour therapy offer 'most promise' for medium- and long-term benefits for many psychosocial outcomes. Intervention offers benefits across a range of outcomes and no single intervention model benefits all. It is important to offer therapies that are useful both in individual and group format, as some patients will prefer the latter where social comparison processes are a powerful part of therapeutic benefit. Patients with existential concerns, often more evident in those with advanced cancers, may need access to therapy that helps them reduce fear of death, put their life in perspective and resolve important life issues as death approaches.

Despite this view that a range of therapy methods is needed to meet varying patient needs, evidence on the benefits of some therapy models is stronger than others. There is good evidence that therapy based on cognitive behavioural methods helps prevent the development of anxiety and depression amongst cancer patients and promotes recovery in those already depressed.[12,22,25] More recently, the NICE[26] review of 'Depression in Adults with a Chronic Physical Health Problem' recommended the use of group CBT, individual CBT and computer-delivered CBT. CBT is the treatment of choice for depression in patients with chronic health problems given the weight of evidence on efficacy. While there is some evidence for the effectiveness of combined antidepressant treatment and CBT in clinically depressed patients, the NICE review concluded that there was uncertainty about benefit in the medium term and the potential for interactions (of antidepressants) with medications prescribed for physical health problems 'is a concern'.

There is a need also to be more creative in the methods of delivering psychological intervention. Patients may find it difficult to comply with an intervention that demands attendance beyond routine hospital appointments and participation rates in face-to-face psychotherapy can vary from 15–82% with a median of 35%.[27] More recently there has been a move towards use of technology. Cognitive behaviour therapy for managing health problems has been successfully adapted for the Internet.[28] The NICE Technology Appraisal Guidance[29] on computer-delivered cognitive behavioural therapy (CCBT) concluded that preliminary evidence supports the use of CCBT in the management of depression and some anxiety disorders in the mental health setting. Telephone outreach and computer-based CBT is likely to improve access and benefits to cancer patients, though clinical trial evidence is at an early stage.[30,31]

In summary, there have been a number of reviews of psychological intervention for cancer patients and their families[32] and an emphasis recently on the idea that one size does not fit all.[10] The need to continue to collect evidence using the randomized clinical trial methodology remains an important goal. There will be increasing pressure to conduct and report outcome studies using well-defined criteria as described by the Consolidated Standards of Reporting Trials (CONSORT) statement.[33] The National Cancer Research Institute's report on 'Supportive and Palliative Care Research in the UK'[34] highlights among its conclusions a 'major lack of consensus on which outcome measure is most appropriate for particular situations. This lack of consensus is holding the field back. It makes systematic reviews... very difficult'. Ellwood and colleagues[35] have argued for consideration of an 'empirically supported treatment' (ESP) approach with a distinction between efficacy research and effectiveness research and the need to consider how evidence is obtained.

Types of formal psychological intervention: What is out there?

The International Psycho-Oncology Society (IPOS) has a set of online lectures (see www.ipos-society.org) on a range of topics including psychological intervention. These lectures are available in a number of languages*. IPOS has also produced a handbook of psychotherapies used with cancer patients and their families (see Watson and Kissane (2011) recommended further reading). The scope of the IPOS handbook is broad and often the therapies described are manualized. Therapies in the IPOS handbook include: cognitive behavioural therapies (CBT), supportive–expressive, meaning-centred psychotherapy, psycho-educational intervention, family-focused grief therapy, guided writing, narrative therapy, mindfulness-based therapy, reconstructing meaning and cognitive-analytic therapy and motivational interviewing. Other approaches focus on specific problems or groups of patients such as sexual dysfunction, intimacy-enhancing therapy, therapy with paediatric patients and their families, therapy for families at genetic risk and therapy for families where a parent has cancer, as well as programmes aimed at the needs of the elderly.

In the United Kingdom there has been a strong tradition of focusing on cognitive behavioural therapies. More recently, the UK National Institute for Health and Clinical Excellence (NICE)[26] review of 'Depression in Adults with a Chronic Physical Health Problem' (CG91) recommended the use of CBT. The review concluded that [Section 7.5] '... the most substantial evidence base (for moderate to severe depression) is for CBT'. This is the treatment of choice for depression in patients with chronic health problems given the weight of evidence on efficacy. This evidence-based NICE recommendation needs to be balanced against the need to provide a range of intervention options depending on patient need and what patients want. There is still a need to clarify what works for which type of cancer patient, which problem, and where in the cancer trajectory it works. For psycho-oncologists the challenge is how to produce a coherent and convincing body of evidence to support the implementation of tailored psychological therapies for cancer patients and their families. We are not there yet but have made some very significant progress over the last two decades.

Major issues

As the literature on psychological intervention has matured a number of issues and controversies have emerged.

Conclusions on efficacy?

Lepore and Coyne[36] outlined problems in the quality of the reviews and meta-analyses of evidence on psychological intervention. They argue that many reviewers fail to apply rigorous standards by which to judge quality of evidence; a situation likely to improve as it becomes a requirement within clinical trials to use stringent criteria set out by the CONSORT guidelines. However, indicators on the efficacy of psychological intervention (such as CBT which has passed stringent review criteria in the adult mental health arena) are favourable overall. Controversies in evaluating the data on efficacy are complicated by a lack of effectiveness data, that is, that there is no compelling case for provision to the typical cancer patient in the usual (non-research) clinical setting.[36,37] This is a good distinction to make.

The issue that emerges with some consistency in relation to efficacy of psychological therapies is that they work best with patients who have high psychological needs. Effect sizes in trials of formal psychological therapy are generally shown to be greater if the patients have more presenting symptoms. There are strong arguments in favour of targeting *more complex* formal interventions to those most in need and not to all patients routinely. The design of clinical trials should reflect this by determining what problem needs to be addressed and then targeting those patients with that problem. Coyne and colleagues[38] focus on the notion of selectivity and they make the point that the cost of providing psychological therapy service might be better justified if they were targeted to patients with high needs. Presumably they mean the provision of formal psychological therapies. In supporting one of their conclusions they are, however, selective about the evidence they cite. They state: 'There is rather consistent evidence that cancer patients prefer more support and communication from oncology clinical staff rather than mental health professionals and interventions designed to increase their access to quality, understandable information about their condition and its treatment to counselling and psychotherapy', that is, it is improved information-giving that is primarily preferred. They omit to point out that the supporting citations for this statement derive from studies solely with men. It may not be appropriate to conclude that patients prefer interventions from their cancer doctor focused on information needs when the evidence for this conclusion is derived only from male patients. However, this does highlight the point that less is known about the needs of men in terms of psychological intervention. As few of the overviews in the literature of psychological therapy bring out issues linked to the psychological needs of men, we are left with unclear direction on what to provide for men who, anyway, will be less often referred to, or will ask for access to, formal psychological therapies and mental health professionals. There is a need to explore and clarify what would be helpful to men; they are not immune to distress but may want to tackle it, in general, in different ways from women. Conclusions about the efficacy of psychological intervention may differ depending on whether or not an analysis or review of the evidence is made according to gender. This issue receives far less attention in discussions about the efficacy data.

Psychiatric versus psychological models

An important issue, rarely addressed in the psycho-oncology literature, relates to the common use of psychiatric models in the care of people with cancer. Historically medical models use an illness framework to conceptualize issues. The study of prevalence rates of morbidity by Derogatis and colleagues[3] was an example whereby emotional and behavioural reactions to cancer, which appeared to be signs of not coping with stress, were described according to the criteria used in the Diagnostic and Statistical Manual of Psychiatric Disorders. *Not coping became a mental disorder*. The impact has been to stigmatize some cancer patients and make it more difficult to push aside the barriers to them seeking and receiving psychological therapies. More important has been the effects on how psychological intervention was conceptualized and developed. The majority of cancer patients do not have formal psychiatric disorders; mental illness of known biological aetiology is not significantly greater for cancer patients than in the general population and many of the struggles cancer patients experience are best conceptualized in psychological not psychiatric terms. Once this becomes acknowledged, then interventions can move to a model of therapy that is explained through psychological processes and can use appropriate methods to focus on these. Some patients will benefit from mainstream psychiatric care but, for the majority, a psychological approach is likely to be better received by the patients themselves and more effective in helping them manage the difficulties that arise. In the past we have borrowed from mainstream psychiatric treatment models and diagnostic criteria but these have gradually evolved to tailored therapies for cancer patients and the need to develop intervention that meets the specific needs of patients with a serious life-threatening medical disorder rather than a mental illness.

Does psychological intervention do harm?

The issue of whether psychological intervention does harm is rarely tackled in psycho-oncology. However, just as measuring benefits of psychotherapy can be tricky, so is assessment of harm. Negative outcome results are rarely published and the number of clinical trials making comparison between different types of psychotherapy within psycho-oncology is still not sufficient. Boisvert and Faust[39] make a point in relation to mainstream psychotherapy that could be applied to psycho-oncology which is that 'If we are going to look at a list of treatments that are effective, then it makes sense to look at treatments that could potentially do harm.' Taking aside what we might consider as obvious psychological harm which may be caused by some methods, it is sometimes overlooked that harm can come from providing the wrong type of therapy thereby potentially preventing patients from making progress. Progress in therapy when used in everyday clinical practice needs to be monitored so that patients not making progress can be identified and appropriate actions taken.[40] Lambert[41] suggests regular monitoring of progress across psychological therapy sessions and likens it to monitoring of vital signs in order to clarify whether psychotherapy is going in the right direction.

While good clinical trial evidence, based on manualized treatments, is a necessary step in the establishment of credibility and benefits of an intervention, the application to daily practice (i.e. effectiveness), is important to ascertain. This can be achieved by ensuring that clinical staff use well-established methods to ensure their therapy continues to benefit those most in need. These processes include:

- regular monitoring of patient progress;
- the need for staff supervision to be routinely available;
- the need for discussions of complex cases with qualified colleagues;
- development of the practice of sharing of formulations and training in new therapy approaches;
- continuing professional development through formal and informal training.

These are an important part of provision of psychological therapy where therapists can be accountable and is good clinical governance. A well-functioning service is one where not only does the individual therapist feel supported in their work but also where each has a good idea of what other therapists, working alongside them, are doing. For those who are interested there is, within the mental health literature, some useful debate focusing on possible harm caused by psychological therapies.[42,43]

Is psychological intervention cost-effective?

There has been little emphasis, until recently, on the costs of psychological therapies for cancer patients. In many instances cancer treatment services are under increasing pressure to limit the costs of oncology treatments as new and expensive drugs are developed. There will be increasing pressure to provide data on the advantages of providing formal psychological intervention in terms of benefits linked to reduced health care utilization. Lemieux and colleagues[44] found that for metastatic cancer patients who were more distressed there was a non-significant decrease in health care utilization costs in favour of those provided with a psychosocial intervention, whereas Mandelblatt and colleagues[45] point out that health care costs tend to increase as psychological intervention intensity increases. Others have suggested more indirect benefits given the evidence that depressed cancer patients are more likely to be non-adherent to cancer drug therapies.[46] Simpson and colleagues[47] found that in a randomized controlled study, a brief group psycho-educational intervention for breast cancer patients, when compared to a waitlist control group saved health care system costs. Psychological therapy provision might have cost implications which are outweighed by the benefits in terms of reduced health care outcomes and utilization, but this needs to be clearly proven. While the cost of psychological therapies may be small in comparison to cancer drugs, there will be an increasing need to assess cost–benefits and justify psychological care on health economic grounds.

Conclusions and summary

A psychological intervention is defined here as *a formal evidence-based therapy with a clear theoretical basis and well-defined techniques developed for, or adapted to, the specific requirements of cancer patients and their families*. A formal psychological intervention approach needs to include associated guidelines, preferably be manualized, and should provide recommendations on who delivers the therapy and what level of skill is required to do this to the highest possible standard. Importantly, the intervention will have been developed for cancer patients and/or their families/partners and the evaluations of efficacy and effectiveness will be based on use within this medical cohort. There exist a number of formal psychological therapies that are strongly theoretically derived; however, evidence on effectiveness remains problematic. Professionals in psycho-oncology continue to struggle to produce trials using the standards required and accepted elsewhere in oncology. Progress will require a shift in the way we do research which will likely mean a move to the style of large clinical cooperative groups oncologists have already formed. For patients there is a need to ensure they are offered the most effective psychological care and are protected from therapies that may provide either little benefit or may cause harm.

Clinical case

The following clinical case aims to illustrate the possible scenarios which may occur if the UK NICE four-tier stepped care model is used. In practice patients do not necessarily have to pass through every one of the four levels of stepped care and may miss out levels depending on the initial assessment.

Managing anxiety

The NICE stepped care model is illustrated in this two-part case study.

The patient Anna is fictitious.

Anna presented at clinic prior to commencing her radiotherapy and when taken through some of the details of what was involved by the clinic nurse became distressed. Anna was able to say that she had a fear of medical procedures and was not sure if she could cope with being in an enclosed space.

Level 1 Intervention

At this point the nurse asked about the history of these fears. What might make things worse and what might make things better based on the patient's prior experience (i.e. problem formulation). The nurse then clarified with the patient what the specific fears were relating to radiotherapy and what the patient's preconceptions were about what might happen.

The nurse was able to ascertain that the patient had a fear both that radiotherapy was harmful and that she would be locked in the radiotherapy suite and unable to get out. She felt that if she panicked and moved during the treatment this would cause her serious harm.

The nurse, following discussion with the radiotherapist, was able to arrange for the patient to visit the radiotherapy suite and be talked through the procedure. The patient was seen by the radiographer who encouraged the patient to use some relaxation methods and also emphasized that more specific help was available. The clinical staff normalized the situation by saying this was not an uncommon problem.

Level 2 Intervention – Escalation Up

After visiting the radiotherapy suite the patient remained anxious and was offered training sessions in some relaxation skills which could be applied by direct experience by visiting the radiotherapy suite with the clinical nurse specialist offering relaxation training in situ. The patient did not want to take a short-acting anxiolytic as she had had adverse prior experience with these drugs.

Level 3 Intervention – Escalation Up

As none of this worked the patient was offered some sessions with a clinical psychologist who, using both systematic desensitization and CBT to deal with cognitive distortions, was able to help the patient find methods to alleviate her procedural-related fears.

Clinical case (continued)

Managing depression

The patient Mary is fictitious

Mary presented at clinic prior to commencing her radiotherapy and when taken through some of the details of what was involved by the clinic nurse became distressed. Mary was able to say that she felt hopeless about the therapy succeeding and did not see the point of continuing. She thought there was no point in going on as she could not see a future.

Level 1 Intervention

At this point the nurse asked about these feelings. The aim was to clarify how long the patient had felt hopeless, to what extent she felt low in her mood and whether she was feeling adequately supported (i.e. problem formulation). She also talked to Mary about what support she would like to have and what was available to enable to her to find the care she needed. The nurse asked the patient if she would like more time to talk about how she was feeling saying that it was not unusual to have these feelings. They decided it might help for her to talk to the clinical nurse specialist on the team providing her cancer care.

Level 2 Intervention – Escalation Up

The clinical nurse specialist (CNS) was subsequently able to provide some simple supportive listening. The CNS was able to learn that not only had the patient been feeling hopeless but she lived alone, felt unsupported and was under the impression that her cancer, which was at an early stage, was untreatable and could not be cured. The CNS considered that the patient might be moderately depressed in mood.

The CNS was able to clarify what Mary understood about her prognosis and correct errors in the patient's thinking. She was offered the opportunity to speak to her oncologist about her prognosis if this would be helpful.

She was also offered the opportunity for some specialist counselling given the provisional view that Mary might be depressed in mood.

Level 3 Intervention – Escalation Up

With the patient's consent, the CNS referred her to an on-site counsellor. The counsellor assessed Mary's needs and decided that she had a mild to moderate level of depression and offered her some sessions of supportive counselling aimed at giving her the opportunity to ventilate her worries; something Mary had been unable to do in her everyday life.

Level 4 Intervention – Escalation Up

While the counsellor observed that the therapy she provided was helpful with some of the patient's problems, she was aware that Mary was not making enough progress and needed a more specific structured therapy. She therefore asked the patient if she would like to be provided with some sessions from a clinical psychologist who could offer a therapy such as cognitive behavioural therapy.

The clinical psychologist made an assessment of Mary's needs and was able to determine that a cognitive behavioural therapy would be appropriate but Mary also required help with sleep problems including provision of a short course of medication. Mary also consulted the psychiatrist who provided an assessment and advice on her psychotropic medication needs. The clinical psychologist and psychiatrist discussed the provision of care to the patient and also offered suggestions to the clinical team on how Mary might best be supported during her radiotherapy.

Key points

- Support and assess patients: listen, acknowledge distress, be compassionate, respectful and empathic. Normalize feelings, give information, avoid premature reassurance.
- Establish nature and level of distress, clarify any issues that may reduce distress. Inform of the availability of

psychological care services and refer IF the patient is interested. If time is limited, consider whether the patient can come back at a less busy time.

- Routinely assess for psychological/emotional problems as it helps develop clinical assessment skills and de-stigmatizes coping difficulties and emotional problems for patients.
- Patients need access to a range of interventions in terms of type of therapy and the context for delivery, that is, individual, couples, family or group according to need.
- Patients will wait for clinicians to show interest in their emotional problems so responsibility lies with clinicians to ask.
- Less complex psychological problems can be managed using effective communication skills.
- More complex and enduring problems need to be assessed to clarify what level of intervention is needed.
- Patients with well-managed psychological problems do better in terms of improved quality of life, better adherence to treatment and reduced use of medical consultations and community services.
- Psychological intervention needs to be tailored to cancer patients' needs and not borrowed from mainstream psychiatry.

Acknowledgements

*The translation of the IPOS online lectures was made possible by a grant from the European School of Oncology.

Suggested further reading

Watson M., Kissane D. (eds) (2011) *Handbook of Psychotherapy in Cancer Care*, Wiley-Blackwell.

Burton M., Watson M. (1998) *Counselling People with Cancer*, John Wiley & Sons, Ltd, Chichester.

UK National Institute for Health and Clinical Excellence (NICE) (2004) Improving Supportive and Palliative Care for Adults with Cancer; www.nice.org.uk

USA Distress Management Clinical Practice Guidelines in Oncology (2003); www.nccn.org

Australian Clinical Practice Guidelines for the Psychosocial Care of Adults with Cancer (2003); www.nhmrc.gov.au/publications

UK National Cancer Survivorship Initiative Vision (2010); www/dh.gov.uk/publications

References

1. Massie J.M. (2004) Prevalence of depression in patients with cancer. *Journal of the National Cancer Institute Monograph*, 32, 57–71.
2. Zabora J.R., BrintzenhofeSzoc K., Curbow B. *et al.* (2001). The prevalence of psychological distress by cancer site. *Psycho-Oncology*, 10, 19–28.
3. Derogatis L.R., Morrow G.R., Fetting J. *et al.* (1983) The prevalence of psychiatric disorders among cancer patients. *Journal of the American Medical Association*, 249, 751–757.
4. Van't Spijker A., Trijsburg R.W., Duivenvoorden H.J. (1997) Psychological sequelae of cancer diagnosis: A meta-analytical review of 58 studies after 1980. *Psychosomatic Medicine*, 59, 280–293.
5. Special Issue on Screening for Distress (2011) *Psycho-Oncology*, 20(6), June.
6. Hodges L., Walker J., Kleiboer A. *et al.* (2011) What is a psychological intervention? A meta-review and practical proposal. *Psycho-Oncology*, 20, 470–478.
7. Manne S.L., Andrykowski M.A. (2006) Are psychological interventions effective and accepted by cancer patients? *Annals of Behavioral Medicine*, 32, 98–103.
8. Strupp H. (1978) Psychotherapy research and practice: An overview, in *Handbook of Psychotherapy and Behavior Change*, 2nd edn (eds S. Garfield, A. Begin), John Wiley & Sons, Inc., New York.
9. National Institute for Health and Clinical Excellence (NICE) (2004) Cancer service guidance (CSGSP): Improving supportive and palliative care for adults with cancer; http://www.nice.org.uk/csgsp (last accessed December 2011).
10. Zimmerman T., Heinrichs N., Baucom D. (2007) Does one size fit all? Moderators in psychosocial interventions for breast cancer patients: A meta-analysis. *Annals of Behavioral Medicine*, 34, 225–239.
11. Moorey S., Cort E., Kapari M. *et al.* (2009) A cluster randomized controlled trial of cognitive behaviour therapy for common mental disorders in patients with advanced cancer. *Psychological Medicine*, 39, 713–23.
12. Pitceathly C., Maguire P., Fletcher I. *et al.* (2009) Can a brief psychological intervention prevent anxiety or depressive disorders in cancer patients?

A randomised controlled trial. *Annals of Oncology*, 20, 928–934.

13. Muriel A.C., Hwang V.S., Kornblith A. *et al.* (2009) Management of psychosocial distress by oncologists. *Psychiatric Services*, 60, 1132–1134.
14. Detmar S.B., Aaronson N.K., Wever L.D. *et al.* (2000) How are you feeling? Who wants to know? Patients' and oncologists' preferences for discussing health-related quality-of-life issues. *Journal of Clinical Oncology*, 18, 3295–3301.
15. Butow P.N., Brown R.F., Cogar S. *et al.* (2002) Oncologists' reactions to cancer patients' verbal cues. *Psycho-Oncology*, 11, 47–58.
16. Fors E.G., Bertheussen G.F., Thune I., Juvet L.K. *et al.* (2010) Psychosocial interventions as part of breast cancer rehabilitation programs? Results from a systematic review. *Psycho-Oncology*, Epub Sept 6.
17. Naaman S.C., Radwan K., Fergusson D., Johnson S. (2009) Status of psychological trials in breast cancer patients: A report of three meta-analyses. *Psychiatry*, 72, 50–69.
18. Newell S.A., Sanson-Fisher R.W., Savolainen N.J. (2002) Systematic review of psychological therapies for cancer patients: Overview and recommendations for future research. *Journal of the National Cancer Institute*, 94, 558–584.
19. Rehse B., Pukrop R. (2003) Effects of psychosocial interventions on quality of life in adult cancer patients: Meta-analysis of 37 published controlled outcome studies. *Patient Education and Counselling*, 50, 179–186.
20. Uitterhoeve R.J., Vernooy M., Litjens M. *et al.* (2004) Psychosocial interventions for patients with advanced cancer – a systematic review of the literature. *British Journal of Cancer*, 91, 1050–62.
21. Moyer A., Sohl S.J., Knapp-Oliver S.K. *et al.* (2009) Characteristics and methodological quality of 25 years of research investigating psychosocial interventions for cancer patients. *Cancer Treatment Reviews*, 35, 475–484.
22. Greer S., Moorey S., Baruch J.D. *et al.* (1992) Adjuvant psychotherapy for patients with cancer: A prospective randomised trial. *British Medical Journal*, 304, 675–680.
23. Moorey S., Greer S., Bliss J., Law M.A. (1998) A comparison of adjuvant psychological therapy and supportive counselling on patients with cancer. *Psycho-Oncology*, 7, 218–228.
24. Pitceathly C., Maguire P., Fletcher I. (2003) Preventing psychological morbidity amongst newly diagnosed cancer patients: The impact of a 3-session intervention. *Psycho-Oncology*, 12, 832 [Abstract].
25. Osborn R., Demoncada A., Feuerstein M. (2006). Psychosocial interventions for depression, anxiety, and quality of life in cancer survivors: Meta-analyses. *International Journal of Psychiatry in Medicine*, 36, 13–34.
26. National Institute for Health and Clinical Excellence (NICE) (2009) Depression in Adults with a Chronic Physical Health Problem: Treatment and management, October 2009. National Clinical Practice Guideline Number 91. National Collaborating Centre for Mental Health commissioned by the National Institute for Health and Clinical Excellence.
27. Owen J.E., Klapow J.C., Roth D.L. *et al.* (2004) Improving the effectiveness of adjuvant psychological treatment for women with breast cancer: The feasibility of providing online support. *Psycho-Oncology*, 13, 281–292.
28. Cuijpers P., van Straten A., Andersson G. (2008) Internet-administered cognitive behavior therapy for health problems: A systematic review. *Journal of Behavioral Medicine*, 31, 169–177.
29. National Institute for Health and Clinical Excellence (NICE) (2002) Technology Appraisal No. 51. Computerised Cognitive Behaviour Therapy, October.
30. Donnelly J.M., Kornblith A.R., Fleishman S. *et al.* (2000) A pilot study of interpersonal psychotherapy by telephone with cancer patients and their partners. *Psycho-Oncology*, 9, 44–56.
31. DuHamel K.N., Mosher C.E., Winkel G. *et al.* (2010) Randomized clinical trial of telephone-administered cognitive-behavioral therapy to reduce post-traumatic stress disorder and distress symptoms after hematopoietic stem-cell transplantation. *Journal of Clinical Oncology*, 28, 3754–3761.
32. Meyer T.J., Mark M.M. (1995) Effects of psychosocial interventions with adult cancer patients: A meta-analysis of randomized experiments. *Health Psychology*, 14, 101–108.
33. Moher D., Schulz K.F., Altman D.G. for the CONSORT group (2001) The CONSORT statement: Revised recommendations for improving the quality of reports of parallel-group randomised trials. *The Lancet*, 357, 1191–1194.
34. Supportive and Palliative Care Research in the UK: Report of the NCRI Strategic Planning Group on Supportive and Palliative Care (2004); www.ncri.org.uk (accessed January 2012).
35. Ellwood A.L., Carlson L.E., Bultz B.D. (2001) Empirically supported treatments: Will this movement in the

field of psychology impact the practice of psychosocial oncology? *Psycho-Oncology*, 10, 199–205.

36. Lepore S.J., Coyne J.C. (2006) Psychological interventions for distress in cancer patients: A review of reviews. *Annals of Behavioral Medicine*, 32, 85–92.
37. Coyne J., Kagee A. (2001) More may not be better in psychosocial interventions for cancer patients. *Health Psychology*, 20, 458.
38. Coyne J., Lepore S., Palmer S. (2006) Efficacy of psychosocial interventions in cancer care: Evidence is weaker than it looks. *Annals of Behavioral Medicine*, 32, 104–110.
39. Boisvert C.M., Faust D.F. (2007) Practicing psychologists' knowledge of general psychotherapy research findings. *Professional Psychology: Research and Practice*, 37, 708–716.
40. Roth A., Fonagy P. (2004) *What Works for Whom? A Critical Review of Psychotherapy Research*, The Guilford Press, New York.
41. Lambert M. (2007) What have we learned from a decade of research aimed at improving psychotherapy outcome in routine care. *Psychotherapy Research*, 17, 1–14.
42. Lilienfeld S.O. (2007) Psychological treatments that cause harm. *Perspectives on Psychological Science*, 2, 53–70.
43. Rhule D. (2005) Take care to do no harm. *Professional Psychology*, 36, 618–625.
44. Lemieux J., Topp A., Chappell H. *et al.* (2006) Economic analysis of psychosocial group therapy in women with metastatic breast cancer. *Breast Cancer Research and Treatment*, 100, 183–190.
45. Mandelblatt J.S., Cullen J., Lawrence W.F. *et al.* (2008) Economic evaluation alongside a clinical trial of psycho-educational interventions to improve adjustment to survivorship among patients with breast cancer. *Journal of Clinical Oncology*, 26, 1684–1690.
46. Kissane D.W., Gabsch B., Clarke D. *et al.* (2007) Supportive-expressive group therapy for women with metastatic breast cancer: Survival and psychosocial outcome from a randomized controlled trial. *Psycho-Oncology*, 16, 277–85.
47. Simpson J.S.A., Carlson L.E., Trew M.E. (2001) Effect of group therapy for breast cancer on healthcare utilization. *Cancer Practice*, 9, 19–26.

CHAPTER 9
Psychopharmacological Interventions

Seema M. Thekdi[1], *María Elisa Irarrázaval*[2] *and Laura B. Dunn*[3]
[1]Department of Psychiatry, MD Anderson Cancer Center, Houston, TX, USA
[2]Mental Health Unit, Fundación Arturo López Pérez Oncologic Center, Santiago, Chile
[3]Department of Psychiatry, University of California, San Francisco, CA, USA

Introduction

Pharmacological interventions, when used carefully and monitored appropriately, can play an important role in the treatment of cancer patients suffering from a variety of psychiatric and psychological symptoms and syndromes. Although there remains a limited database from which to draw conclusions about the efficacy of any specific medication class for cancer patients,[1] it is notable that, one study found that half of women with breast cancer were prescribed some type of psychotropic medication.[2] It is likely that many patients are being prescribed these medications by their primary care physicians or oncologists.[3,4]

Therefore, those practising in cancer settings should be aware of the major drug classes, indications for their use, and important cautions regarding the use of these medications. This chapter addresses the indications, risks and benefits of the major classes of medications in oncology patients.

Background

The experience of being diagnosed with and treated for cancer can be quite overwhelming and may precipitate depressive, anxiety and other psychiatric symptoms. Ideally each cancer patient would have the opportunity to pursue psychotherapy or supportive counselling to sort through emotions and manage such symptoms. However, rapid control of psychiatric symptoms for the sake of cancer treatment compliance, safety and quality of life often necessitates the initiation of appropriate psychopharmacotherapy. In addition, cancer and its treatment cause physiological disturbances that may underlie the development of both psychological and physical cancer symptoms, and these symptom clusters often overlap.[5] Psychotropics have utility in managing emotional distress, cancer symptoms and treatment side-effects. Medication management of psychiatric symptoms is a valuable part of the overall psychosocial care of the cancer patient.

Major issues

Often the primary oncology team will be in the best position to identify mental health symptoms and untoward treatment side-effects due to frequency of contact. Educating the patient about the potential benefits of a mental health referral, coordinating the evaluation with other medical appointments, and reducing stigma by normalizing the need for psychosocial support are very helpful in completing a referral.

During an evaluation for psychopharmacological intervention, the mental health clinician will assess target symptoms that include both psychiatric and cancer symptoms (Table 9.1). Cancer patients may be more open to utilizing psychotropics if they find

Clinical Psycho-Oncology: An International Perspective, First Edition. Edited by Luigi Grassi and Michelle Riba.

Table 9.1 Drug classes and target symptoms in oncology settings.

Drug Classes Commonly Used
Antidepressants
Anxiolytics
Hypnotics
Anticonvulsant mood stabilizers
Antipsychotics
Psychostimulants
Target Psychiatric Syndromes/Symptoms
Depression
Anxiety
Sleep disturbance
Appetite disturbance
Cognitive dysfunction
Substance abuse
Psychosis
Target Cancer or Treatment Symptoms
Fatigue
Nausea
Pain
Dyspnoea
Hot flushes
Anorexia/cachexia
Hiccups

benefit in both of these domains. Often the patient will experience improvement in some symptoms quickly, such as sleep disturbance or anxiety. Ongoing compliance with the medication brings additional benefits within a few weeks, such as improvement in depressive symptoms.

Encouraging patients to accept medications for the treatment of psychiatric symptoms is one of the most challenging tasks in psycho-oncology. Societal attitudes toward psychotropic medication use vary widely. Stigma related to psychiatric and psychological symptoms such as depression and anxiety remains high in most countries and cultures. Awareness of the underlying stigma and shame that patients may feel about accepting help in the form of medication will serve the clinician well. Validating these concerns, and gently encouraging patients to care for themselves as a whole person, as a person with human responses to the stress of cancer and its treatment, and as a family member, can help foster more acceptance of the need for treatment.

It is also critical to understand that it may require more than one visit with a psychiatrist for a patient to accept help in the form of medications. If the clinical situation permits (e.g. so long as the patient's psychiatric status is not life-threatening or otherwise extremely urgent), then providing information and giving patients time to consider their options, rather than pressuring the patient, may make a tremendous difference. Drawing analogies between the use of medications for chronic conditions, and the need to treat all aspects of the disease, as well as the important connections between mind and body, are also strategies to help patients come to terms with the need for psychotropic treatments.

Analysis of the evidence

Antidepressant medications in the oncology setting

Antidepressants and stimulants: overview

The use of antidepressants in patients with cancer is as effective as in patients with other major medical illnesses.[1,6,7] The choice of antidepressant medication should be informed by most common side-effects, the potential benefits of these side-effects for specific cancer treatment-related symptoms, the likelihood of serious adverse events, the lethality of the medication in the case of a suicide attempt (e.g. tricyclic antidepressants), and the potential for drug–drug interactions. See Table 9.2 for details of mechanisms and dosing for the most commonly used antidepressant and stimulant medications, as well as clinically relevant information for the cancer setting.

Some side-effects may be of particular concern to specific patient populations. That many antidepressants induce weight gain may be particularly relevant to patients with breast and some gynaecological cancers, where obesity and weight gain negatively affect cancer prognosis.[8] The relevance of this issue for other cancers is a subject of current investigation. Therefore, in terms of weight gain, fluoxetine, sertraline, duloxetine, or bupropion are first-choice agents if weight gain is the primary concern. However, drug–drug interactions,

Table 9.2 Antidepressant use in psycho-oncology settings.

Drug	Mechanism of action	Dosing (mg/day)	Clinical pearls, side-effects, and precautions
SSRIs			• Decrease platelet aggregation • Serotonin syndrome can occur • Associated with hyponatraemia • May cause headache, gastrointestinal disturbance, sexual dysfunction, insomnia, restlessness
Fluoxetine	SSRI	10–80	• Minimal risk of discontinuation syndrome due to long half-life • Once weekly formulation available at 90 mg • Inhibits conversion of tamoxifen to active metabolite • High potential for drug–drug interactions via CYP450 enzymes
Sertraline	SSRI	25–200	• Few drug–drug interactions • Gastrointestinal side-effects common
Paroxetine	SSRI	5–60	• Inhibits conversion of tamoxifen to active metabolite • High potential for drug–drug interactions via CYP450 enzymes • High risk of discontinuation syndrome due to short half-life • Weight gain, sedation, dry mouth
Citalopram	SSRI	10–40	• Few drug-drug interactions
Escitalopram	SSRI	10–20	• S-enantiomer of citalopram • Few drug–drug interactions
SNRIs			• Monitor blood pressure regularly • Decrease platelet aggregation • Serotonin syndrome can occur • Associated with hyponatraemia • May cause headache, gastrointestinal disturbance, sexual dysfunction, insomnia, restlessness
Venlafaxine	SNRI	37.5–300	• Least likely to interact with tamoxifen metabolism • Used for neuropathic pain and hot flushes • Increased blood pressure at higher doses • High risk of discontinuation syndrome
Desvenlafaxine	SNRI	50	• Metabolite of venlafaxine
Duloxetine	SNRI	20–60	• Used for neuropathic pain and hot flushes • Sedative effects • Hepatotoxicity risk, monitor liver function tests • Urinary retention.
Tricyclics			• Use low dose range in cancer setting for neuropathic pain and migraines, and as sleep aid • Potentially fatal in overdose • Anticholinergic side-effects common (constipation, dry mouth) • Risk of anticholinergic toxicity, including delirium • Risk of orthostatic hypotension, cardiac arrhythmias • Weight gain and sedation frequent
Amitriptyline	SNRI	25–150	• Sedating profile
Imipramine	SNRI	25–150	• Activating profile
Clomipramine	SNRI	25–150	• Activating profile • Parenteral administration forms

(Continued)

Table 9.2 (*Continued*)

Drug	Mechanism of action	Dosing (mg/day)	Clinical pearls, side-effects, and precautions
Atypicals			
Mirtazapine	Presynaptic α2 blockade	7.5–45	• Sleep aid and appetite stimulant • Antiemetic properties • Minimal sexual dysfunction • Rare risk of agranulocytosis, monitor white blood cell count and absolute neutrophil count • Increases lipids • Contraindicated in phenylketonuria • Available in orally dissolvable formulation
Bupropion	NDRI	75–450	• Reduces seizure threshold • Inhibits conversion of tamoxifen to active metabolite • Minimal sexual dysfunction • Useful for smoking cessation • Does not decrease platelet aggregation like serotonergic agents • Central nervous system stimulating effect • Insomnia, headache
Trazodone	SARI	25–250	• Non-habit-forming sleep aid • Minimal sexual dysfunction • Priapism rare side-effect • Avoid post-myocardial infarction • Anxiolytic effect

SSRI, serotonin reuptake inhibitor; SNRI, serotonin and norepinephrine reuptake inhibitor; NDRI, norepinephrine and dopamine reuptake inhibitor; SARI, serotonin antagonist and reuptake inhibitor.

as described below and in Tables 9.2 and 9.3, must also be considered as part of any psychopharmacological strategy.

Major drug interactions with antidepressants[9–12]

Drug–drug interactions are crucial issues for the field of psycho-oncology (Table 9.3). As most cancer patients are taking several other drugs concurrently – including antiemetic, analgesic, chemotherapeutic and other drugs – the psychopharmacologic evaluation must include a thorough screening for possible drug–drug interactions.[7,9] In a recent study of 297 cancer patients, almost 50% were prescribed a drug combination that could result in a potential major drug interaction with antidepressants.[9]

Key drug interactions that the psycho-oncologist should be aware of include:

1 Serotonin syndrome: some drugs including codeine, hydrocodone, oxycodone and tramadol, metoclopramide, fentanyl, ondasentron, triptans (the latter are common in drugs for migraine headaches) have some serotonergic action and can interact with any selective serotonin reuptake inhibitor (SSRI). This interaction can trigger a serotonin syndrome (characterized by muscle rigidity, confusion or other mental status changes, agitation and autonomic instability). The antineoplastic agent procarbazine is a monoamine oxidase inhibitor, as are the antimicrobials isoniazid and linezolid. These agents should not be combined with antidepressants.

2 Interactions with anticoagulants: concurrent use of SSRIs or serotonin-norepinephrine reuptake inhibitors (SNRIs) and anticoagulants may increase the risk of bleeding due to potential cytochrome P450 (CYP) inhibition by antidepressants, with a

Table 9.3 Pharmacological issues in antidepressant use. Reproduced from Miller *et al.*[15], with permission from Sage.

Drug	Reduced dose in renal disease?	Reduced dose in hepatic disease?	Reduced dose in elderly?	Major P450 CYP enzymes involved in metabolism	Drug–drug interactions
Fluoxetine	In severe disease	Yes	Yes	2D6, 1A2, 2C19	++++
Sertraline	No	Yes	Yes	2D6	+
Paroxetine	Yes	Yes	Yes	2D6, 3B6, 2C19	++++
Citalopram	In severe disease	Yes	Yes	3A4, 2C19, 2D6	+
Escitalopram	In severe disease	Yes	Yes	3A4, 2C19, 2D6	+
Venlafaxine	In severe disease	50% reduction	Yes	4A4, 2D6	++
Desvenlafaxine	50% reduction in severe disease	No	No	3A4	+
Bupropion	Yes	Yes, avoid use in cirrhosis	No	2B6 (and inhibits 2D6)	+++
Duloxetine	Yes	Do not use	Lower initial dose	1A2, 2D6	++
Mirtazapine	Yes	Yes	Yes	1A2, 2D6, 3A4	++
Trazodone	No	Yes	Yes	2B6, XX	++
Amitriptyline	No	Yes	Yes	3A4, 2C9, 2D6	++++
Imipramine	No	Yes	Yes	2C19	++++

AD, antidepressant; CYP, cytochrome

resulting increase in anticoagulant plasma levels. Serotonergic antidepressants also decrease platelet aggregation, resulting in prolonged bleeding time.

3 Tamoxifen metabolism and antidepressants: tamoxifen is used as adjuvant therapy to reduce the risk of breast cancer recurrence in women with estrogen receptor positive tumours. Tamoxifen's metabolism to endoxifen, its active metabolite, is impeded by antidepressants that inhibit cytochrome P450 2D6 (CYP2D6). It is therefore recommended to treat women with antidepressants with the lowest potential to inhibit CYP2D6. In addition, those patients with a specific CYP2D6 genetic polymorphism who are slower tamoxifen metabolizers are at higher risk. Antidepressants recommended for women on tamoxifen are venlafaxine, desvenlafaxine, escitalopram and citalopram.[10,11] Fluoxetine, paroxetine and sertraline are the strongest CYP2D6 inhibitors, and should therefore be avoided in women taking tamoxifen. Less is known about the potential CYP2D6 inhibitory effects of the other antidepressants (duloxetine, mirtazapine and bupropion).

4 Other drug–drug interactions: antidepressant-related enzymatic inhibition of hepatic metabolic pathways may reduce the clearance of antipsychotic drugs (e.g. haloperidol, quetiapine and risperidone). The effects of certain analgesic medications may also be reduced by antidepressant induction of specific enzymatic pathways. Again, coadministration of antidepressants and other medications requires monitoring for potential drug–drug interactions.

Indications for antidepressants in oncology settings

Psychiatric disorders should be diagnosed by a trained clinician. As in any clinical psychiatric evaluation, a full history of symptoms should be taken, as patients may have underlying psychiatric disorders (e.g. bipolar disorder) that have not been diagnosed or treated. The time course and precipitating factors of presenting symptoms also will help direct treatment, including the form and focus of psychotherapeutic interventions.

- Major depressive disorder (MDD): all antidepressants described later can be used.

• Post-traumatic stress disorder (PTSD): sertraline and paroxetine are FDA-approved for the treatment of PTSD.
• Panic disorder: drugs approved by the FDA for the treatment of panic disorder include fluoxetine, paroxetine, sertraline and the SNRI venlafaxine.
• General anxiety disorder: antidepressants commonly used include fluoxetine, paroxetine, escitalopram, sertraline, venlafaxine, imipramine and duloxetine.

Antidepressants can also be useful for the treatment of other symptoms in cancer patients, including hot flushes, pain, anorexia, sleep disturbance and fatigue.

• Management of hot flushes in breast cancer survivors: bupropion, venlafaxine, paroxetine, fluoxetine and citalopram have been used, and desvenlafaxine is being studied. It is important to consider cautions regarding specific medications for women taking tamoxifen.
• Chronic and neuropathic pain: amitriptyline, duloxetine and venlafaxine are the most commonly used, generally in combination with other pain medications.
• Anorexia and cachexia: amitriptyline, imipramine and mirtazapine can be useful.
• Sleep disturbance: paroxetine, trazodone, mirtazapine and amitriptyline can be beneficial in patients with sleep disturbance. Moreover, this can help reduce the use of concomitant benzodiazepines.
• Cancer-related fatigue: psychostimulants and stimulating antidepressants, such as methylphenidate, modafinil and bupropion, can be useful for cancer-related fatigue,[13] although there are relatively few clinical trials examining the efficacy of these medications in this setting.

Antidepressant classes and medications

Several different antidepressant classes are useful in oncology: SSRIs, SNRIs, tricyclics (TCAs) and the 'atypical antidepressants'. Only the MAO-Is are not used in this setting, because of their multiple drug–drug interactions.[9] All of these antidepressants, with the exception of bupropion, produce their effects by altering neuronal transmission pathways mediated by serotonin, norepinephrine, or both. Anxiolytic and sedating properties of antidepressants will appear earlier (in the first week), while the antidepressant effects take longer (2–8 weeks) to manifest. For anxiety disorders, all SSRIs and SNRIs can be used, with clomipramine as a second-line treatment. Efficacy studies have shown similar overall response rates across antidepressant medications. When 'response' is defined as 50% improvement on symptom scales, approximately 60–70% of persons on antidepressants have a favourable response, compared to 35% on placebo.[9]

SSRIs inhibit the reuptake of serotonin in the synaptic cleft. They have no significant effect upon norepinephrine and, with the exception of sertraline, little effect upon dopamine. Although there is variability in the receptor affinity and specificity of the SSRIs, none has been proven to be clearly more effective than another. SSRIs may also interact with other drugs that have serotonergic properties, including non-psychotropic medications such as narcotics, to precipitate serotonin syndrome. Symptoms of serotonin syndrome typically include restlessness, hyperreflexia, muscle twitches, tremor and autonomic dysfunction. More severe intoxication can progress to seizures and coma.[7]

Distinguishing features among the SSRIs include rates and types of adverse side-effects, and the degree and types of cytochrome P450-related metabolism and inhibition that can lead to drug–drug interactions (Table 9.3). Both paroxetine and fluoxetine cause elevation of many drugs levels by inhibiting their metabolism in the liver. Citalopram, escitalopram and sertraline are all metabolized through the 3A4, 2C19 and 2D6 pathways but have a low likelihood of drug–drug interactions (Table 9.3). Many SSRIs can inhibit the clearance of benzodiazepines. All of the SSRIs can cause nausea, diarrhoea, headache, insomnia, nervousness, fatigue and sexual dysfunction, but sertraline has the highest rates of gastrointestinal side-effects, and fluoxetine, of sexual side-effects. Their use is also associated with an increased risk of haemorrhage from the gastrointestinal tract, especially in combination with NSAIDs. Concurrent use of SSRIs and anticoagulants may also increase the risk of bleeding. They can also induce the syndrome of inappropriate secretion of antidiuretic hormone (SIADH), and/or hyponatraemia. Finally, sudden cessation of SSRIs can induce an abstinence syndrome with sensory disturbances, pronounced dizziness and other symptoms. The short half-life of some medications (paroxetine and venlafaxine) makes symptoms more likely to appear when stopped suddenly, therefore very gradual tapers are recommended. The very long half-life of the active metabolites of fluoxetine results in a much lower risk of symptoms. The other SSRIs have an intermediate risk of abstinence syndrome between those two extremes.

SNRIs inhibit the reuptake of both serotonin and norepinephrine, with varying selectivity for serotonin. The most common side-effects are headache, somnolence, dizziness, insomnia, nausea, dry mouth, constipation, anorexia and weakness. Concurrent use of SNRIs and anticoagulants may also increase the risk of bleeding. Venlafaxine is associated with an increased risk of hypertension, therefore blood pressure must be monitored in patients taking this medication. Desvenlafaxine appears to have a better metabolic profile with fewer drug–drug interactions and fewer side-effects than venlafaxine. In addition, as desvenlafaxine has no anticholinergic effects, it may be a first choice medication in elderly cancer patients or in those with other comorbid medical conditions. Duloxetine is distinguished by its FDA-approved indication for the treatment of painful diabetic neuropathy, fibromyalgia and back pain. Its sedative effect may be helpful for oncology patients, but its metabolic profile should be considered. Duloxetine predisposes to urinary retention, which may be helpful to incontinent patients but may cause problems in other patients.

Tricyclic antidepressants (TCAs) inhibit the reuptake of serotonin while acting directly on various serotonin receptors. A second mechanism of action involves inhibition of norepinephrine transport. They also block muscarinic, histamine (HI) and α1- and α2-adrenergic receptors, and cholinergic receptors, resulting in a wide variety of generally unwanted side-effects (Table 9.2). TCAs are commonly associated with side-effects that may be problematic in medically ill patients, such as orthostatic hypotension, weight gain, sedation, cardiac arrhythmias, anticholinergic delirium, seizures and lethal overdose. Side-effects statistically more likely to occur in TCAs compared to SSRIs include dry mouth, blurred vision, dizziness, constipation and tremor. SSRIs are more likely than TCAs to cause nausea, diarrhoea, insomnia and headache. Nevertheless, the side-effect profiles of the SSRIs and SNRIs are generally preferred to the side-effects of the TCA antidepressants. The TCAs have thus become second-choice treatments for depression. However, they can be useful for specific situations, such as for pain, persistent diarrhoea, anorexia/weight loss and sleep problems. TCAs can be lethal in overdose, therefore suicidality must be carefully assessed on an ongoing basis in any patient on a TCA.

On the other hand, the lower cost of TCAs is a principal reason for their greater use in some countries. Imipramine and amitriptyline are the most commonly used. An electrocardiogram must be performed to detect cardiac arrhythmias or cardiac conduction abnormalities. Because of the pharmacological and toxicological profiles of this class of medications, they have a greater number of major drug–drug interactions. Furthermore, they are not recommended in elderly patients because of their anticholinergic activity.[14]

Atypical antidepressants include trazodone, mirtazapine and bupropion. Trazodone is a relatively weak SSRI, with little norepinephrine or dopamine effects. The major side-effects of trazodone are sedation and orthostatic hypotension. Priapism is an infrequent but serious side-effect. It should be used with caution in combination with other sedatives. Trazodone has shown mixed results in clinical trials, with apparently inferior performance in severely depressed patients, although evidence supports its use for anxiety and insomnia.[15] Given its limitations, trazodone is used primarily as a sleep aid, but should be used with caution in older patients or others at risk for orthostatic hypotension or falls.

Mirtazapine produces its effect by increasing both norepinephrine and serotonin levels. It is a potent antihistamine and has considerable adrenergic and muscarinic antagonist activity. The major side-effects include sedation, constipation, dry mouth, dizziness and weight gain. It can rarely produce agranulocytosis, therefore it is recommended to monitor ANC/WBC. It also increases lipids and weight, the latter being a useful side-effect for underweight patients, or those with decreased appetite. This unique antidepressant possesses antiemetic properties due to serotonin-3 receptor blockade, and it is associated with a lower incidence of sexual dysfunction than SSRIs. Bupropion – unique among the antidepressants for its mechanism of action (inhibition of the dopamine reuptake) – may have side-effects that include dizziness, headache, insomnia, nausea and dry mouth. Bupropion increases the risk of seizure and is therefore contraindicated in epileptic patients. Of note, its efficacy in aiding in smoking cessation makes it a potentially valuable medication for smokers diagnosed with cancer.

Special considerations regarding antidepressants in oncology settings

Brain tumour patients: in brain tumour patients, who are at an increased risk of seizures, antidepressants with the least effect on the seizure threshold are recommended, namely, citalopram, escitalopram and sertraline.

Palliative care patients: for a rapid onset of antidepressant action in palliative care, one option is to begin with a psychostimulant such as methylphenidate, dextroamphetamine, or modafinil.[15] Psychostimulants have a rapid onset of action and high response rates. Psychostimulants side-effects may include agitation, confusion, paranoia and insomnia. About one week later, an SSRI can be added and may eventually replace the psychostimulant. Venlafaxine, duloxetine and mirtazapine are second-choice antidepressants for these patients.

Elderly patients:[16] cancer is mainly a disease of the elderly. As a result of increased life expectancy, in Europe and in the United States, over 60% of new cancer cases and over 70% of cancer deaths occur in people >65 years. Several factors need to be considered in antidepressant prescribing for older patients: the higher incidence of other chronic diseases, primarily cardiovascular disease and diabetes; the use of concomitant medications and therefore a higher risk of drug–drug interactions; and the risk of impaired renal and hepatic function. In addition, elderly patients are at higher risk of delirium, particularly with the use of multiple anticholinergic medications. Medications with anticholinergic activity, such as TCAs, have a negative effect on cognitive performance among older adults. SSRIs or, in some cases, SRNIs are therefore the first-choice antidepressants at this age even though they may be at greater risk of developing hyponatraemia. Patients taking diuretics or who are otherwise volume-depleted, may be at greater risk. Electrolyte monitoring is recommended. As always with elderly patients, the logic of starting low and going slow applies to the use of antidepressants as well.

Recommended screening, monitoring, and cautions for patients (see also Tables 9.2 and 9.3)

In at-risk patients (elderly, or patients with diabetes, hypertension, or other comorbid cardiovascular disease):

1 Renal function (BUN or creatinine clearance, if necessary). Adjust dosage as needed.
2 Liver function (hepatic transaminases, conjugated and unconjugated bilirubin). Adjust dose as needed.
3 Electrolyte levels to check blood sodium level. (SSRI side-effect)
4 Platelets and white blood cell count. Coagulation tests may be required to detect any coagulation problem in patients with ecchymosis or other bleeding problems (SSRIs or SNRIs). White blood cell count may be monitored in patients administered mirtazapine for agranulocytosis.
5 Monitor blood pressure in patients on SNRIs.
6 Electrocardiogram in patients on TCAs.
7 Glycaemic control in non-insulin-dependent diabetic patients on SSRIs.

Cautions that should be communicated to patients: as in the general population, it is important to bear in mind the risk of increased suicidal thoughts and behaviours during the acute phases of treatment with antidepressants, particularly in children and adolescents. As a major depressive episode may be the initial presentation of bipolar disorder, attention must be given to the potential appearance of a mixed/manic episode in patients at risk for bipolar disorder. The development of a potentially life-threatening serotonin syndrome or neuroleptic malignant syndrome (NMS)-like reactions have been reported with SNRIs and SSRIs alone, so it is important to recognize these symptoms promptly: mental status changes (e.g. agitation, hallucinations, coma), autonomic instability (e.g. tachycardia, labile blood pressure, hyperthermia), neuromuscular aberrations (e.g. hyperreflexia, incoordination) and/or gastrointestinal symptoms (e.g. nausea, vomiting, diarrhoea). The risk of discontinuation symptoms if antidepressants are abruptly stopped must be communicated to patients.

Interference with psychomotor performance: any psychoactive drug may impair judgment, thinking or motor skills. Cognitive function, impaired memory, sedation and dizziness can appear at the beginning of any antidepressant treatment. Therefore, patients should be cautioned about operating hazardous machinery including automobiles, until they are reasonably certain that the antidepressant does not affect their ability to engage in such activities. Seizures can appear especially with the use of: clomipramine, amitriptyline, buproprion, fluoxetine and paroxetine. Patients should be advised of the risk of orthostatic hypotension and syncope, especially during the period of initial use and subsequent dose escalation with SNRI drugs. In patients with narrow-angle glaucoma, TCAs, mirtazapine, paroxetine, venlafaxine and duloxetine cannot be prescribed.

Antipsychotic medications in the oncology setting

Indications for antipsychotic use in oncology settings

Antipsychotics have great utility in the management of psychiatric conditions as well as non-psychiatric symptoms and treatment side-effects occurring in cancer patients.[17]

Delirium

Delirium, also referred to as encephalopathy, is associated with excessive mesolimbic dopamine activity. Therefore, the management of delirium often involves the use of antipsychotics to control agitation, maintain sleep-wake cycle, prevent self-harm and reduce distress caused by confusion and hallucinations. While the search for an underlying medical cause of delirium is of key importance, antipsychotics may facilitate the more rapid return of cognitive function and sensorium.[18]

Selection of an antipsychotic agent in the delirious patient is determined by route of administration, side-effects and medical comorbidities of the patient (see Table 9.4). Haloperidol continues to be the gold standard in the treatment of delirium

Table 9.4 Antipsychotic use in psycho-oncology settings.

Medication	Dosing (mg/day)	Route of administration	EPS	Sedation	Weight gain	Anticholinergic	Orthostatic hypotension
Haloperidol	0.5–15	PO, IV, IM, OS, long-acting IM	xxx	x	x	x	x
Chlorpromazine	10–100	PO, IV, IM, OS, PR	xx	xxx	xxx	xx	xxx
Risperidone	0.25–2	PO, OS, ODT, long-acting IM	xx	x	xx	0	xx
Olanzapine	2.5–10	PO, IM, ODT, long-acting IM	x	xx	xxx	xx	x
Quetiapine	12.5–200	PO	0	xx	xx	xx	xx
Ziprasidone	20–80	PO, IM	x	x	0	0	x
Aripiprazole	2.0–30	PO, IM, ODT, OS	x	0	0	0	0

EPS, extrapyramidal symptoms; PO, oral; IV, intravenous; IM, intramuscular; ODT, oral disintegrating tablet; QTc, QT interval corrected for heart rate; PR, per rectum; OS, oral solution.
0 = Very low risk; x = Low risk; xx = Moderate risk; xxx = High risk

because it can be administered intravenously (IV), which is very useful in the critical care setting and when oral administration is not possible. It is important to keep in mind that IV dosing of haloperidol is twice as potent as oral. Atypical antipsychotics, particularly risperidone, olanzapine, quetiapine, ziprasidone,[19] and aripiprazole,[20] are being utilized more often in the medical setting with good results.[21] However, experience with the newest agents (paliperidone, asenapine, iloperidone and lurasidone) remains very limited. Clozapine is not generally used in the cancer population due to its unique toxicities, specifically agranulocytosis and decreased seizure threshold. Although intramuscular (IM) dosing of several antipsychotics is available, this route is less preferable in cancer patients who are at risk for developing haematomas due to impaired coagulation and thrombocytopenia.

Psychosis

Whether due to a primary psychotic illness or one that results from a medical condition or drug, antipsychotics are the treatment of choice for delusions, hallucinations and thought disorganization. Brain tumours, paraneoplastic encephalitis and psychomotor seizures are examples of medical causes of secondary psychosis that occur in the oncology setting.[22] Glucocorticoid steroids are commonly prescribed to cancer patients, and these medications are associated with substantial risk of neuropsychiatric side-effects. In particular, irritability, sleep disturbance, mania and psychosis can result from the administration of acute, high dose corticosteroids. These symptoms respond well to antipsychotic treatment.[23]

Anxiety and sleep disturbance

Antipsychotics may substitute or augment benzodiazepines for control of acute anxiety symptoms in situations such as procedures, contact isolation, etc. As benzodiazepines may be relatively contraindicated or ineffective in patients with substance use disorders, atypical antipsychotics may be useful for the management of anxiety and insomnia in these patients.[24] Anxious patients at risk for delirium or respiratory depression from benzodiazepines may also benefit from administration of a low dose, sedating atypical antipsychotic.[25]

Depression

In major depressive disorder, several atypical antipsychotics including quetiapine, aripiprazole, olanzapine and risperidone are effective as antidepressant augmentation.[26] This strategy may be useful in psycho-oncology as well, particularly in patients with pre-existing major depressive disorder exacerbated by cancer diagnosis and treatment. There are no studies, however, specifically examining the use of antipsychotic augmentation for depression in cancer patients.

Nausea

Pharmacological treatment of chronic nausea in the cancer patient includes metoclopramide and the phenothiazine antiemetics, prochlorperazine and promethazine. Serotonin-3 receptor antagonists are more useful in chemotherapy-induced nausea. The antipsychotics haloperidol and chlorpromazine may also be used for chronic or opioid-induced nausea.[27] It is important to remember the additive pharmacodynamic effects of antipsychotics when combined with these antiemetics in terms of extrapyramidal reactions, anticholinergic side-effects, sedation and cardiotoxicity (see below).[28]

Hiccups

Although not first line, chlorpromazine and haloperidol are part of the treatment algorithm for intractable hiccups due to central dopamine antagonism in the hypothalamus.[29]

Classification of antipsychotics

Antipsychotics, often referred to as neuroleptics, are divided into two main classes: first generation (typical) antipsychotics and second generation (atypical) antipsychotics. Among the typical antipsychotics, haloperidol and chlorpromazine are the most commonly used in the medical setting. Haloperidol is classified as a high-potency antipsychotic, referring to its high affinity for dopamine-2 (D_2) receptors. Chlorpromazine, the first drug found to have antipsychotic properties in 1952, is a low-potency typical antipsychotic. Although useful in certain situations, it is not administered first line due to numerous side-effects and precautions. Atypical agents differ from typical antipsychotics due to lower affinity for D_2 receptors and greater affinity for serotonin ($5HT_{2A}$) receptors, resulting in a more favourable side-effect profile (see below).[30]

Side-effects and safety monitoring

Extrapyramidal reactions

Antipsychotic dopamine-2 receptor blockade in the nigrostriatal pathway causes the development of extrapyramidal symptoms (EPS). Such side-effects include rigidity, tremor, bradykinesia and dystonia. Akathisia, a subjective sense of restlessness and inability to sit still, is a type of EPS that can be hard to distinguish from psychomotor agitation due to hyperactive delirium. It is not uncommon for patients to experience akathisia when antipsychotics are combined with antiemetics. Generally, EPS subside when the offending medication is withdrawn, but tardive dyskinesia may persist for months or years. Propranolol or clonazepam may be used to treat akathisia. Anticholinergics or diphenhydramine may be effective for acute dystonia.[31]

With the exception of high dose risperidone, atypical antipsychotics rarely cause EPS because they have greater affinity for serotonin-2A receptors, which attenuates the dopamine-2 blockade in the nigrostriatal pathway. When the need arises to use antipsychotics in elderly patients with high risk for EPS, these agents are preferred. However, the black box warning of increased risk of death in elderly patients with dementia-related psychosis underscores the importance of discontinuing these medications when no longer indicated.[32]

Neuroleptic malignant syndrome (NMS)

NMS is a rare, potentially life-threatening syndrome arising from excessive dopamine blockade in the brain. Cancer patients are at increased risk because dehydration, malnutrition, and iron deficiency are all risk factors for NMS.[33] Antipsychotics coadministered with metoclopramide or the phenothiazine antiemetics compound the risk further. Clinical presentation of this syndrome involves muscle rigidity, fever, autonomic instability, delirium and diaphoresis. Laboratory evaluation reveals elevated creatine phosphokinase and possibly leukocytosis. Renal function may be compromised due to rhabdomyolysis. After discontinuing the offending medication, management requires intensive support measures such as hydration and cooling, circulatory and respiratory support, and perhaps the use of bromocriptine or dantrolene.

Cardiotoxicity

The degree of alpha-1-adrenergic blockade differs between antipsychotics. Chlorpromazine, quetiapine, risperidone and olanzapine have the highest risk of causing orthostatic hypotension and syncope. These agents enhance the hypotensive effects of antihypertensives, and they should be avoided in patients with congestive heart failure. QTc prolongation is a cardiac side-effect of antipsychotics that may precipitate a potentially fatal arrhythmia, torsades de pointes, due to blockade of cardiac potassium channels. Intravenous haloperidol, ziprasidone and quetiapine have the greatest effect on QTc interval, but olanzapine does not typically have a clinically significant effect on QTc interval.[34] An electrocardiogram should be obtained at baseline and at regular intervals while administering antipsychotics to a delirious, medically compromised patient. The American Psychiatric Association Practice Guideline for Delirium suggests a QTc interval of 450 milliseconds or a 25% increase in QTc as the threshold for discontinuing or reducing the dose of the antipsychotic medication. Risk factors for QTc prolongation include congenital QTc prolongation, a family history of sudden death, and use with other QTc prolonging medications. Caution should be exercised when prescribing antipsychotics in patients with pre-existing heart disease, and magnesium and potassium should be monitored along with other electrolytes.

Endocrine and metabolic side-effects

The metabolic side-effects of atypical antipsychotics are very troublesome in the context of long-term use in psychiatric patients. These include weight gain, insulin resistance and atherogenic dyslipidaemia. Of those agents used more commonly in the cancer setting, olanzapine, quetiapine and risperidone pose the greatest risk.[35] When using these medications long term, body mass index (BMI), fasting glucose, lipid profiles, and blood pressure should be monitored.

The more highly dopamine-2 receptor blocking antipsychotics, haloperidol and risperidone, may cause elevation of prolactin via the tuberoinfundibular dopamine pathway. Long-term consequences of hyperprolactinemia include amenorrhoea, gynecomastia, galactorrhea, sexual dysfunction and osteoporosis.

Both typical and atypical antipsychotics are known to cause the syndrome of inappropriate secretion of antidiuretic hormone (SIADH). The increased retention of water by the renal tubule causes hyponatraemia and high urine osmolality. Clinical symptoms manifest as weakness, lethargy, delirium and headache. Of note, small cell carcinoma of the lung and brain tumours are also associated with SIADH.[36]

Sedation

Atypical antipsychotics vary in terms of their sedative potential, largely due to histamine-1 antagonism, with olanzapine and quetiapine being the most sedating, and aripiprazole and ziprasidone the least.[37] Sedative properties can be beneficial for a cancer patient struggling with insomnia, but can exacerbate the feeling of fatigue and anergia. When sedating antipsychotics are combined with other CNS depressants, such as opioids and benzodiazepines, respiratory depression can result in increased risk for aspiration.

Seizure

At higher doses, antipsychotics can decrease seizure threshold. As far as agents used in the medical setting, chlorpromazine, olanzapine and quetiapine have a higher risk than haloperidol and risperidone.[38] Cancer patients with CNS disease are at increased risk of this adverse effect, as are those prescribed corticosteroids.

Haematological

Agranulocytosis is more commonly associated with the use of clozapine and low-potency typical antipsychotics. However, neutropenia, aplastic anaemia and thrombocytopenia have been observed with most atypical antipsychotics. Given the myelosuppression occurring with many chemotherapy regimens, this adverse effect must be given consideration.

Hepatic

Mild elevations in the liver transaminases and alkaline phosphatase may occur with administration of antipsychotics. Phenothiazines may rarely cause cholestatic jaundice.

Anticholinergic

Chlorpromazine, quetiapine and olanzapine have the greatest antimuscarinic action of the antipsychotics used in the medical setting. Particularly when combined with other anticholinergic agents, these drugs may cause delirium, constipation, dry mouth and urinary retention.[34]

Drug–drug interactions (pharmacokinetics)

Like many psychotropics, antipsychotics interact with other medications via the cytochrome P450 enzyme system because they both inhibit and are metabolized by these isoenzymes.[39] For example, several antipsychotics are metabolized by CYP1A2, CYP2D6 and CYP3A4. At the same time, haloperidol inhibits CYP2D6 and CYP3A4, and dexamethasone (commonly prescribed in cancer patients) induces these isoenzymes. The picture becomes even more complicated when antidepressants, anticonvulsants, antimicrobials and other drugs are prescribed. The interactions are extensive, and clinicians are advised to utilize one of many online drug interaction programmes when adding an antipsychotic to a cancer patient's complex medication regimen.

The metabolism and clearance of antipsychotics are affected in cases of renal and hepatic dysfunction, and dose adjustments may be necessary. As a general rule in the oncology setting, dosing should start low and be gradually and cautiously titrated. The half-life of antipsychotics varies from 2–75 hours, depending on the drug. However, half-life is not necessarily clinically important when gauging duration of action because CNS levels of antipsychotics remain high much longer than serum levels, as does receptor binding.

Anxiolytics and hypnotics: use in the oncology setting

Anxiolytics

Beyond the use of the antidepressant medications (SSRIs and SNRIs) for the management of anxiety, benzodiazepines can play a useful role in helping the anxious cancer patient. All benzodiazepines have potential side-effects of sedation, dizziness, incoordination, as well as the potential for tolerance and abuse or dependence. The shortest acting benzodiazepine (alprazolam), in particular, can cause rebound anxiety and has a higher risk of abuse and dependence. Its use should therefore be limited to rare situations (e.g. one-time administration for procedures), and in most cases other benzodiazepines can be used instead.

Other side-effects that may be problematic include bradycardia and respiratory depression (particularly with lorazepam, diazepam), drug–drug interactions (particularly alprazolam and triazolam), impaired memory or disorientation, and the potential for withdrawal symptoms if the medication is stopped abruptly. It is critical that benzodiazepines not be given routinely or lightly to patients for 'sleep' or 'anxiety' without a thorough evaluation for underlying or contributing factors and syndromes, as these symptoms are not disorders. A clear indication, treatment plan, monitoring and follow-up schedule, and (in most cases) plan for eventual tapering and discontinuation, should be part of the management plan for all patients prescribed benzodiazepines.

Hypnotics

Insomnia occurs frequently in the context of cancer, affecting 30–50% of cancer patients.[40] Sleep hygiene education, cognitive-behavioural therapy, relaxation training and other non-pharmacological approaches are the first-line treatment for insomnia. Hypnotics should not be prescribed routinely for 'sleep difficulties' without first taking a detailed sleep hygiene, depression, anxiety, substance use history, as well as assessing for possible sleep apnoea. Often, underlying psychiatric or medical conditions, environmental factors, habits and other factors are contributing to the initiation and maintenance of a sleep problem.

After assessment, however, if a short-term hypnotic is prescribed, those hypnotics that act on the GABAergic system are preferred. Most have short half-lives except for the extended release formulations. The most common side-effects are: headache, dizziness, dry mouth, metallic taste and hallucinations. They can cause withdrawal symptoms; in particular, cessation after prolonged use can lead to rebound and more difficult to treat insomnia. Commonly used hypnotics in the cancer setting are: zopiclone (dose: 7.5 mg), eszopiclone (dose: 1–3 mg), zaleplon (dose: 5–20 mg), zolpidem (dose: 5–10 mg), and zolpidem CR (6.25–12.5 mg). These drugs aid in sleep induction and maintenance for the short-term management of insomnia. There is no evidence that one hypnotic drug is more effective than another.[41] Moreover, there are few comparative trials of the effects of anxiolytics for sleep, with no clear evidence of one agent being more effective than another for short-term management of insomnia.

All hypnotics are metabolized in the liver, therefore dose adjustments are necessary in patients with hepatic insufficiency. Zaleplon is metabolized by CYP3A4, therefore drugs that inhibit CYP3A4 may predispose patients to drug–drug interactions.[42] The potential for other drug–drug interactions exist, therefore checking the most current online databases is prudent when prescribing these medications.

Anticonvulsants and mood stabilizers: use in the oncology setting

Lithium, anticonvulsants and atypical antipsychotics are used in bipolar disorder for mood stabilization. Due to drug interactions and toxicities, lithium is seldom used in the medically ill patient. However, anticonvulsants are frequently prescribed to cancer patients for seizure prophylaxis and neuropathic pain. In such patients, these agents may be preferred over the atypical antipsychotics when mood stabilization and impulse control issues need to be addressed since a single agent can serve multiple purposes.

Divalproex sodium and carbamazepine are indicated for mania in bipolar disorder, and they can be helpful in manic-spectrum presentations induced by steroids or brain tumours.[43] Side-effects include bone marrow suppression, ataxia, gastrointestinal disturbance, weight gain and hepatotoxicity. It is important to note that both agents interact with the metabolism of other drugs via the cytochrome P450 enzyme system. Levetiracetam is an anticonvulsant frequently used in the cancer setting, but relative to the other antiepileptic drugs, it is associated with depression, irritability and even self-harm.[44] If a cancer patient experiences such adverse effects from this agent, a switch to another anticonvulsant is advised.

Data has been weak regarding the mood stabilizing properties of gabapentin and pregabalin, but these anticonvulsants are used for neuropathic pain in cancer and may have anxiolytic and sedative effects.[45] These agents have very minimal drug–drug interactions. Lamotrigine is indicated for prevention of depressive episodes in bipolar disorder and may be used for seizure control in the cancer setting. It is associated with a rash that may progress to the rare, but life-threatening, Stevens-Johnson syndrome.

Cultural implications

The availability to the general public of medications to treat psychiatric syndromes and symptoms differs markedly from country to country. In many regions, mental health providers are in short supply.[46] Therefore, each professional needs to be aware of country- and region-specific issues regarding access. Knowledge about specific available medications (e.g. tricyclic antidepressants where those are most readily available) should be more extensively pursued depending on the specific circumstances.

In the United States and Europe, generic medication quality is certificated by bioequivalence studies, so these generics can help patients already burdened with medical expenses due to cancer. However in other countries, generic medications may not be as well regulated, and quality and efficacy may be affected.

Natural remedies and homeopathy are utilized widely around the globe, such as in Ayurvedic and Chinese medicine. There are many medicinal plants that may alleviate symptoms in cancer patients, but these supplements may have pharmacokinetic and pharmacodynamic interactions that place patients at risk for adverse effects. It is essential that providers prescribing psychotropics screen for use of non-allopathic remedies that may be commonly available in their region.[47]

Another factor with potential clinical impact on prescribing practices of many psychotropics is the differential frequency of cytochrome P450 enzyme allelic variants. For instance, Asians and Africans more commonly have reduced function or non-functional 2D6 alleles compared to European Caucasians.[48] This affects the rate of metabolism of several medications discussed above, and the practitioner is advised to adjust dosing and be more vigilant for dose-related side-effects in these specific populations.

Finally, in much of the world people are still reluctant to see a psychiatrist, but they may be more open to taking an antidepressant prescribed by their general practitioner or oncologist. Thus another important task for psychiatrists is to educate other medical specialists about diagnosing and treating psychiatric disorders.

Conclusions

In patients who have been carefully evaluated by a trained clinician and whose symptoms warrant pharmacological intervention, the first task often involves encouraging patients to accept medications. Despite a limited database about the efficacy of specific medications and medication classes for the treatment of psychiatric syndromes in cancer patients, it appears safe to say that psychotropic medications are as effective in cancer patients as in patients with other major medical illnesses. Common side-effects, the likelihood of serious adverse events, the route of administration, and the potential for drug–drug interactions, are all factors that should be considered when selecting a medication, given that most oncology patients are taking numerous other medications. Relief of psychiatric symptoms in patients with cancer can usually be achieved and is well worth the effort, as these symptoms have a serious negative effect on patients' overall quality of life.

Summary

Antidepressants have a number of important indications in cancer patients. The choice of medication should be dictated by the side-effect profiles (e.g. weight gain) and potential drug–drug interactions (e.g. tamoxifen and certain antidepressants) of the medications in the context of the individual patient's presenting symptoms. Antidepressant medications can be useful for managing other common symptoms seen in cancer patients. There are limited clinical trials examining antidepressant efficacy in cancer populations, however, so this is an area in need of further study.

Antipsychotics are primarily used for the management of delirium, but they may be beneficial for other symptoms as well, including insomnia and anxiety. Caution regarding potential drug–drug interactions is warranted, however, and clinicians can efficiently check for these interactions using an online program. Benzodiazepines are clinically useful for the management of specific phobias (e.g. radiation mask), but the use of the shorter acting benzodiazepines should be restricted and monitored closely. Ongoing use of benzodiazepines by cancer patients after treatment is an area in need of study. Insomnia affects a large proportion of cancer patients. Sleep hygiene education, other non-pharmacological strategies, and the short-term use of hypnotic medications may all play a role in the management of sleep difficulties.

Clinical case

A 67-year-old female with metastatic breast cancer to chest wall, status post-radical mastectomy with lymph node dissection, chemotherapy and radiation treatment, was admitted to the hospital for acute altered mental status. Symptoms began 24 hours prior to admission and included disorientation, forgetfulness and decreased level of consciousness. Her past medical history was significant for hypertension and hyperlipidaemia. Although she had no significant psychiatric, substance abuse, or dementia history prior to her cancer diagnosis two years ago, the patient had been treated for depression, anxiety and sleep disturbance by her oncologist over the course of her cancer treatment with amitriptyline 75 mg PO qhs and lorazepam 1 mg PO bid as needed for anxiety with good symptomatic response. A few days ago, her primary care physician added diphenoxylate with atropine PRN for diarrhoea and a scopolamine patch for chronic nausea.

A full medical workup revealed no evidence of infection, metabolic disturbance, or acute neurological or cardiac event. Anticholinergic-induced delirium quickly became the working diagnosis, and scopolamine, diphenoxylate with atropine, and amitriptyline were discontinued. Lorazepam, which the patient took rarely, was also discontinued. Haloperidol 1 mg IV q 6 hrs PRN was started for agitation and disorientation, and the patient received three doses per day. The patient's QTc on electrocardiogram and electrolytes were monitored daily.

The patient's mental status returned to baseline within 48 hours, and haloperidol was discontinued. Mirtazapine was substituted for amitriptyline to target her depression, anxiety, sleep disturbance and nausea. An alternative antidiarrhoeal and antiemetic were suggested by the oncology team with fewer anticholinergic properties, and the patient was discharged back to her home.

Key points

- Pharmacological treatment is an important component of the overall psychosocial care of the cancer patient.
- Successful referral for psychiatric evaluation involves patient education, addressing stigma, and practical issues in coordinating care.
- Psychiatric medications are helpful in the treatment of depression, anxiety, insomnia, appetite disturbance and cognitive disorders in the cancer setting.
- Psychotropics may also be beneficial for related cancer symptoms and cancer treatment side-effects, including fatigue, nausea, hot flushes and neuropathic pain.
- When prescribing in this population, the clinician must be aware of the many drug–drug interactions,

as well as altered metabolism and clearance in cases of hepatic or renal disease.

- Cancer patients exhibit heightened sensitivity to medication side-effects, and doses should be titrated gradually with frequent monitoring.

Key references

Bostwick J.M. (2010) A generalist's guide to treating patients with depression with an emphasis on using side effects to tailor antidepressant therapy. *Mayo Clinic Proceedings*, 85, 538–550.

Braun I.M, Pirl W.F. (2010) Psychotropic medications in cancer care, in *Psycho-Oncology*, 2nd edn (eds J. Holland, W. Breitbart, P. Jacobsen *et al.*), Oxford University Press, New York, pp. 378–385.

Carroll J.K., Kohli S., Mustian K.M. *et al.* (2007) Pharmacologic treatment of cancer-related fatigue. *Oncologist*, 12(suppl 1), 43–51.

Grassi L., Nanni M.G., Uchitomi Y., Riba M. (2011) Pharmacotherapy of depression in people with cancer, in *Depression and Cancer* (eds D.W. Kissane, M. Maj, N. Sartorius), World Psychiatric Association, pp. 151–176.

Henry N.L., Stearns V., Flockhart D.A. *et al.* (2008) Drug interactions and pharmacogenomics in the treatment of breast cancer and depression. *American Journal of Psychiatry*, 165, 1251–1255.

Lee B.N., Dantzer R., Langley K.E. *et al.* (2004) A cytokine-based neuroimmunologic mechanism of cancer-related symptoms. *Neuroimmunomodulation*, 11, 279–292.

Muriel A.C., Hwang V.S., Kornblith A. *et al.* (2009) Management of psychosocial distress by oncologists. *Psychiatric Services*, 60, 1132–1134.

Pirl W.F. (2004) Evidence report on the occurrence, assessment, and treatment of depression in cancer patients. *Journal of the National Cancer Institute Monographs*, 32, 32–39.

Robinson M.J., Owen J.A. (2005) Psychopharmacology, in *Textbook of Psychosomatic Medicine* (ed. J.L. Levenson), American Psychiatric Publishing, Inc., pp. 871–914.

Sheehan J.J., Sliwa J.K., Amatniek J.C. *et al.* (2010) Atypical antipsychotic metabolism and excretion. *Current Drug Metabolism*, 11, 516–525.

Savard J., Morin C.M. (2001) Insomnia in the context of cancer: A review of a neglected problem. *Journal of Clinical Oncology*, 19, 895–908.

Suggested further reading

An excellent and detailed overview of psychotropic medications, by Braun and Pirl, can be found in the most recent edition of the textbook *Psycho-Oncology*.[28]

A thorough review of pharmacological management of depression in cancer patients, by Grassi, Nanni, Uchitomi and Riba, can be found in the book *Depression and Cancer*.[49]

An overview of the management of psychiatric symptoms in the palliative care setting, by Breitbart, can be found in the *Oxford Textbook of Palliative Medicine*.[25]

A thorough overview of delirium and its management, by Maldonado, can be found in *Critical Care Clinics*.[18]

A review of the use of neuroleptics in supportive care is provided by Mazzocato in *Supportive Care in Cancer*.[17]

A review of antidepressant use, strategies and prescribing principles is found in an excellent and accessible review article by Bostwick.[50]

An excellent review, available in French only, of the specific uses of antidepressants in oncology, was written by Reich.[51]

References

1. Pirl W.F. (2004) Evidence report on the occurrence, assessment, and treatment of depression in cancer patients. *Journal of the National Cancer Institute Monographs*, 32, 32–39.
2. Coyne J.C., Palmer S.C., Shapiro P.J. *et al.* (2004) Distress, psychiatric morbidity, and prescriptions for psychotropic medication in a breast cancer waiting room sample. *General Hospital Psychiatry*, 26, 121–128.
3. Muriel A.C., Hwang V.S., Kornblith A. *et al.* (2009) Management of psychosocial distress by oncologists. *Psychiatric Services*, 60, 1132–1134.
4. Hu X.H., Bull S.A., Hunkeler E.M. *et al.* (2004) Incidence and duration of side effects and those rated as bothersome with selective serotonin reuptake inhibitor treatment for depression: Patient report versus physician estimate. *Journal of Clinical Psychiatry*, 65, 959–965.
5. Lee B.N., Dantzer R., Langley K.E. *et al.* (2004) A cytokine-based neuroimmunologic mechanism of cancer-related symptoms. *Neuroimmunomodulation*, 11, 279–292.
6. Reich M. (2008) Depression and cancer: Recent data on clinical issues, research challenges and treatment

approaches. *Current Opinion in Oncology*, 20, 353–359.

7. Kim H.F., Fisch M.J. (2006) Antidepressant use in ambulatory cancer patients. *Current Oncology Reports*, 8, 275–281.
8. McTiernan A., Irwin M., Vongruenigen V. (2010) Weight, physical activity, diet, and prognosis in breast and gynecologic cancers. *Journal of Clinical Oncology*, 28, 4074–4080.
9. Lal L.S., Zhuang A., Hung F. *et al.* (2011) Evaluation of drug interactions in patients treated with antidepressants at a tertiary care cancer center. *Supportive Care in Cancer*, Apr 26:Epub ahead of print.
10. Henry N.L., Stearns V., Flockhart D.A. *et al.* (2008) Drug interactions and pharmacogenomics in the treatment of breast cancer and depression. *American Journal of Psychiatry*, 165, 1251–1255.
11. Irarrazaval M.E. (2011) Tamoxifen and antidepressants: Antagonists in breast cancer prevention? *Revista Medica de Chile*, 139, 86–93.
12. DeSanty K.P., Amabile C.M. (2007) Antidepressant-induced liver injury. *The Annals of Pharmacotherapy* [Review], 41, 1201–1211.
13. Carroll J.K., Kohli S., Mustian K.M. *et al.* (2007) Pharmacologic treatment of cancer-related fatigue. *Oncologist*, 12(suppl 1), 43–51.
14. Fischer D.J., Villines D., Kim Y.O. *et al.* (2010) Anxiety, depression, and pain: Differences by primary cancer. *Supportive Care in Cancer*, 18, 801–810.
15. Miller K.E., Adams S.M., Miller M.M. (2006) Antidepressant medication use in palliative care. *The American Journal of Hospice and Palliative Care*, 23, 127–133.
16. Campbell N., Boustani M., Limbil T. *et al.* (2009) The cognitive impact of anticholinergics: A clinical review. *Clinical Interventions in Aging*, 4, 225–233.
17. Mazzocato C., Stiefel F., Buclin T., Berney A. (2000) Psychopharmacology in supportive care of cancer: A review for the clinician: II. Neuroleptics. *Supportive Care in Cancer*, 8, 89–97.
18. Maldonado J.R. (2008) Delirium in the acute care setting: Characteristics, diagnosis and treatment. *Critical Care Clinics*, 24, 657–722, vii.
19. Girard T.D., Pandharipande P.P., Carson S.S. *et al.* 2010) Feasibility, efficacy, and safety of antipsychotics for intensive care unit delirium: The MIND randomized, placebo-controlled trial. *Critical Care Medicine*, 38, 428–437.
20. Boettger S., Breitbart W. (2005) Atypical antipsychotics in the management of delirium: A review of the empirical literature. *Palliative and Supportive Care*, 3, 227–237.
21. Grover S., Mattoo S.K., Gupta N. (2011) Usefulness of atypical antipsychotics and choline esterase inhibitors in delirium: A review. *Pharmacopsychiatry*, 44, 43–54.
22. Damek D.M. (2009) Cerebral edema, altered mental status, seizures, acute stroke, leptomeningeal metastases, and paraneoplastic syndrome. *Emergency Medicine Clinics of North America*, 27, 209–229.
23. Warrington T.P., Bostwick J.M. (2006) Psychiatric adverse effects of corticosteroids. *Mayo Clinic Proceedings*, 81, 1361–1367.
24. Rowe D.L. (2007) Off-label prescription of quetiapine in psychiatric disorders. *Expert Reviews of Neurotherapeutics*, 7, 841–852.
25. Breitbart W., Chochinov H., Passik S. (2004) Psychiatric symptoms in palliative medicine, in *Oxford Textbook of Palliative Medicine*, 3rd edn (eds D. Doyle, G. Hanks, N. Cherny, K. Calman), Oxford University Press, New York, p. 749.
26. Komossa K., Depping A.M., Gaudchau A. *et al.* (2010) Second-generation antipsychotics for major depressive disorder and dysthymia. *Cochrane Database Systematic Review*, 12, CD008121.
27. Fadul N. (2008) Chronic nausea, in *The MD Anderson Supportive and Palliative Care Handbook*, 3rd edn (eds A. Elsayem, E. Bruera), UT Printing and Media Services, Houston, TX, pp. 45–51.
28. Braun I.M., Pirl W.F. (2010) Psychotropic medications in cancer care, in *Psycho-Oncology*, 2nd edn (eds J. Holland, W. Breitbart, P. Jacobsen *et al.*), Oxford University Press, New York, pp. 378–385.
29. Smith H. (2009) Hiccups, in *Palliative Medicine* (eds D. Walsh, A.T. Caraceni, R. Fainsinger *et al.*), Saunders Elsevier, Philadelphia, PA, pp. 894–897.
30. Stahl S. (2000) *Essential Psychopharmacology*, 2nd edn, Cambridge University Press, New York.
31. Janicak P.G., Davis J.M., Preskorn S.H., Ayd F.J. (1997) *Principles and Practice of Psychopharmacology*, 2nd edn, Lippincott Williams & Wilkins, Philadelphia, PA.
32. Dorsey E.R., Rabbani A., Gallagher S.A. *et al.* (2010) Impact of FDA black box advisory on antipsychotic medication use. *Archives of Internal Medicine*, 170, 96–103.
33. Kawanishi C., Onishi H., Kato D. *et al.* (2005) Neuroleptic malignant syndrome in cancer treatment. *Palliative and Supportive Care*, 3, 51–53.
34. Haddad P.M., Sharma S.G. (2007) Adverse effects of atypical antipsychotics : Differential risk and clinical implications. *CNS Drugs* 21, 911–936.
35. Drici M.D., Priori S. (2007) Cardiovascular risks of atypical antipsychotic drug treatment. *Pharmacoepidemiology and Drug Safety*, 16, 882–890.

36. Meulendijks D., Mannesse C.K., Jansen P.A. *et al.* (2010) Antipsychotic-induced hyponatraemia: A systematic review of the published evidence. *Drug Safety*, 33, 101–114.
37. Tandon R. (2002) Safety and tolerability: How do newer generation "atypical" antipsychotics compare? *Psychiatric Quarterly*, 73, 297–311.
38. Robinson M.J., Owen J.A. (2005) Psychopharmacology, in *Textbook of Psychosomatic Medicine* (ed. J.L. Levenson), American Psychiatric Publishing, Inc., Washington, DC, pp. 871–914.
39. Sheehan J.J., Sliwa J.K., Amatniek J.C. *et al.* (2010) Atypical antipsychotic metabolism and excretion. *Current Drug Metabolism*, 11, 516–525.
40. Savard J., Morin C.M. (2001) Insomnia in the context of cancer: A review of a neglected problem. *Journal of Clinical Oncology*, 19, 895–908.
41. Dundar Y., Boland A., Strobl J. *et al.* (2004) Newer hypnotic drugs for the short-term management of insomnia: A systematic review and economic evaluation. *Health Technology Assessment*, 8, iii-x, 1–125.
42. Hesse L.M., von Moltke L.L., Greenblatt D.J. (2003) Clinically important drug interactions with zopiclone, zolpidem and zaleplon. *CNS Drugs*, 17, 513– 532.
43. Grunze H.C. (2010) Anticonvulsants in bipolar disorder. *Journal of Mental Health*, 19, 127–141.
44. Andersohn F., Schade R., Willich S.N., Garbe E. (2010) Use of antiepileptic drugs in epilepsy and the risk of self-harm or suicidal behavior. *Neurology*, 75, 335–340.
45. Eisenberg E., River Y., Shifrin A., Krivoy N. (2007) Antiepileptic drugs in the treatment of neuropathic pain. *Drugs*, 67, 1265–1289.
46. Ghodse H. (2003) Pain, anxiety and insomnia – a global perspective on the relief of suffering: Comparative review. *British Journal of Psychiatry*, 183, 15–21.
47. Vaidya A.D., Devasagayam T.P. (2007) Current status of herbal drugs in India: An overview. *Journal of Clinical Biochemistry and Nutrition*, 41, 1–11.
48. Bradford L.D. (2002) CYP2D6 allele frequency in European Caucasians, Asians, Africans and their descendants. *Pharmacogenomics*, 3, 229–243.
49. Grassi L., Nanni M.G., Uchitomi Y., Riba M. (2011) Pharmacotherapy of depression in people with cancer, in *Depression and Cancer* (eds D.W. Kissane, M. Maj, N. Sartorius), World Psychiatric Association, pp. 151–176.
50. Bostwick J.M. (2010) A generalist's guide to treating patients with depression with an emphasis on using side effects to tailor antidepressant therapy. *Mayo Clinic Proceedings*, 85, 538–550.
51. Reich M. (2010) Les antidepresseurs en oncologie: Specificités et particularités. *Psycho-Oncology*, 4, 51–64.
52. Iosifescu D.V. (2007) Treating depression in the medically ill. *Psychiatric Clinics of North America*, 30, 77–90.

CHAPTER 10
Rehabilitation

Anja Mehnert[1] *and Uwe Koch*[2]
[1]Psycho-Oncology and Palliative Care Research Group, Department of Medical Psychology, University Medical Centre Hamburg Eppendorf, Hamburg, Germany
[2]Medical Faculty, Hamburg University, University Medical Centre Hamburg Eppendorf, Hamburg, Germany

Cancer survivorship

Progress in various cancer treatments has markedly improved the prognosis and life expectancy for many cancer patients during recent years, though cancer is still one of the leading causes of morbidity and mortality worldwide. An estimated 3 191 600 cancer cases were diagnosed in Europe in 2006.[1] The most common form of cancers was breast cancer (13.5% of all cancer cases), followed by colorectal cancers (12.9%) and lung cancer (12.1%). Over the past decades a considerable amount of research has shown the significant emotional and social impact of cancer and its treatment on patients and their families.[2] Like most people suffering from chronic illness, cancer patients experience distress caused by a number of problems that arise during the course of the illness and effect different areas of a patient's life. Specific problems that existed prior to the cancer diagnosis as well as the initial level of distress may also play a role in coping and psychological adjustment to the disease. In addition to a variety of physical symptoms such as pain, fatigue and disabilities, sources of distress also include: strain on the partner and the family; emotional, existential and spiritual concerns; a range of social, financial and occupational problems as well as long-term dependence on medical and social care facilities.

A typical in- or outpatient cancer patient suffers from 5–10 distressing symptoms that are directly associated with a lower quality of life.[3] Prevalent symptoms are pain, fatigue, nausea, sleep problems and cognitive dysfunctions. Functional limitations include limitations of the shoulder–arm mobility, lung functions, the voice and speech functions, sexual function and incontinence.

The psychological burden includes anxiety and particularly fears of recurrence or disease progression, feelings of helplessness and hopelessness, depression, problems due to changes in the body image, self-concept and self-esteem, and identity problems. The causes of psychological problems are multiple, but often conditioned by the life-threatening illness and the uncertainty about the disease process as well as autonomy and loss of control. Stress in family and social relationships resulting from uncertainty about social roles and tasks such as giving up social functions or new social dependencies such as a longer-term dependence on medical care facilities.

Previous studies using self-report screening measures have reported distress, anxiety and depression in on average one quarter to one third of cancer survivors with levels up to 50% following diagnosis and treatment.[4,5] However, lower prevalence rates were reported in studies using structured clinical interviews for DSM or ICD. While high levels of psychosocial distress have been found within the first year post diagnosis, there is evidence for an improvement in distress, psychosocial well-being and quality of life in long-term

Clinical Psycho-Oncology: An International Perspective, First Edition. Edited by Luigi Grassi and Michelle Riba.

survivors,[6] even though research has shown no improvement or even a decline in physical and/or mental health, specifically in older patients.[7]

The International Classification of Functioning, Disability and Health (ICF)

Since the early 1980s, continuous efforts have been made by the World Health Organization (WHO) to provide a cross-cultural definition of disability and chronic diseases through the establishment of a disease consequence model. The WHO has defined rehabilitation as 'the use of all means aimed at reducing the impact of disabling and handicapping conditions and at enabling people with disabilities to achieve optimal social integration'.[8] Thus, the (re-)integration of individuals with disabilities, chronic health conditions, diseases and handicaps into the society and working life is one important aspect of participation according to the International Classification of Functioning, Disability and Health (ICF).[8]

The ICF is a classification of health and health-related domains. A health condition is a global term for disease, disorder, injury or trauma, and may also include other circumstances, such as ageing and stress. Health conditions are coded using ICD-10. The ICF domains are classified from body, individual and societal perspectives by means of two lists: a list of body functions and structure, and a list of domains of activity and participation. Body functions are the physiological (and psychological) functions of body systems, and body structures are anatomical parts of the body. Impairments are problems in body function or structure such as a significant deviation or loss (including somatic and mental disorder).

Activity is defined as the execution of a task or action by an individual. Thus, activity limitations are difficulties an individual may have in executing various activities. Participation is involvement in a life situation including family and social life, community life, working life. Hence, participation restrictions are problems an individual may experience in involvement in life situations. Figure 10.1 shows the ICF model of functioning and disability. Since an individual's functioning and disability occurs in a context, the ICF also includes context factors such as person-related and environmental factors. Personal factors comprise demographic characteristics such as age, education, and gender, and individual features of the patient's character. Environmental factors include the physical, social and attitudinal environment in which people live and conduct their lives.

The ICF dimensions and the ICF core sets for various diseases allow the classification of limitations and restrictions in different areas of a patient's life. Thus, they provide the opportunity to initiate purposeful and target-oriented actions and interventions to overcome individual barriers. The provision of interventions through cancer rehabilitation services and ambulant follow-up care facilities will help patients to return to work. Main goal is the promotion of participation in society and working life as well as self-determination of a patient with

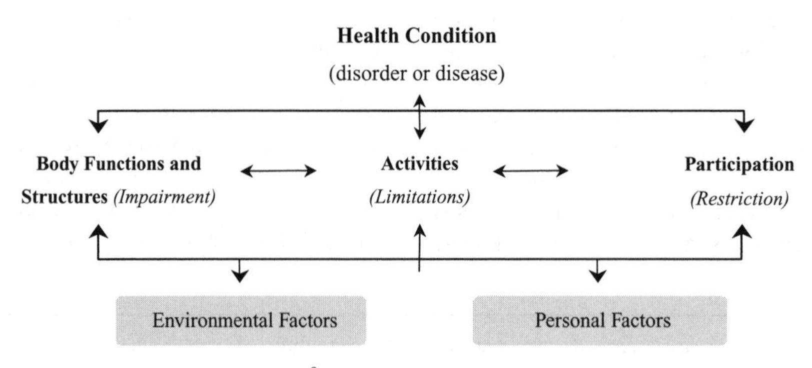

Figure 10.1 Model of functioning and disability.[8]

disabilities and impairments or threat of disabilities and impairments. Possible aims within the area of occupational reintegration include return to work, study or training, the development of a new scope of work and activities, part-time work, the promotion of changes and adaptation of the job and job requirements as well as the place of work in consultation with the patient, the employer and co-workers.

Clinical case study

For a 47-year-old patient with breast cancer, for example, the health condition is coded using ICD-10 (e.g. breast cancer C50). The patient might experience a variety of impaired body functions and structures due to the cancer and cancer treatments. Impaired body functions, for example, include pain and sensation of pain, functions of the lymph nodes, sleep functions, body image, emotional functions, energy and drive functions, and sensations related to the skin. Impaired body structures could comprise the structure of the immune system or the structure of areas of the skin. Activity limitations and participation restrictions for this breast cancer patient as a consequence of the health condition and the impaired functions and structures then possibly will include handling stress and other psychological demands, lifting and carrying objects, hand and arm use as well as preparing meals, doing housework, participation in community life and employment. Environmental factors possibly will contain facilitators such as friends and family as well as health professionals, and barriers such as individual's attitudes of acquaintances, peers, colleagues, neighbours and community members.

Objectives and the concept of cancer rehabilitation

Due to the changing age structure of the population, changes in working conditions and advances in acute medical care, there has been a significant increase in cancer and other chronic diseases over the last decades.[9,10] Given the changing disease spectrum, the demands on the medical health care have altered considerably and the importance of rehabilitation has been significantly enhanced.[11] Rehabilitation of people with illness or disabilities aims to eliminate or reduce the impact of chronic illness, disability or a specific acute event, and to maintain the patient's optimal physical, sensory, intellectual, psychological and social functional levels.

Rehabilitation provides people with disabilities with the tools they need to attain independence and self-determination. Rehabilitation focuses on all three levels of functional health, namely reduction of damage to body functions and structures, as well as aiming to maintain, restore or promote activity and participation. Thus, rehabilitation serves to prevent an impending disability or the aggravation of existing physical damage. It should help people with (incipient) diseases and disabilities, to cope with their illness and its consequences, and to participate independently as much as possible in normal family life, work and society. If a full rehabilitation is not feasible, the goal is to reduce the impact of disability on the mentioned areas of life to a minimum. Insofar as possible, rehabilitation is aimed at relieving symptoms, stabilizing the current health and functional state in those patients with disease progress, slowing the progression, preventing maladaptation and relapse, and the acquisition of compensatory services with or without technical aids.

Despite the common objectives of different countries with regard to the goals of rehabilitation, the rehabilitation concepts differ considerably.[12] Differences are found with respect to the provision of rehabilitation services, the accessibility and funding opportunities or the cost of rehabilitation.[12] Important principles of many rehabilitation programmes are a biopsychosocial understanding of illness and disability, the earliness of initiation of rehabilitation measures, the assurance of the continuity of rehabilitative treatment, and a tailored rehabilitation plan. Figure 10.2 shows cancer rehabilitation as a systematic process as it is realized in Germany.

Medical rehabilitation involves the improvement of work ability, activities and participation. Physiotherapy, occupational therapy (counselling and training in dealing with functional disorders, in particular training in activities of daily living) and speech therapy (treatment of voice, speech, and swallowing difficulties) are important aspects of medical rehabilitation.

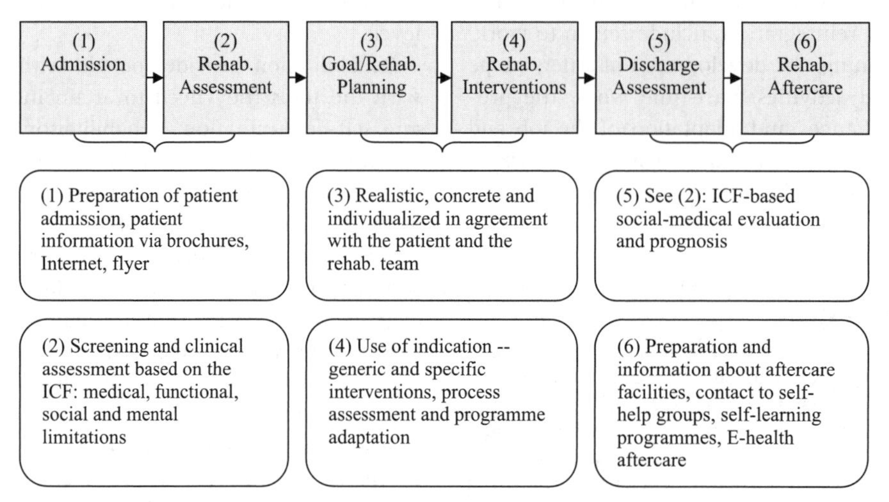

Figure 10.2 Model of the cancer rehabilitation process in Germany.

Previous research has indicated the significance of work in cancer survivorship. The motivation to continue work during treatment or to return to work after treatment completion seems strong in many cancer patients who are physically able.[13,14] Vocational and educational rehabilitation measures include the promotion of reintegration into working life and vocational adjustment. Typical interventions contain education, training, retraining or job promotion, or with a longer-term perspective, the facilitation of a (higher) education such as a college or university degree. Vocational rehabilitation services are usually held close to home, but can also be performed in specific rehabilitation facilities. Vocational rehabilitation does not necessarily focus on the acquisition of skills for a new employment, often the requirements for the professional reintegration of a patient are most likely given, if it is possible, by adjustment assistance (e.g. concrete changes in the workplace) that enables patients to continue their previous activity.

Psychological aspects of rehabilitation

According to the ICF model, psychological treatment or psychosocial support is an integral component of any comprehensive rehabilitation. Rehabilitation psychology builds on knowledge and research of clinical psychology, neuropsychology, psychiatry, psychosomatic medicine, health psychology, behavioural medicine and organizational psychology.

Central topics of psychological assessment in rehabilitation include the identification of psychosocial distress, psychological and psychosomatic symptoms and disorders, illness behaviour and coping strategies, and performance and functional ability in daily life and work. Furthermore, subjective well-being, quality of life, risk factors, individual and social protective factors such as the availability of social resources and motivation are recognized. The psychological assessment not only determines the type of distress severity, the time of onset and the course or chronicity of distress, but is also important to distinguish psychosocial distress and mental disorders using diagnostic systems such as DSM or ICD. The psychological assessment in rehabilitation includes a variety of clinical psychological assessment methods such as exploration and interview, observation, screening questionnaires and testing procedures. Meanwhile, an additional series of rehabilitation-specific diagnostic tools are available.

Indication and rehabilitation motivation

The indication for psychological support is based on the level of psychosocial distress, the individual, family and professional life situation, and the patient's motivation. The presence of a mental disorder is generally an indication for psychotherapeutic and psychopharmacological treatment if necessary. Psychological interventions in the context of rehabilitation do not only focus on distinct mental disorders, but also on a variety of typical psychological problems such as self-esteem issues, fatigue, partnership or family problems.

Furthermore, disease- and disability-related psychological interventions such as patient education and health promotion may be indicated. The cause of psychological support in rehabilitation is, however, not only dependent on the situation of the individual patient, but often also on the availability of appropriate care services. In addition to the initial screening and diagnosis it is also important during the course or at the end of the rehabilitation programme to implement a distress screening, evaluate the effectiveness of interventions and make an assignment to further follow-up measures.

Prerequisite for the success of any psychological intervention is sufficient motivation on the part of the individual patient. The motivation for rehabilitation includes aspects such as distress, hope for a good outcome, attitude and knowledge about rehabilitation, active participation and a willingness to change lifestyle, health behaviour and illness concepts.[11] Motivation for psychological counselling or psychotherapy, however, refers specifically to psychosocial and psychological aspects such as psychological distress, stress reduction and relaxation, desire for self-reflection, disease concepts and hope for an overall enhancement of the treatment by psychotherapy. Some of the patients with cancer and other chronic physical illnesses have a strong somatic disease-oriented approach and a rather passive attitude towards changes of risky health behaviours and unhealthy lifestyle aspects. These patients require special efforts with regard to motivation and participation particularly in psychological interventions.

The Transtheoretical Model of Change by Prochaska and DiClemente[15] provides a comprehensive understanding of a patient's motivation and readiness to make changes that helps clinicians also to anticipate possible barriers during the rehabilitation process. The Transtheoretical Model describes behaviour changes as a process that consists of different stages: during the first stage ('pre-contemplation stage'), patients do not consider any health behaviour changes, because they do not evaluate their behaviour as potentially harmful or have previously failed in making any significant behaviour changes (e.g. to quit smoking). In the second stage ('contemplation stage') patients are concerned with the idea of a behavioural change, pondering possible benefits and barriers to change. In the third stage ('preparation stage') patients are preparing to take action and might experiment with minor behaviour changes. The actual behaviour changes take place during the fourth stage ('action stage'), and in the fifth stage ('maintenance stage') maintenance strategies must be developed to stabilize long-term behaviour change. The transition from one stage to another can be facilitated and supported by psychological interventions tailored and adapted to the particular stage. This model also suggests that not only the motivation of a patient is crucial, but the fit between the situation of the individual patient and the activities offered within a rehabilitation programme.

Psychological interventions during rehabilitation

Psychological interventions in the rehabilitation can be differentiated according to the following criteria: (a) target group (patient, partner, family, social environment); (b) cause (including disease management, illness behaviour, partnership, mental disorders, role problems, job integration); (c) type of intervention (counselling, psychotherapy, patient education, health promotion); (d) intensity (frequency, treatment dose and duration); and (e) setting (individual, partner or group offers). The differentiation of the individual psychological interventions that play a role in the rehabilitation succeeds only partially because they overlap in content and methodology. However, they can be divided into psychological counselling and psychotherapy as well as health promotion, psychoeducation and patient education.

Psychological counselling is a method of problem-based care for patients undergoing rehabilitation and is indicated for all problems in the context of adaptation to the illness or disability. Psychological counselling may be initiated by the patient, at the initiative of a rehabilitation team member or based on a distress screening at the beginning of the rehabilitation programme. Typical circumstances for psychological counselling are problems in adapting to the cancer and disease consequences, problems in family life, occupational and social environment. Other events include psychological crises during the course of rehabilitation, rehabilitation motivation and low cooperation (compliance), maladaptive illness concepts or existing fears of therapeutic measures. Psychological counselling is usually supportive and involves of one or more patient–counsellor contacts. The involvement of partners, relatives and relevant others in the context of the counselling may also be useful.

Psychotherapy is indicated mainly within the rehabilitation of cancer survivors with comorbid mental disorders such as depression, post-traumatic stress disorder and anxiety disorders. The realization of psychotherapeutic interventions depends to a considerable extent on the indicative focus of the rehabilitative institution. A variety of studies show high psychological distress and impaired quality of life among cancer survivors and patients with other chronic physical health conditions.[16–18]

Although meta-analytical findings support the usefulness of psychosocial interventions for improving quality of life in cancer patients,[19] only very few studies have focused on psychological interventions in cancer rehabilitation. Furthermore, in many rehabilitative institutions and facilities, only brief psychotherapy can be realized due to time constraints and the limited available treatment capacity for systematic psychological treatments. Thus, psychological services are often pursuing the most likely target, to motivate a patient to enter psychotherapeutic treatment after rehabilitation. In addition, other important rehabilitative goals are to reduce emotional distress, provide support in family and social reintegration, as well as to regain the ability to work.

Health promotion, patient education and psychoeducation

Health promotion, patient education and psychoeducation are aimed at improving the quality of life for patients. Information and education about the disease, its causes, treatment options and their subsequent problems reduce health-risk behaviours, enhance coping skills and strengthen individual and social protective factors.[20] Health promotion is based on the principles of the Ottawa Charter, WHO.[21] It aims to create the social, environmental, structural and individual requirements for a health-promoting lifestyle. This understanding is based on a multidimensional, positive definition of health: health is understood not as a state, but as a process that develops in the interaction of an active trading, self-determined individual and their social environment.

Patient education and health promotion are usually based on elaborated manuals, training and treatment programmes that focus on the typical complaints and problems of cancer patients (e.g. fatigue, chronic pain, cognitive dysfunctions, anxiety and depression). Patient education and psychoeducation cover issues that are specific to a particular disease and those that concern the general problems of chronic diseases.

Key components of patient education are the increase in knowledge and the development of a disease and change model, enhanced body awareness, the communicating of self-management skills; measures to prevent relapse as well as the promotion of a healthy lifestyle and of social skills to mobilize social support.

The multiprofessional rehabilitation team

Chronic diseases and disabilities generally require rehabilitation and care that goes beyond the medical treatment and includes a variety of therapeutic approaches.[22] Comprehensive rehabilitation programmes contain interdisciplinary diagnosis and therapy to integrate somatic, functional, occupational and psychosocial activities into an individual rehabilitation plan. The need for medical therapy, nursing care, physiotherapy, speech therapy, occupational therapy, social work, psychosocial counselling and education requires the collaboration of various vocational and professional groups. Team size and team composition will vary depending on the population to be treated and the treatment plan as well as the equipment of the rehabilitation facility.

Since interdisciplinarity is regarded as an important quality of rehabilitation, collaboration between the different disciplines is a key demand. Otherwise, inadequate collaboration can adversely affect the treatment process and the success of the rehabilitation. Furthermore, different expectations and perceptions of the rehabilitation goals among members of the team can lead to uncertainty, noncompliance and discontinuation of the therapy.

Rehabilitation research

Rehabilitation is based on knowledge and research of various disciplines (such as oncology, cardiology and neurology) and the findings of that research. Such interdisciplinary, general science of rehabilitation is only at the beginning of its development.[11] Important and priority areas of research involve the aetiology, the course and prognosis of chronic diseases, disabilities and their consequences, rehabilitation-specific assessment measures, and the development and evaluation of rehabilitative interventions. The tasks of the health services research include the integration of rehabilitation into the individual health care system, clarification of needs and vulnerability, the clarification of access to rehabilitation programmes (availability of rehabilitative services) and economic evaluation of rehabilitative interventions.

Important criteria for the evaluation of the efficacy and success of a rehabilitative programme are the following:

– *medical indicators* (such as diagnosis, disease duration, severity, comorbidity, prognosis, functional capacity);
– *sociomedical indicators* (such as performance at work, performance levels, social consequences);
– *socioepidemiological indicators* (such as social integration, return to work);
– *insurance-related indicators* (such as work ability, degree of disability, invalidity);
– *subjective indicators and quality of life* (such as well-being, symptom distress, anxiety, depression, coping skills, patient satisfaction); and
– *health-economic indicators* (such as medical expenses, lost work time).

With the operationalization and assessment of indicators, measurement instruments are divided into generic and disease- or treatment-specific tools. While disease- or treatment-specific instruments can be used among disease-related (e.g. cognitive impairments) or population-related (e.g. breast cancer) groups, generic measures are used to assess characteristics such as global health or daily activities independent of the disease status of a patient.

Given these heterogeneous criteria and rehabilitation objectives, outcome research is faced with the question, based on which indicators should be decided, of whether the rehabilitation and treatment objectives have been met. Thus, it is important that all individuals involved in the rehabilitation process (patients, staff, institutions, experts) agree on the treatment goals. Rehabilitation outcome furthermore will depend on the temporal distance to the programme. This should be considered with regard to the timing of outcome measurements (catamneses, follow-ups). Depending on the diagnosis and treatment goals, levels of success can be measured in the short term (at the end of the rehabilitation measure: e.g. improved well-being, reduction of nicotine consumption, lower serum cholesterol), medium term (within one year: e.g. return to work, abstinence after alcohol abuse), or long term (after several years: complete remission and ability to work).

It is therefore imperative to determine the viable therapeutic goals in advance, and to measure the degree of goal achievement to the date on which the effect of the measure may have had an impact and relevance. Controlled and randomized intervention studies represent the best research method. Quasi-experimental or naturalistic designs are, however, often realized primarily for the purposes of cumulative evidence, which is considered an alternative.

Key points

- Given the population growth and associated changes of disease spectrum and the advances in medicine, the importance of rehabilitation will continue to grow.
- Rehabilitation is aimed at reducing the impact of disabling and handicapping conditions and at enabling people with disabilities to achieve optimal social integration.
- Current approaches for more effective rehabilitative interventions include patient empowerment and participation, early and detailed evaluation of rehabilitation needs, stronger orientation towards return to work, and the implementation of cancer survivorship programmes and rehabilitative services.
- Rehabilitative treatment should be better geared to the living environment of people with disabilities and chronic diseases, and the effects of the disease consequences in everyday life.
- The integration of people with disabilities and chronic illnesses into society shows itself in participation and in the meeting of their needs.

References

1. Ferlay J., Autier P., Boniol M. *et al.* (2007) Estimates of the cancer incidence and mortality in Europe in 2006. *Annals of Oncology*, 18, 581–592.
2. Holland J.C. (2002) History of psycho-oncology: Overcoming attitudinal and conceptual barriers. *Psychosomatic Medicine*, 64, 206–221.
3. Chang V.T., Hwang S.S., Feuerman M., Kasimis B.S. (2000) Symptom and quality of life survey of medical oncology patients at a Veterans Affairs medical center: A role for symptom assessment. *Cancer*, 88, 1175–1183.
4. Burgess C., Cornelius V., Love S. *et al.* (2005) Depression and anxiety in women with early breast cancer: Five-year observational cohort study. *British Medical Journal*, 330, 702–706.
5. Zabora J., BrintzenhofeSzoc K., Curbow B. *et al.* (2001) The prevalence of psychological distress by cancer site. *Psycho-Oncology*, 10, 19–28.
6. Helgeson V.S., Tomich P.L. (2005) Surviving cancer: A comparison of 5-year disease-free breast cancer survivors with healthy women. *Psycho-Oncology*, 14, 307–317.
7. Ganz P.A., Guadagnoli E., Landrum M.B. *et al.* (2003) Breast cancer in older women: Quality of life and psychosocial adjustment in the 15 months after diagnosis. *Journal of Clinical Oncology*, 21, 4027–4033.
8. World Health Organization (WHO) (2001) *ICF – International Classification of Functioning, Disability and Health*, WHO, Geneva.
9. Sant M., Allemani C., Santaquilani M. *et al.* (2009) EUROCARE-4 Survival of cancer patients diagnosed in 1995–1999. Results and commentary. *European Journal of Cancer*, 45, 931–991.
10. Mehnert A., Volkert J., Wlodarczyk O., Andreas S. (2001) Psychische Komorbidität bei Menschen mit chronischen Erkrankungen im höheren Lebensalter unter besonderer Berücksichtigung von Krebserkrankungen. *Bundesgesundheitsblatt*, 54, 75–82.
11. Bengel J., Koch U. (eds) (2000) *Grundlagen der Rehabilitationswissenschaften*, Springer, Berlin.
12. Hellbom M., Bergelt C., Bergenmar M. *et al.* (2011). Cancer rehabilitation: A Nordic and European perspective. *Acta Oncologica*, 50, 179–186.
13. Mahar K.K., BrintzenhofeSzoc K., Shields J.J. (2008) The impact of changes in employment status on psychosocial well-being: A study of breast cancer survivors. *Journal of Psychosocial Oncology*, 26, 1–17.
14. Mehnert A. (2011) Employment and work-related issues in cancer survivors. *Critical Reviews in Oncology/Hematology*, 77, 109–130.
15. Prochaska J., DiClemente C. (1992) Stages of change the modification of problem behaviors, in *Progress Behavior Modification* (eds M. Hersen, R. Eisler, P. Miller), Sage, Newbury Park, CA, pp. 184–218.
16. Baumeister H., Hutter N., Bengel J., Härter M. (2011) Quality of life in medically ill persons with comorbid mental disorders: A systematic review and meta-analysis. *Psychotherapy and Psychosomatics*, 80, 275–286.
17. Mitchell A.J., Chan M., Bhatti H. *et al.* (2011) Prevalence of depression, anxiety, and adjustment disorder in oncological, haematological, and palliative-care settings: A meta-analysis of 94 interview-based studies. *The Lancet Oncology*, 12, 160–174.

18. Mehnert A., Koch U. (2008) Psychological comorbidity and health-related quality of life and its association with awareness, utilization, and need for psychosocial support in a cancer register-based sample of long-term breast cancer survivors. *Journal of Psychosomatic Research*, 64, 383–391.
19. Rehse B., Pukrop R. (2003) Effects of psychosocial interventions on quality of life in adult cancer patients: Meta-analysis of 37 published controlled outcome studies. *Patient Education and Counseling*, 50, 179–186.
20. Faller H., Reusch A., Meng K. (2011) Innovative Schulungskonzepte in der medizinischen Rehabilitation. *Bundesgesundheitsblatt*, 54, 444–450.
21. World Health Organization (WHO) (1986) *Ottawa Charter for Health Promotion*, WHO, Geneva.
22. Ruppert L., Stubblefield M., Stiles J., Passik S.D. (2010) Rehabilitation medicine in oncology, in *History of Psycho-Oncology: Overcoming attitudinal and conceptual barriers* (ed. J. Holland), Oxford University Press, New York, pp. 460–463.

PART 2
Special Populations

CHAPTER 11

Pediatric Psycho-oncology

Margaret L. Stuber[1] *and Elizabeth M. Strom*[2]

[1]Jane and Marc Nathanson Professor, David Geffen School of Medicine, UCLA, Los Angeles, CA, USA

[2]Medical student, University of Illinois at Chicago College of Medicine, Dixon, IL, USA

Introduction

Since 1986, the American Academy of Pediatrics (AAP) has had specific guidelines regarding treatment facilities for childhood cancer. These guidelines, which were most recently updated in 2004 and reaffirmed in 2009, suggest that paediatric cancer should be managed using the types of 'facilities available only at a tertiary center'.[1] Thus, childhood cancer in the United States is almost always treated in the large paediatric oncology centres. Within these centres, it is expected that treatment of the child involves 'Board-certified pediatric subspecialists available to participate actively in all areas of the care of the child with cancer, including anesthesiology, intensive care, infectious diseases, cardiology, neurology, endocrinology and metabolism, genetics, gastroenterology, *child and adolescent psychiatry*, nephrology, and pulmonology' (p. 1833, emphasis added).[1] Additionally, the AAP guideline states that the 'pediatric hematologist/oncologist must be assisted by skilled nurses, social workers, pharmacists, nutritionists, and psychologists who specialize in pediatric oncology' (p. 1834).[1] Thus, these guidelines convey not only the expectation, but also the necessity, of involving clinical social workers, psychologists, and child and adolescent psychiatrists in the care of children with cancer.

As these guidelines for childhood cancer treatment have been modified, so too has the role of psychiatric care in paediatric oncology. Prognosis for paediatric cancer has improved immensely; 80% of patients are expected to have long-term survival from childhood cancers.[2] Thus, despite the fact that significant life threat is indeed still present, the primary focus of psychiatric concern has shifted from dying and bereavement to coping and survivorship.

This chapter will provide a background about the current situation in paediatric oncology and associated psychiatric issues. It will consider the normal developmental context in which children understand cancer and treatment. Specific common psychological and psychiatric problems of child cancer patients and their families associated with initial diagnosis and treatment of the malignancy will be discussed as well as long-term effects on the psychological health of adult survivors of childhood cancer. The chapter will conclude with consideration of interventions for survivors, parents and siblings.

Background

Every year, more than 14 000 children (ages 0–19) in the United States are diagnosed with cancer.[3] Although this affects less than 1% of children, the approximate 2000 deaths each year make cancer the leading cause of death from disease in children.[3,4] Of these childhood cancers, leukaemia is the most prevalent, accounting for approximately 34% of cases and also the most deaths; acute

Clinical Psycho-Oncology: An International Perspective, First Edition. Edited by Luigi Grassi and Michelle Riba.

lymphocytic leukaemia is the most common type of leukaemia. Brain and other nervous system tumours make up about 21% of cases and are the second most common childhood cancer. Neuroblastomas, Wilms' tumours, lymphomas, rhabdomyosarcomas, retinoblastomas and osteosarcomas each account for 3–7% of paediatric oncology cases.

Fortunately, all of these cancers have a relatively positive prognosis that has improved significantly since the mid 1970s. Among children aged 10–14 years, the five-year relative survival rate increased from 58.9% for those diagnosed in 1975–1977 to 80.8% for those patients diagnosed in 1999–2005.[2] This figure is representative of the overall five-year survival rate average of 80%, which ranges from 66% (rhabdomyosarcoma) to 95% (Hodgkin's lymphoma) for specific cancer sites.[2] Thus, despite the relatively large incidence of deaths resulting from malignancy and the anguish and uncertainty that often follow a cancer diagnosis, the probability of long-term survival is encouraging.

Just as the type and prognosis for oncology in children are distinct from adults, the psychological issues and care needed for paediatric oncology patients are different from those for adults. Unlike adults, diagnosis and treatment for children take place during a time of physical, cognitive, behavioural and social development.[5] Interference with any of these developmental processes may impact both acute and long-term psychological outcomes. Acutely, some psychological symptoms may appear as a response to the stress that a cancer diagnosis and treatment inflict, whereas other symptoms may be a direct physical effect of the treatment itself.[6] Subclinical levels of depression and anxiety are common in children with cancer, as they are in any child with a medical condition. Delirium, possibly resulting from chemotherapy or drug treatment, is also a psychiatric risk factor in these patients that must be monitored closely.[7] Parents may also suffer from acute psychological distress. For example, Patiño-Fernández *et al.* found that 'nearly all' parents report subclinical symptoms of acute stress (SAS) following their child's cancer diagnosis, and that many meet criteria for acute stress disorder.[8] The mental health of parents is of particular importance because the ability of parents to adjust following their child's cancer diagnosis has been shown to play a significant role in the well-being of the child.[9]

The average survivor of childhood cancer can expect to live another 66 years, during which the focus of life may include education, social experiences, employment, marriage, fertility and a variety of other issues that are generally less significant in the lives of older adults.[5,10] Success in these aspects of life may impact long-term psychological health and quality of life and must be considered when counselling survivors of paediatric cancer. Additionally, treatment and the associated stress may have direct effects, including post-traumatic stress disorder, which is reported to be associated with functional impairment and/or clinical distress in 9% of adult survivors of childhood cancer.[11] Studies analysing the quality of life of adult survivors of childhood cancer will be discussed later in the chapter.

Psychological care of a child cancer patient therefore must address familial function, potential disturbance of developmental milestones, and long-term psychological and physical sequelae. The following sections will provide more information about the acute and long-lasting psychological effects of childhood cancer and offers data to guide those working in paediatric oncology.

Developmental issues

The response of a child or adolescent and family to a cancer diagnosis and treatment must always be considered within a developmental context. 'Normal' responses of a pre-school-age child would obviously be interpreted very differently if seen in an adolescent. Similarly, the supports children need from the family will differ with the age of the paediatric patient. A full explanation of child development is beyond the scope of this chapter. The Pediatric Medical Traumatic Stress Toolkit for Health Care Providers offers a detailed set of instructions as to how to help hospitalized children of different ages. It can be found at http://www.nctsnet.org/trauma-types/pediatric-medical-traumatic-stress-toolkit-for-health-care-providers.[12] In this section we will discuss some common issues seen in caring for paediatric oncology patients of varying ages.

Infants and toddlers

Adult cancer patients are often worried about the future. Children, however, especially very young children, live primarily in the present. Infants and toddlers respond primarily to whether or not they are currently feeling safe and comfortable. Explanations of why you have to do something will not matter. What matters is that procedures are done with as much comfort and safety as is possible.

For very young children, most of the focus for caregivers should be on the family, with the goal of allowing the child to maintain a secure attachment to the primary caregiver(s). Attachment is a term used to describe the reciprocal relationship a child has with a caregiver which ideally provides the child with a secure base from which to explore the world and predictable support when distressed.[13] However wonderful the relationship is between a child and the medical staff, it does not (and should not) substitute for the relationship with the family.

In the mid twentieth century, parents were seen as problematic to have in the hospital with their children. They took up space, brought in microbes, and sometimes interfered with care. More recent efforts to provide a place for a family member to stay with a child in the hospital have been very helpful in providing children with predictable access to their parents.[14] One recent study found that having a place for parents to sleep in a Paediatric Intensive Care Unit reduced the anxiety of the parents.[15] However, a depressed or severely anxious family member will have a difficult time providing a secure and dependable base for a child. Parents can also be very helpful with children undergoing procedures, but only if they are able to remain calm and focused on supporting the child. In the section on the family below we will discuss specific interventions for parents.

The first three years are a time of very rapid growth and development, which can and should continue despite cancer. Development of language, fine motor skills and social interactions can be encouraged, even if illness and treatment limits use of many gross motor skills for these children. Young children need to be touched and, if possible, held and cuddled.[16] Providing them with a language rich environment (such as parents talking, reading, or singing to them) will allow them to continue to develop.

Transitional objects, like a pillow or blanket, can be comforting reminders of home and family. It can be challenging to keep such items clean enough for immunosuppressed patients, particularly with children who are inclined to throw objects on the floor. It can, however, be quite soothing for children, even if the blanket needs to be autoclaved periodically.

Pre-schoolers

The pre-schooler is a common paediatric patient, as the most common age group for paediatric leukaemia is 3 to 6 years. This is a time of rapid acquisition of language. However, articulation may be problematic, resulting in the frequent scenario of a mother providing interpretation of what her frustrated four year old is trying to tell the doctor. Causal reasoning is also not well developed in children of this age, who are in what Piaget referred to as Pre-operational Thinking. Also known as 'magical thinking' this type of cognition may assume temporal association to be causal association. For example, a child may think that they got an infection because they watched a scary, late-night movie, when they had heard a parent say that the movie 'wasn't good for you'. It is easy to over-estimate the understanding of an articulate five year old, who may accurately parrot back what has been explained to them. However, a little probing will often reveal that the understanding is very superficial, and could be subject to significant misinterpretation.[17]

Anxiety is a common issue for pre-school-age oncology patients. It is very difficult for them to understand why adults who seem otherwise to be nice people are sticking needles in them, giving them things that make them throw up, or making them go to the hospital. It is even more difficult to understand why their parents appear to be colluding with these people who are hurting and frightening them.

Hospitals are uncomfortable for most adults, but can be terrifying for young children. The lack of a regular routine, unfamiliar foods, and waking up in a strange bed can lead to dysregulated children, who are not sleeping or eating as would be desired. Having a familiar adult sleep nearby and available during the day is important, as is having foods which are healthy but familiar.

Separation anxiety is a pathological level of this type of developmental anxiety. It is defined as a 'developmentally inappropriate and excessive anxiety concerning separation from home or from those to whom the individual is attached'.[18] This means that, for young children who have not previously been away from home overnight, it is not uncommon for children to have nightmares or intrusive thoughts that a loved one (usually parent) is in danger, as well as physical symptoms of increased autonomic arousal such as headaches, abdominal pain, or nausea. As mentioned above, familiar toys, pillows, or blankets can help, but having a (calm) parent or loved one nearby on a predictable basis is the best way to address this type of anxiety. Severe anxiety, or separation anxiety in older children, may require additional intervention.

School-age children

By the age of 6 or 7 children are able to think about the world in a more logical way. Children between ages 7 and 11 often deal with cancer by asking many questions, and seeking to understand how the various machines work. However, their thinking can be quite concrete, and they may miss the abstract interpretation of events.[19] For this reason, it is important to avoid euphemisms with school-age children. For example, insomnia is likely to result from an explanation that another child 'fell asleep and never woke up'. They also have difficulty understanding multiple factors in causation, making it harder to explain complex explanations, such as why the same medication will not work for everyone.

School-age children are less dependent on their parents than younger children, and more invested in being with, and similar to, other children. Missing school is a problem for them, as school is their social world. Returning to school bald, or with a central line, is also problematic, as they do not know how to explain it to the other children, who may find their appearance frightening. Providing consultation to schools to help them explain what has happened can help transform a returning cancer survivor from a target to a sort of local hero.

This growing role of friends makes 'cancer camps' a valuable adjunct for school-age children. Children are allowed to do something 'normal' like be away from home in a setting in which worried parents can know there is appropriate medical care. Scars, baldness and amputations are common, and do not set the child apart as odd. Natural conversations can spring up between children, at the child's pace and comfort level, resulting in increased understanding of the illness and treatment as well as increased sense of well-being.[20]

Adolescents

Cognitive development has advanced to the point of abstract reasoning by about age 11. The cognitive challenges with adolescents have less to do with logic than with judgment. A high school student is capable of understanding that chemotherapy can help cure the cancer, but also has negative consequences. That same individual, however, may truly believe that it would be better to die than to lose her hair. The prefrontal or executive portion of the brain is generally not fully mature until the mid twenties, leaving the strong emotions of the developing brain inadequately balanced for fully adult decision-making. Deciding how much to weigh irrational but powerful opinions in treatment decisions can be difficult for the team, particularly as the patient approaches the legal age of majority.

The role of patient is also in conflict with the developmental goals of adolescence. The teen years are a time of adjusting to the body, emotional and role changes of puberty, and beginning to establish an identity which is separate from the family. Typically adolescents are gradually given more and more independence as they mature. Cancer takes them out of their social world, and makes them dependent again. Parents are once again involved in intimate body functions, and the new body with which they were starting to feel comfortable is again changed.[21]

Adolescents are more inclined to think about the future in their response to cancer and treatment than younger children. They also have a greater appreciation of the significance of potential side-effects of treatment such as infertility, or the meaning of risk for recurrence or second malignancies. However, with their sense of identity still emerging, they are generally reluctant to become identified with the cancer. This can extend to not wanting friends to visit them in the hospital, or to participate in adult approaches to support, such as cancer groups.[22] More useful approaches are camps or other social events which focus on 'normal' teen activities, and allow cancer to come up as an incidental, rather than central, part of who they are.

Psychiatric disorders

Paediatric oncology patients and their families are quite resilient, and most make a successful adjustment to the diagnosis and treatment.[6] However, there are some problems that rise to the level of a psychiatric disorder, and require intervention.

Traumatic stress symptoms

Both acute stress disorder (ASD) and post-traumatic stress disorder (PTSD) include symptoms of hyperarousal (elevated heart rate, amplified startle responses, hypervigilance), avoidance of reminders, and intrusive thoughts of the event which was traumatic.[18] ASD differs from PTSD in three ways: it is time-limited (no less than 2 days, no more than 4 weeks), acute (within 4 weeks of the traumatic event), and involves dissociative amnesia, numbing, depersonalization, derealization, or a feeling of being dazed. As with many disorders, ASD and PTSD may manifest somewhat differently in children than in adults, such as with agitated and disorganized behaviour, particularly in response to a perceived threat. These symptoms are similar to those seen in children with depression, anxiety or delirium. A study comparing 76 medically children to 31 otherwise traumatized children found that intrusion symptoms were of most utility when assessing stress responses in medically ill children.[23]

Although anxiety and acute stress responses are relatively commonly seen in paediatric oncology, it is more difficult to say anything certain about PTSD. Studies of children and adolescents who are at least 2 years in remission after end of cancer treatment have had mixed results, finding symptoms of PTSD but not significantly elevated levels of full PTSD criteria compared to healthy controls.[24] This is quite different from what is seen in young adult long-term survivors of childhood cancer, as is detailed below. Perhaps the most interesting aspect of the development of traumatic stress symptoms in childhood cancer patients is that the symptoms are correlated with the child's perception of life threat or treatment intensity, and not with the data-based prognosis given by the oncology physician or nurse. Less surprising is that parental anxiety is associated with child anxiety, which is related to the child's appraisal.[25]

Level of family functioning also appears to be related to risk for PTSD in adolescents. A study of 144 adolescent cancer survivors 1 to 12 years post cancer treatment (M = 5.3 years) and their parents found that 47% of the adolescents, 25% of mothers, and 30% of fathers reported poor family functioning on the Family Device. Adolescents whose families were perceived as functioning poorly were five times as likely to report symptoms consistent with PTSD on a structured diagnostic interview.[26]

Anticipatory anxiety, phobias and conditioned anxiety

It is common for a child (or parent) to be said to be 'afraid of needles'. Rarely, however, is this fear a true phobia, which is defined as an intense and unreasonable fear of specific objects or situations, even when they are not posing any immediate danger.[18] After the first experience with a painful injection or bone marrow aspiration even a young child may develop a conditioned response to stimuli reminiscent of the event. Vomiting in response to the smell of chemotherapy, or in the care on the way to receive chemotherapy are also conditioned responses. Other symptoms that may appear to be phobic are better understood as responses to traumatic reminders, such as elevated heart rate and agitation when someone in a white coat enters the room. Developmental understanding of the body may also account for the level of fear, such as the three year old who really thinks he is going to exsanguinate when an IV comes out.

Delirium

The literature on delirium in children in general is quite limited, but suggests that delirium is less common in children than adults.[27] A 2010 article reviewed the literature from 1980 to March 2009, and found data on only 217 child and adolescent patients with definite delirium and 136 with 'probable delirium'.[28] For example a study of 1027 consecutive psychiatric consultations in a children's hospital over four years yielded a diagnosis of delirium in only 84 patients. Many of the symptoms are similar in children and adults, including impaired alertness, apathy, anxiety, disorientation and hallucinations. However, sleep-wake disturbance, fluctuating symptoms, impaired attention, irritability, agitation, affective lability and confusion appear to be more common in children, while impaired memory, depressed mood, speech disturbance, delusions and paranoia were more often seen in adults.[29] A study of 184 patients in the paediatric intensive care unit, ages 1–17 years over 3.5 years, found that the Paediatric Anaesthesia Emergence Delirium Scale (PAED) could be successfully administered to 93.5% of the patients and had a sensitivity of 91% and a specificity of 98% (AUC 0.99) compared to the 'gold standard' clinical interview.[30] However, diagnosis of delirium in infants and very young children remains difficult.[31,32]

Depression

Although depression is a common symptom, very few children with cancer appear to meet diagnostic criteria for depression. Only 3 of 41 adolescents on active cancer treatment were in the moderate or extremely elevated range for depression on the Beck Youth Inventory II (BYI II) Depression and Anxiety scales, and only 2 were in the moderate or extremely elevated range for anxiety, compared to published norms.[33] However, it can be surprisingly difficult to determine whether or not a medically ill child has a major depressive illness.[34] Alterations in sleep or appetite are not unusual when a child is in the hospital or receiving cancer treatment. It can be difficult to determine if a child has anhedonia or is bored and unable to do what he or she really wants to do. Chemotherapy and radiation can cause fatigue and result in social withdrawal. A recent study found that a lower cut-off score on the Children's Depression Inventory of 11 and above, rather than 13 or 20, correctly identified 80% of those with depression out of 125 medically ill children, with a specificity of 70%.[34]

Long-term issues for adult survivors

Although modern paediatric oncology treatment is very effective, it is still very toxic, with long-term as well as acute adverse effects, some of which only emerge 5–10 years after successful treatment ends.[35] Two thirds of childhood cancer survivors will have at least one of these 'late effects', and one fourth of those complications are severe or life-threatening.[36] Predictors of late effects include age at time of treatment, and the type of treatment received.[37] Specific exposure-based health screening guidelines have been developed by the Children's Oncology Group (COG), which coordinates the treatment protocols and outcome data collection for childhood cancer centres across the United States.[36] These clinical guidelines are informed by ongoing epidemiological studies such as the Childhood Cancer Survivors Study.[38] The CCSS is a longitudinal cohort study that tracks the health status of survivors of childhood cancer diagnosed between 1970 and 1986 and treated at collaborating centres across the United States and Canada. This study, funded by the National Cancer Institute over the past 15 years, has greatly improved our understanding of long-term survival after childhood cancer. The initial sample included 20 691 long-term survivors of childhood cancer identified for the original cohort. Even with 3058 (14.8%) lost to follow-up, this has provided data on many issues having to do with survival of childhood cancer.[38] A similar longitudinal cohort study of almost 18 000 childhood cancer survivors has been established in Great Britain[39] and will provide an opportunity to compare biological and psychological outcomes across treatment settings and protocols.

Psychological distress and quality of life

Although there is a great deal of interest in the long-term psychosocial outcome of childhood cancer survivors, the research until recently has been sparse and plagued with methodological problems, resulting in varied outcomes.[40] Some studies which meet quality criteria suggest that survivors report lower psychological well-being, mood, liveliness, self-esteem, and motor and physical functioning, as well as increased anxiety, problem behaviours and sleeping difficulties. Other reputable studies note that survivors reported high self-worth, good behavioural conduct, and improved mental health and social behaviour.[41] A Swiss study found that childhood cancer survivors, on average, have less psychological distress than a normative population but that the proportion of survivors at risk for high psychological distress is disproportionally large.[42] A comparison of 167 US childhood cancer survivors to 170 healthy controls found they did not differ in terms of psychological distress or health-related quality of life, although survivors did endorse less adaptive health beliefs.[43] Another United States study found that 73 long-term (mean 20 years off therapy) survivors of childhood acute lymphoblastic leukaemia were significantly *less* likely to report symptoms of depression on the Beck Depression Inventory than 146 healthy controls. Survivors and controls also did not differ significantly on a General Health Questionnaire assessment of mental distress.[44] Even when they report symptoms, very few seem to seek treatment. A German study of 820 adolescent cancer survivors found that 184 survivors reported clinically relevant symptoms of post-traumatic stress, anxiety and/or depression on standardized instruments. However, of these distressed teens only 12.0% received psychosocial care and 13.6% took psychotropic medication.[45]

Clinicians have been concerned that these encouraging findings may be the result of a response bias. This suspicion was supported by a study of quality of life reports of 107 adult (mean age 31.85) survivors of childhood cancer. Although the survivors reported quality of life ratings similar to normative groups, the survivors scored significantly higher on the Self-Deception Enhancement Scale (SDE) than norms. The SDE was significantly correlated with the scores on the two quality of life measures, suggesting a systematic tendency to under-report difficulties.[46]

Using the data of the much larger Childhood Cancer Survivor Study (CCSS) of psychological quality of life, health-related quality of life (HRQOL) and life satisfaction, it was possible to look at distribution of symptoms, rather than just comparing group means. The CCSS found that a significant proportion of survivors reported more symptoms of global distress and poorer physical, but not emotional, domains of HRQOL. Most survivors (with the exception of brain tumour survivors) reported good present and expected future life satisfaction. Correlated with psychological distress and poor HRQOL were female sex, lower educational attainment, unmarried status, annual household income less than US$20 000, unemployment, lack of health insurance, presence of a major medical condition, and treatment with cranial radiation and/or surgery.[5]

Post-traumatic growth, perceived positive impact, and benefit finding

A growing area of interest has been post-traumatic growth, perceived positive impact, or benefit finding. Survivors have reported that there were positive changes after the cancer experience which were associated with a higher quality of life.[47] Changes reported included improvements in the way they treat others and make friends, the way their family and others treat them, the quality of their schoolwork and behaviour, and their plans for the future.[48] One theoretical construct for understanding positive change out of adversity is post-traumatic growth, in which a traumatic event alters a person's worldview, resulting in personal growth. This would suggest a potential association between post-traumatic stress and post-traumatic growth. Another perspective is that an event can be seen as creating burdens or benefits.[49] A study of 79 Dutch paediatric oncology patients using the revised Benefit/Burden Scale for Children (BBSC) found that reported burden of the cancer was orthogonal to reported benefits of the cancer.[50]

A third perspective comes from the Childhood Cancer Survivors Study (CCSS) which examined Perceived Positive Impact of the cancer experience on young adult survivors of childhood cancer using self-reports from 6425 survivors and 360 siblings on a modified version of the Post-traumatic Growth Inventory (PTGI). Survivors reported Perceived Positive Impact more commonly than siblings, and more often in female and non-White survivors. Predictors higher Perceived Positive Impact were being female or non-White, exposure to at least one intense therapy, a second malignancy or cancer recurrence, diagnosis at an older age, and fewer years since diagnosis.[51]

Suicidal ideation

Although it is encouraging to know that so many long-term childhood cancer survivors are doing well and even seeing positives in the cancer experience, not all of the CCSS data have been so hopeful. In an assessment of suicidal ideation, survivors were more likely to report thoughts of suicide over the previous week than siblings (7.8% vs. 4.6%, OR: 1.79). Suicidal ideation was positively correlated with a primary central nervous system malignancy, depression, pain and poor global health ratings. After controlling for depression and type of cancer, suicidal ideation remained significantly related to poor current physical health.[52]

Post-traumatic stress disorder

Post-traumatic stress disorder (PTSD) in response to childhood cancer has been a focus of research since the Diagnostic and Statistical Manual IV[18] when the diagnosis was redefined to include medical illness as a potential precipitant of PTSD.[24,53,54] The largest study to date is from the CCSS, and includes 6542 survivors and 368 siblings. Survivors were over four times as likely to report symptoms consistent with a full diagnosis of PTSD as the sibling controls (9% vs. 2%). PTSD in survivors was positively correlated with an educational level of high school or less, being unmarried, having an annual income below US$20 000, and being unemployed. Intensive treatment was also associated with an increased risk of PTSD (OR: 1.36 [95% CI, 1.06–1.74]).[11] This study used a very strict definition of PTSD. The percentage of young adult childhood cancer survivors defined as having PTSD obviously depends on the criteria used to define PTSD for the study. However, risk factors for PTSD and correlations with PTSD also vary with the definition used, making it difficult to compare studies.[55] However, it is clear that the vast majority of childhood cancer survivors do not have PTSD, despite life threat and adverse late effects. The concern is that there is a subset of survivors who have PTSD and also are not doing well in terms of the usual developmental tasks of young adulthood, such as completing school, being employed, and finding life partners.

> **Case study**
>
> Carlos is an 18-year-old long-term survivor of ALL. He comes to the paediatric oncologist saying that he is about to go to college and needs to get some information. His parents moved to the United States from Mexico before he was born, but most of his extended family is still in Mexico. His parents were so afraid when he was diagnosed that they did not discuss his diagnosis or treatment with any of the family in Mexico. They stopped socializing with the family that was in the United States, as they felt the family thought the cancer was their fault, or wanted them to seek non-medical interventions. He is hesitant to speak with his parents about his illness or treatment, as it still upsets them to talk about it. As a result, he has very little understanding of his medical history, or if there is any follow-up care that he needs. He is embarrassed to admit that one of his biggest questions is about his fertility. 'Well, I can't ask my parents, can I?'

Families of paediatric patients and survivors

Parents

Parents of paediatric oncology patients also report traumatic responses to cancer diagnosis and treatment in the acute phase. Over half of 129 mothers and 40% of 72 fathers of 138 newly diagnosed paediatric oncology patients met DSM-IV diagnostic criteria for ASD.[8] A recent Swedish longitudinal study of 107 mothers and 107 fathers of children on active treatment for cancer, administering the PTSD Checklist (Civilian) at one week, two months and four months after the child's diagnosis, found somewhat lower prevalence of symptoms, but little decrease over time. At 1 week post-diagnosis 33 % of the parents reported symptoms consistent with ASD, with the prevalence decreasing to 28% at 2 months, and 22% at 4 months. As in all studies to date, mothers reported a higher number of symptoms than fathers.[56] Another study compared 27 parents of childhood cancer survivors (mean age = 25.6 y) and 28 parents of current paediatric cancer patients (mean age = 10.2 y) on, or within 1 year of, active treatment, and found no significant differences in psychological functioning, post-traumatic stress symptoms, and adjustment to the disease experience. However, parents of children on active treatment did report more objective and family burden (e.g. financial cost, time off from work, less time with family members), and more anger associated with the illness experience.[57]

These findings are consistent with earlier studies. A survey of 63 mothers and 42 fathers of childhood leukaemia survivors found that 39.7% of the mothers and 33.3% of the fathers reported symptoms consistent with a severe level of post-traumatic stress.[58] Analysis of surveys of mothers and fathers from 331 families of childhood cancer survivors found that trait anxiety was the strongest predictor of PTSD in the parents. Other significant contributes were perceived life threat, perceived treatment intensity, and social support. Objective medical data about diagnosis or treatment was not a significant independent contributor to post-traumatic stress symptoms.[59]

This discrepancy between how the oncologists viewed the situation and how parents view the situation was also seen in a recent study of parental optimism. Four hundred and eleven parents of children on active cancer treatment were surveyed. Parental optimism was associated with an absence of depression, parental education, and the parents' perception of the child's prognosis. Correlation between the parents' and the oncologists' view of the child's prognosis were low. Optimism was hypothesized to be a trait of the parent which predicted resiliency, as trait anxiety had been found to be associated with PTSD.[60]

Interventions for parental distress are important not only for the well-being of the parents. A prospective study of 55 childhood cancer survivors and 60 healthy peer controls got data during the active treatment phase, and then after subjects turned 18 years old. Mother and father reports of initial parent distress were associated with their reports of young adult distress at follow-up for both survivors and controls. Intensity of initial treatment and late effects as rated by health care professionals moderated the association between parent and young adult distress in the cancer survivors.[61]

Siblings

There is limited data on the siblings of children under active treatment for cancer and childhood cancer survivors. A recent review found 19 published articles that suggested that aspects of psychosocial health were impacted by doubts, worries and memories. In some cases these were associated with behavioural problems, depression, somatic complaints and PTSD.[62] A survey of parents from 86 families found that parents felt that their healthy children were likely to have problems due to cancer diagnosis of their sibling, and that the current support offered was not adequate.[63] Specific issues identified in another study of parental perception of siblings' needs were losses arising from the illness experience, behavioural challenges and adaptation, and parent–sibling communication.[64]

The Childhood Cancer Survivors Study (CCSS) has significantly increased the amount of data available on siblings of young adult survivors from the 1970s and 1980s in the United States and Canada, since it used siblings as a matched control group for their investigations. A review of these studies demonstrated that siblings appeared to be doing quite well, particularly relative to their affected siblings.[5] CCSS studies report that the prevalence of PTSD in siblings of young adult survivors is 2%[11] and that suicidal ideation is reported by 4.6% of siblings.[52] We also know that siblings are less likely to see a perceived positive impact of the cancer experience than survivors.[50]

Therapeutic interventions

Survivors

Specific psychosocial supports, including social work and Child Life or Child Development professionals, are a part of all paediatric oncology centres, following the recommendations of the American Association of Pediatrics.[18] These are provided to all paediatric oncology patients and their families, most of whom are stressed but adjust well. The services are generally focused on education and support of families and patients, using materials like the Medical Traumatic Stress Toolkit,[12] available through the National Child Traumatic Stress Network website at www.nctsn.org. Because they are the norm, there are few rigorous studies of the utility of these services. One study with adolescents found that the participating adolescents had an overall decrease in the level of distress when compared with a waitlist control group, and improvements in body image and anxiety about psychosexual issues.[65] Another study which used a web-based resource for families of children newly diagnosed with cancer found a disappointing level of use, with most hits on the peer discussion groups.[66] These virtual groups appear to be more acceptable to adolescents than in-person support groups, and are worthy of exploration.

Targeted interventions for pain and distress have been better studied. According to the Cochrane Central Register of Controlled Trials, distraction and hypnosis have the largest impact on self-reported pain, and cognitive behavioural interventions have the largest effect size on other reported and behavioural measures of distress in children undergoing needle-related procedures.[67] A review of the literature in paediatric oncology found 32 research articles suggesting that the use of mind–body interventions such as hypnosis, distraction and imagery can be helpful for managing procedure-related pain, anxiety and distress.[68]

Family-focused interventions

Weekend camps have been the most common types of family-focused interventions. Family camps can accommodate families of varying sizes and children of various ages in a casual and comfortable setting, with adequate medical support. They help reduce the sense of isolation commonly experienced by parents of childhood cancer patients on active treatment, increase the sense of normalcy for the children, and are well received by families.[69]

A more targeted family intervention has also been tested, based on a post-traumatic stress model with apparently beneficial results.[70] However, these types of interventions are expensive in terms of professional time. A promising screening tool may help to target future interventions to those families at highest risk, for maximum benefit. The Psychosocial Adaptation Tool provided risk classifications which were stable over time, with almost two thirds of the families remaining at the same level of risk across the first 4 months of cancer treatment. Families classified at higher levels of psychosocial risk at diagnosis had more distress, more family problems and greater psychosocial service use 4 months into treatment.[71]

Case study

Jasmine, a 13-year-old girl, born in the United States to parents who had emigrated from Romania, was diagnosed with osteogenic sarcoma in her right femur. Her father was very well educated, with a master's degree in engineering, and was fluent in English. He taught maths at a local high school and taught night classes at the community college. Her mother had some college education, but did not speak fluent English, and she was primarily at home with Jasmine and her four younger siblings. Jasmine's mother was very frightened, as everyone she had ever known with cancer had died. She felt overwhelmed making important medical decisions, as the doctors seemed to expect her to do when she was in the hospital or clinic with Jasmine. She felt that such decisions should be made by her husband, who spoke better English and was more educated, but he was often unreachable during the day. This created tension between the parents as her husband felt his job was to keep employed so they had money and medical insurance. Jasmine and her family got a lot of their support from the local Catholic Church. When a hospital chaplain visited, Jasmine confessed she was wrestling with why this had happened to her, feeling she must have sinned. She also worried that she would never get married, as she would be so ugly after an amputation.

Siblings

Services for siblings have focused on enhancing coping skills and increasing knowledge and understanding of the medical situation. A review of studies of interventions for siblings found significant improvements in depressive symptoms, health-related quality of life and medical knowledge.[72] An example is a summer camp for siblings that used projective measures (the Human Figure Drawing and the Kinetic Family Drawing-Revised) and found that the siblings' emotional distress scores decreased significantly after camp compared to pre-camp measures.[73]

Psychopharmacology

The goals for intervention for children undergoing the long and often painful treatment of cancer have been similar for the past 20 years: to maximize comfort and minimize pain, using both non-pharmacological and pharmacological interventions, including preparation and support of the child and family, with consideration of the developmental age of the child.[74] However, the pharmacological recommendations have changed somewhat over the years. Pre-medication with benzodiazepines, once used routinely for paediatric procedures, is now of questioned benefit.[75] Diagnostic imaging is done without sedation when possible, and agents such as chloral hydrate, barbiturates and benzodiazepines are being replaced by etomidate, propofol and dexmedetomidine.[76]

However, there is a very limited evidence base to guide psychopharmacology in paediatric oncology, and most of it is without controls and with small samples sizes. For example, fluvoxamine was found to be well tolerated in a five-week, open-label study of 100 mg orally per day, with a significant decrease in symptoms of depression and anxiety.[77] Low-dose haloperidol has been found to be effective in treating symptoms of sleep–wake cycle disturbance, agitation, lability of affect, and impairments of orientation, attention and short-term memory in 45 paediatric oncology patients with delirium.[78] A practical treatment algorithm has been published for the use of medications to treat delirium in paediatric oncology, based on subtypes of delirium which have been identified. Hyperactive and hypoactive/mixed types of delirium appear to have differential response to haloperidol and risperidone.[79]

Despite the sparse research literature, specific serotonin reuptake inhibitors (SSRIs) are frequently prescribed by paediatric oncologists. One major paediatric oncology centre surveyed 40 of their oncologists and found that half of the oncologists prescribed SSRIs for their patients. Most of these prescriptions were given during the first year of treatment. Common reasons for the prescriptions were the perception that the patient was sad, anxious, or had a major depressive disorder.[80] In a subsequent survey of 151 paediatric oncologists from 9 children's cancer centres, 71% of the oncologists reported prescribing SSRIs for their patients. Only 28% reported monitoring patients on SSRIs at the intervals recommended by the FDA for children and adolescents, and only 9% reported they assess for suicidal ideation.[81] However, most oncologists would agree that use of psychopharmacology in children under active treatment for cancer requires great care and careful monitoring.[82]

Key points

- Children and families are resilient, even in the face of something as overwhelming as cancer. Given education and support, the vast majority will do well.
- Those who had pre-existing vulnerability, such as children with anxiety disorder or families in conflict, are more likely to have problems with depression, anxiety and PTSD.
- Although some general interventions are useful, specific screening instruments are needed to target intensive interventions to where they are needed.
- Perceived life threat and aspects of intensity of treatment (such as cranial radiation), appear to be predictors of poorer outcome in adulthood.
- There is little evidence for the use of commonly used medications such as SSRIs, haloperidol and risperidone.
- With better survival of childhood cancer, long-term survivors are a major challenge for future medical and psychosocial care.

Acknowledgements

Ms Strom's effort on this chapter was supported by a fellowship from the American Pediatric Society and Society for Pediatric Research.

Suggested further reading

Kreitler S., Arush M.W.B. (eds) (2004) *Psychosocial Aspects of Pediatric Oncology*, John Wiley & Sons, Ltd, Chichester.

Shaw R.J., DeMaso D.R. (eds) (2010) *Pediatric Psychosomatic Medicine*, American Psychiatric Publishing, Inc., Arlington, VA.

Brown R.T., Anonuccio D.O., DuPaul G.J. *et al.* (2008) *Childhood Mental Health Disorders*, American Psychological Association, Washington, DC.

References

1. American Academy of Pediatrics, Section on Hematology/Oncology (2004) Guidelines for Pediatric Cancer Centers: Policy Statement. *Pediatrics*, 113, 1833–1835.
2. American Cancer Society (2010) *Cancer Facts & Figures 2010* at http://www.cancer.org/Research/CancerFactsFigures/CancerFactsFigures/cancer-facts-and-figures-2010 (accessed 24 July 2011).
3. U.S. Cancer Statistics Working Group (2010) *United States Cancer Statistics: 1999–2007 Cancer Incidence and Mortality Data*, Web-based Report, U.S. Department of Health and Human Services, Centers for Disease Control and Prevention and National Cancer Institute, Atlanta; http://apps.nccd.cdc.gov/uscs/ (last accessed January 2012).
4. Linabery A.M., Ross J.A. (2008) Childhood and adolescent cancer survival in the US by race and ethnicity for the diagnostic period 1975–1999. *Cancer*, 113, 2575–2596.
5. Zeltzer L.K., Recklitis C., Buchbinder D. *et al.* (2009) Psychological status in childhood cancer survivors: A report from the Childhood Cancer Survivor Study. *Journal of Clinical Oncology*, 27, 2396–2404.
6. Kurtz B.P., Abrams A.N. (2010) Psychiatric aspects of pediatric cancer. *Child and Adolescent Psychiatric Clinics of North America*, 19, 401–421, x–xi.
7. Apter A., Farbstein I., Yaniv I. (2003) Psychiatric aspects of pediatric cancer. *Child and Adolescent Psychiatric Clinics of North America*, 12, 473–492, vii.
8. Patiño-Fernández A.M., Pai A.L., Alderfer M. *et al.* (2008) Acute stress in parents of children newly diagnosed with cancer. *Pediatric Blood Cancer*, 50, 289–292.
9. Robinson K.E., Gerhardt C.A., Vannatta K., Noll R.B. (2007) Parent and family factors associated with child adjustment to pediatric cancer. *Journal of Pediatric Psychology*, 32, 400–410.
10. Parsons S.K., Brown A.P. (1998) Evaluation of quality of life of childhood cancer survivors: A methodological conundrum. *Medical Pediatric Oncology*, Suppl 1, 46–53.
11. Stuber M.L., Meeske K.A., Krull K.R. *et al.* (2010) Prevalence and predictors of posttraumatic stress disorder in adult survivors of childhood cancer. *Pediatrics*, 125, e1124–1134.
12. Stuber M.L., Schneider S., Kassam-Adams N. *et al.* (2006) The medical traumatic stress toolkit. *CNS Spectrum*, 11, 137–142.
13. Bretherton I. (1997) Bowlby's legacy to developmental psychology. *Child Psychiatry and Human Development*, 28, 33–43.
14. Hardgrove C.B., Kermoian R. (1978) Parent-inclusive pediatric units: A survey of policies and practices. *American Journal of Public Health*, 68, 847–850.
15. Smith A.B., Hefley G.C., Anand K.J. (2007) Parent bed spaces in the PICU: Effect on parental stress. *Pediatric Nursing*, 33, 215–221.
16. Duhn L. (2010) The importance of touch in the development of attachment. *Advances in Neonatal Care*, 10, 294–300.
17. Eiser C. (1984) Communicating with sick and hospitalised children. *Journal of Child Psychology and Psychiatry*, 25, 181–189.
18. American Psychiatric Association (1994) *Diagnostic and Statistical Manual*, APA Press, Washington, DC.
19. Stuber M.L., Nader K.O., Houskamp B.M., Pynoos R.S. (1996) Appraisal of life threat and acute trauma responses in pediatric bone marrow transplant patients. *Journal of Traumatic Stress*, 9, 673–686.
20. Bluebond-Langner M., Perkel D., Goertzel T. *et al.* (1990) Children's knowledge of cancer and its treatment: Impact of an oncology camp experience. *Journal of Pediatrics*, 116, 207–213.
21. Abrams A.N., Hazen E.P., Penson R.T. (2007) Psychosocial issues in adolescent with cancer. *Cancer Treatment Reviews*, 33, 622–630.
22. Stuber M., Gonzalez S., Benjamin H., Golant M. (1995) Fighting for recovery: Group interventions for adolescent with cancer patients and their parents. *The Journal of Psychotherapy Practice and Research*, 4, 286–296.

23. Shemesh E., Annunziato R.A., Newcorn J.H. *et al.* (2006) Assessment of posttraumatic stress symptoms in children who are medically ill and children presenting to a child trauma program. *Annals of the New York Academy of Sciences*, 1071, 472–477.
24. Kazak A.E., Barakat L.P., Meeske,K. *et al.* (1997) Posttraumatic stress symptoms, family functioning, and social support in survivors of childhood leukemia and their mothers and fathers. *Journal of Consulting and Clinical Psychology*, 65, 120–129.
25. Stuber M.L., Kazak A.E., Meeske K. *et al.* (1997) A. Predictors of posttraumatic stress symptoms in childhood cancer survivors. *Pediatrics*, 100, 958–964.
26. Alderfer M.A., Navsaria N., Kazak A.E. (2009) Family functioning and posttraumatic stress disorder in adolescent survivors of childhood cancer. *Journal of Family Psychology*, 23, 717–725.
27. Turkel S.B., Tavaré C.J. (2003) Delirium in children and adolescents. *Journal of Neuropsychiatry and Clinical Neuroscience*, 15, 431–435.
28. Hatherill S., Flisher A.J. (2010) Delirium in children and adolescents: A systematic review of the literature. *Journal of Psychosomatic Research*, 68, 337–344.
29. Turkel S.B., Trzepacz P.T., Tavaré C.J. (2006) Comparing symptoms of delirium in adults and children. *Psychosomatics*, 47, 320–324.
30. Janssen N.J., Tan E.Y., Staal M. *et al.* (2011) On the utility of diagnostic instruments for pediatric delirium in critical illness: An evaluation of the Pediatric Anesthesia Emergence Delirium Scale, the Delirium Rating Scale 88, and the Delirium Rating Scale-Revised R-98. *Intensive Care Medicine*, 37, 1331–1337.
31. Silver G.H., Kearney J.A., Kutko M.C., Bartell A.S. (2010) Infant delirium in pediatric critical care settings. *American Journal of Psychiatry*, 167, 1172–1177.
32. Schieveld J., Staal M., Voogd L. *et al.* (2010) Refractory agitation as a marker for pediatric delirium in very young infants at a pediatric intensive care unit. *Intensive Care Medicine*, 36, 1982–1983.
33. Kersun L.S., Rourke M.T., Mickley M., Kazak A.E. (2009) Screening for depression and anxiety in adolescent cancer patients. *Journal of Pediatric Hematology and Oncology*, 31, 835–839.
34. Shemesh E., Yehuda R., Rockmore L. *et al.* (2005) Assessment of depression in medically ill children presenting to pediatric specialty clinics. *Journal of the American Academy of Child and Adolescent Psychiatry*, 44, 1249–1257.
35. Oeffinger K.C., Mertens A.C., Sklar C.A. *et al.* (2006) Chronic health conditions in adult survivors of childhood cancer. Childhood Cancer Survivor Study. *New England Journal of Medicine*, 355, 1572–1582.
36. American Academy of Pediatrics, Section on Hematology/Oncology, Children's Oncology Group (2009) Long-term follow-up care for pediatric cancer survivors. *Pediatrics*, 123, 906–915.
37. Castellino S.M., Casillas J., Hudson M.M. *et al.* (2005) Minority adult survivors of childhood cancer: A comparison of long-term outcomes, health care utilization, and health-related behaviors from the childhood cancer survivor study. *Journal of Clinical Oncology*, 23, 6499–6507.
38. Robison L.L., Armstrong G.T., Boice J.D. *et al.* (2009) The Childhood Cancer Survivor Study: A National Cancer Institute-Supported Resource for Outcome and Intervention Research. *Journal of Clinical Oncology*, 27, 2308–2318.
39. Reulen R.C., Frobisher C., Winter D.L. *et al.* (2011) British Childhood Cancer Survivor Study Steering Group. Long-term risks of subsequent primary neoplasms among survivors of childhood cancer. *Journal of the American Medical Association*, 305, 2311–2319.
40. McDougall J., Tsonis M. (2009) Quality of life in survivors of childhood cancer: A systematic review of the literature (2001–2008). *Supportive Care in Cancer*, 17, 1231–1246.
41. Wakefield C.E., McLoone J., Goodenough B. *et al.* (2010) The psychosocial impact of completing childhood cancer treatment: A systematic review of the literature. *Journal of Pediatric Psychology*, 35, 262–274.
42. Michel G., Rebholz C.E., von der Weid N.X. *et al.* (2010) Psychological distress in adult survivors of childhood cancer: The Swiss Childhood Cancer Survivor study. *Journal of Clinical Oncology*, 28, 1740–1748. Epub 2010 Mar 1.
43. Kazak A.E., Derosa B.W., Schwartz L.A. *et al.* (2010) Psychological outcomes and health beliefs in adolescent and young adult survivors of childhood cancer and controls. *Journal of Clinical Oncology*, 28, 2002–2007.
44. Harila M.J., Niinivirta T.I., Winqvist S., Harila-Saari A.H. (2011) Low depressive symptom and mental distress scores in adult long-term survivors of childhood acute lymphoblastic leukemia. *Journal of Pediatric Hematology/Oncology*, 33, 194–198.
45. Dieluweit U., Seitz D.C., Besier T. *et al.* (2011) Utilization of psychosocial care and oncological follow-up assessments among German long-term survivors of cancer with onset during adolescence. *Klinische Pädiatrie*, 223, 152–158.

46. O'Leary T.E., Diller L., Recklitis C.J. (2007) The effects of response bias on self-reported quality of life among childhood cancer survivors. *Quality of Life Research*, 16, 1211–1220.
47. Kazak A.E., Stuber M.L., Barakat L.P., Meeske K. (1997) Assessing posttraumatic stress related to medical illness and treatment: The Impact of Traumatic Stressors Interview Schedule (ITSIS). *Families, Systems and Health*, 14, 365–380.
48. Kamibeppu K., Sato I., Honda M. *et al.* (2010) Mental health among young adult survivors of childhood cancer and their siblings including posttraumatic growth. *Journal of Cancer Survivors*, 4, 303–312.
49. Currier J.M., Hermes S., Phipps S. (2009) Brief report: Children's response to serious illness: Perceptions of benefit and burden in a pediatric cancer population. *Journal of Pediatric Psychology*, 34, 1129–1134.
50. Maurice-Stam H., Broek A., Kolk A.M., *et al.* (2011) Measuring perceived benefit and disease-related burden in young cancer survivors: Validation of the Benefit and Burden Scale for Children (BBSC) in the Netherlands. *Supportive Care in Cancer*, 19, 1249–1253.
51. Zebrack B.J., Stuber M.L., Meeske K.A. *et al.* (2011) Perceived positive impact of cancer among long-term survivors of childhood cancer: A report from the childhood cancer survivor study. *Psycho-Oncology*, Mar 22, DOI: 10.1002/pon.1959.
52. Recklitis C.J., Diller L.R., Li X. *et al.* (2010) Suicide ideation in adult survivors of childhood cancer: A report from the Childhood Cancer Survivor Study. *Journal of Clinical Oncology*, 28, 655–661.
53. Hobbie W.L., Stuber M., Meeske K. *et al.* (2000) Symptoms of posttraumatic stress in young adult survivors of childhood cancer. *Journal of Clinical Oncology*, 18, 4060–4066.
54. Bruce M. (2006) A systematic and conceptual review of posttraumatic stress in childhood cancer survivors and their parents. *Clinical Psychology Reviews*, 26, 233–256.
55. Stuber M.L., Meeske K.A., Leisenring W. *et al.* (2011) Defining medical posttraumatic stress among young adult survivors in the Childhood Cancer Survivor Study. *General Hospital Psychiatry*, 33, 347–353.
56. Pöder U., Ljungman G., von Essen L. (2008) Posttraumatic stress disorder among parents of children on cancer treatment: A longitudinal study. *Psycho-Oncology*, 17, 430–437.
57. Hardy K.K., Bonner M.J., Masi R. *et al.* (2008) Psychosocial functioning in parents of adult survivors of childhood cancer. *Journal of Pediatric Hematology Oncology*, 30, 153–159.
58. Stuber M.L., Christakis D.A., Houskamp B., Kazak A.E. (1996) Posttrauma symptoms in childhood leukemia survivors and their parents. *Psychosomatics*, 37, 254–261.
59. Kazak A.E., Stuber M.L., Barakat L.P. *et al.* (1998) Predicting posttraumatic stress symptoms in mothers and fathers of survivors of childhood cancers. *Journal of the American Academy of Child and Adolescent Psychiatry*, 37, 823–831.
60. Fayed N., Klassen A.F., Dix D. *et al.* (2011) Exploring predictors of optimism among parents of children with cancer. *Psycho-Oncology*, DOI: 10.1002/pon.1743.
61. Robinson K.E., Gerhardt C.A., Vannatta K., Noll R.B. (2009) Survivors of childhood cancer and comparison peers: The influence of early family factors on distress in emerging adulthood. *Journal of Family Psychology*, 23, 23–31.
62. Buchbinder D., Casillas J., Zeltzer L. (2011) Meeting the psychosocial needs of sibling survivors: A family systems approach. *Journal of Pediatric Oncology Nursing*, 28, 123–136.
63. Ballard K.L. (2004) Meeting the needs of siblings of children with cancer. *Pediatric Nursing*, 30, 394–401.
64. Sidhu R., Passmore A., Baker D. (2005) An investigation into parent perceptions of the needs of siblings of children with cancer. *Journal of Pediatric Oncology Nursing*, 22, 276–287.
65. Seitz D.C., Besier T., Goldbeck L. (2009) Psychosocial interventions for adolescent cancer patients: A systematic review of the literature. *Psycho-Oncology*, 18, 683–690.
66. Ewing L.J., Long K., Rotondi A. *et al.* (2009) Brief report: A pilot study of a web-based resource for families of children with cancer. *Journal of Pediatric Psychology*, 34, 523–529.
67. Uman L.S., Chambers C.T., McGrath P.J., Kisely S. (2006) Psychological interventions for needle-related procedural pain and distress in children and adolescents. *Cochrane Database Systematic Review*, 4, CD005179.
68. Landier W., Tse A.M. (2010) Use of complementary and alternative medical interventions for the management of procedure-related pain, anxiety, and distress in pediatric oncology: An integrative review. *Journal of Pediatric Nursing*, 25, 566–579.
69. Ruffin J.E., Creed J.M., Jarvis C. (1997) A retreat for families of children recently diagnosed with cancer. *Cancer Practice*, 5, 99–104.
70. Pai A.L., Kazak A.E. (2006) Pediatric medical traumatic stress in pediatric oncology: Family systems

interventions. *Current Opinions in Pediatrics,* 18, 558–562.

71. Kazak A.E., Barakat L.P., Ditaranto S. *et al.* (2011) Screening for psychosocial risk at pediatric cancer diagnosis: The psychosocial assessment tool. *Journal of Pediatric Hematology and Oncology,* 33, 289–294.
72. Prchal A., Landolt M.A. (2009) Psychological interventions with siblings of pediatric cancer patients: A systematic review. *Psycho-Oncology,* 18, 1241–1251.
73. Packman W., Mazaheri M., Sporri L. *et al.* (2008) Projective drawings as measures of psychosocial functioning in siblings of pediatric cancer patients from the Camp Okizu study. *Journal of Pediatric Oncology Nursing,* 25, 44–55.
74. Hockenberry M.J., McCarthy K., Taylor O. *et al.* (2011) Managing painful procedures in children with cancer. *Journal of Pediatric Hematology Oncology,* 33, 119–127.
75. Rosenbaum A., Kain Z.N., Larsson P. *et al.* (2009) The place of premedication in pediatric practice. *Paediatric Anaesthesia,* 19, 817–828.
76. Rutman M.S. (2009) Sedation for emergent diagnostic imaging studies in pediatric patients. *Current Opinions in Pediatrics,* 21, 306–312.
77. Gothelf D., Rubinstein M., Shemesh E. *et al.* (2005) Pilot study: Fluvoxamine treatment for depression and anxiety disorders in children and adolescents with cancer. *Journal of the American Academy of Child and Adolescent Psychiatry,* 44, 1258–1262.
78. Grover S., Malhotra S., Bharadwaj R., Bn S., Kumar S. (2009) Delirium in children and adolescents. *International Journal of Psychiatric Medicine,* 39, 179–187.
79. Karnik N.S., Joshi S.V., Paterno C., Shaw R. (2007) Subtypes of pediatric delirium: A treatment algorithm. *Psychosomatics,* 48, 253–257.
80. Kersun L.S., Kazak A.E. (2006) Prescribing practices of selective serotonin reuptake inhibitors (SSRIs) among pediatric oncologists: A single institution experience. *Pediatric Blood Cancer,* 47, 339–342.
81. Phipps S., Buckholdt K.E., Fernandez L. *et al.* (2011) Pediatric oncologists' practices of prescribing selective serotonin reuptake inhibitors (SSRIs) for children and adolescents with cancer: A multi-site study. *Pediatric Blood Cancer,* Jan 31, DOI: 10.1002/pbc.22788.
82. Kersun L.S., Elia J. (2007) Depressive symptoms and SSRI use in pediatric oncology patients. *Pediatric Blood Cancer,* 49, 881–887.

CHAPTER 12

A Life-stage Approach to Psycho-oncology

Peter Fitzgerald[1], *Rinat Nissim*[2] *and Gary Rodin*[3]

[1]Fellow in Psychosocial Oncology, Princess Margaret Hospital, Toronto, Canada

[2]Department of Psychosocial Oncology and Palliative Care, Princess Margaret Hospital, University Health Network, Toronto, Canada

[3]Department of Psychiatry, University of Toronto; Department of Psychosocial Oncology and Palliative Care, Princess Margaret Hospital; Senior Scientist, Ontario Cancer Institute, Ontario, Canada

Introduction and background

Some cancers, particularly haematological malignancies and cancers of the brain, thyroid and testis, commonly affect younger adults. However, the vast majority of cancers occur in adults aged >50 and more than half of all cancers occur in those aged >65.[1] Further, cancer incidence worldwide has been growing in industrial nations since the middle of the last century because of the steady expansion of this age group. In fact, it has been estimated that the number of such individuals in developed nations will double over the next 25 years.

Age-related differences may affect the nature and course of cancer, the effectiveness and toxicity of treatment and the experience and psychosocial impact of the disease.[2,3] However, it is not possible to identify precise age boundaries that demarcate groups in meaningful ways. Indeed, 'old age' is difficult to define because of variability in the biological, psychosocial and cultural factors that affect the process of ageing. Age 65 has frequently been adopted as an arbitrary point to define people as elderly, although individuals above this age are heterogeneous, both physically and psychologically. A lifespan perspective,[4] in which age is regarded as only a rough proxy for life stage, may be a more useful approach to understanding the impact of cancer and the potential needs of individuals and their families for therapeutic intervention. Such an approach is consistent with the view that adaptation involves balancing the sequential of gains and losses that occur at all stages of the lifespan.

Some have divided the life stages of older adults into the 'young-old', and the 'old-old'. The developmental tasks of the 'young-old' include consideration of retirement, transition to post-retirement roles, and the establishment of new life goals. For those at this life stage who enjoy good health, cancer may be a shocking experience which disrupts a state of relative well-being. By contrast, the 'old-old' may have already experienced a noticeable decline in physical and cognitive function, with reduced social contact because of more limited mobility and the death of family and friends. The cultural and family context of those affected by cancer may also shape the perception of gains and losses at this life stage. For example, the extent to which individuals feel honoured and valued, even when they are elderly and ill, may have a profound effect on the degree of distress and demoralization that is experienced when cancer occurs.

The common tendency to view older adults as a homogeneous group may have obscured the variability in the life stage and needs of this group of cancer patients. For that reason, some have

Clinical Psycho-Oncology: An International Perspective, First Edition. Edited by Luigi Grassi and Michelle Riba.

suggested that frailty, which has only a rough correlation with chronological age, may be a more useful defining characteristic. That term has been used to refer to an increased vulnerability to stressors due to impairments in multiple, inter-related systems that lead to an increased risk for multiple adverse health-related outcomes.[5] In this chapter, we will adopt a life-stage approach, focusing on the impact of cancer on patients in the later stages of life, contrasting their problems and concerns with younger patients and will emphasize strategies to provide optimal care to this group.

The psychological impact of cancer in old age

The process of adjustment to cancer may vary across the adult lifespan, based on normative developmental changes in identity, social roles and responsibilities, emotion regulation and relationships. Knowledge about how older individuals react and experience cancer is scant, although the existing literature suggests that younger adults with cancer experience more cancer-related distress, less satisfaction with quality of life, and more post-traumatic stress symptoms than older adults with cancer. Some studies show that these age differences are most prominent at the time of diagnosis and diminish by 3 months after diagnosis. However, older cancer patients may face particular challenges due to other lifespan changes such as widowhood, social isolation, illness comorbidities, and decline in physical functioning.

Some research indicates that old age may protect from psychological distress because of its association with greater life experience, more time to prepare for illness and disability, more attachment security and a greater capacity to find meaning in life in the face of illness.[6] Others suggest that the different social roles of younger and older persons also shape how they cope with the stress of cancer. In that regard, older adults tend to have fewer competing demands, as they may have often already accomplished more of their financial and child-rearing tasks. In addition, while active problem-solving strategies are more common in younger adults, older individuals tend to be more able to accept realistic goals in the context of the illness and to experience less emotional disturbance. Other factors may also contribute to age differences in distress, including the aggressiveness of the cancer, the intensity of the treatment and the likelihood to develop treatment toxicity. There may also be age-related and generational effects that contribute to greater comfort of younger patients in communicating emotional distress and obtaining social support.

Access to cancer care and psychosocial oncology services

A variety of factors in older cancer patients and in their medical caregivers may contribute to the frequency with which such individuals receive less adequate health care. Older patients are less likely to be screened for cancer, to receive information about treatment options, and to be delivered suboptimal treatment, even after controlling for comorbidities, cancer stage, performance status and socioeconomic status. Moreover, older patients are under-represented in clinical trials, so that less is known about appropriate cancer treatment for this population. Treatment biases based on chronological age have also been documented in relation to pain management and palliative care. For example, Hall *et al.*[7] reported that with each decade of life after the age of 40, patients are less likely to be prescribed opioids; others have reported a reduced likelihood of older patients to receive palliative radiotherapy. In addition, a bias in referrals to psychosocial support has been observed. For example, Ellis *et al.*[8] reported that even amongst those with significant and comparable distress, adults with metastatic cancer age 40 or younger were five times more likely to be referred for psychosocial care than those who are >70 years.

The relative neglect of the needs of older cancer patients may stem from a variety of factors. Such individuals may be less able or less willing to advocate for themselves, may perceive more stigma related to psychosocial care, or may believe that pain and emotional distress are burdens that they

Table 12.1 Comprehensive Geriatric Assessment Measures.

Domain	Instrument	No. of items	Time required (mins)
Function	Activities of daily living	8	5–10
Nutrition	Mini Nutritional Assessment	6	<5
Comorbidity	Cumulative illness rating scale	13	10
Social support	RAND medical social support scale	5	<5
Cognition	Blessed Orientation Memory	6	<5
Depression	Geriatric Depression Scale	15	<5

must bear. Ageism or biases in health care providers regarding the elderly may also contribute to the discrepancy in the provision of services. Medical caregivers who are younger than their patients may be less likely to identify with them and to refer them for psychosocial care. In some cases, there may be unjustified assumptions that older adults would neither want nor tolerate certain interventions. Such attitudes of medical caregivers toward older patients may create a circumstance in which the wishes of older patients for less aggressive care are more readily accepted, and in which older patients may accept less than optimal psychosocial and medical care. Older patients may require additional time and effort dedicated to explain to them the risks and benefits of treatment and to encourage their involvement in decision-making and in obtaining access to support services. Similarly, education regarding symptom control may be of particular value to older adults who may believe that analgesia should be used only when pain is intolerable or that 'good patients' should not complain. Establishing approaches for cancer care that take into account frailty and life stage will become even more important as the population ages.

Assessment considerations

The Comprehensive Geriatric Assessment

Though chronological age often influences medical decision-making, there is considerable variability within the elderly population with regard to biological, psychological and social parameters. A systematic evaluation of functional age is therefore necessary to identify appropriate interventions to facilitate psychosocial well-being and quality of life for the older cancer patient. This can be performed using a multidimensional battery of validated standardized tools, which together is known as the Comprehensive Geriatric Assessment (CGA). The purpose of the CGA is to record the assessment of such geriatric domains as comorbidity, functional status, cognitive and psychological status, medications and social support (see Table 12.1 below for examples of individual measures).

Research has found that the CGA uncovers previously undetected conditions in over half of those who undergo this assessment. Such comorbidities are common in older cancer patients and can affect treatment tolerance, life expectancy, and needs for psychosocial and palliative care. The likelihood of polypharmacy increases with the number of comorbid conditions, which in turn increases the risk of drug interactions with chemotherapy agents. Frail individuals are not only physiologically less able to tolerate a course of rigorous chemotherapy, but they are also at greater risk of social isolation and of having less capacity to communicate emotional distress. The CGA can help clinicians to uncover such factors, which may be relevant to medical decision-making and to quality of life.[9] In many settings, shorter versions of the CGA, such as the 13 item self-report Vulnerable Elders Survey (VES-13), may be more feasible to use for initial screening purposes, as recommended by the National Cancer Comprehensive Network (NCCN) practice guidelines for senior adults. Those who are identified as vulnerable can then be assessed with more comprehensive CGA.

Cognitive assessment and capacity

Older cancer patients are at greater risk to suffer from pre-morbid neurocognitive impairment or to develop this secondary to the disease and its treatment. While cognitive status should be assessed in all individuals attending an oncology service, this is especially important in the elderly, and in those with advanced cancer or brain disease because of their increased risk of delirium or an underlying dementia.

Dementia is characterized by a progressive deterioration in such aspects of cognitive functioning as memory, judgment, language and problem-solving. It may also be manifest in disinhibited or socially inappropriate behaviour, self-neglect, or emotional liability, including 'catastrophic' reactions characterized by overwhelming emotional responses to relatively minor stressors. Prevalence rates of dementia steadily increase from 5–10% in those over the age of 65 to 25–50% in those >80 years. However, it is often undetected in clinical settings, particularly when short-term memory loss is not prominent. The failure to identify underlying dementia in the elderly may lead to an underestimation of the risk of delirium as a complication of chemotherapy, other drug treatment or of radiotherapy to the brain. The routine use of validated screening tools such as the Mini Mental State Examination, the Mini-Cog or the Blessed Dementia Scale may be of great value to identify those with cognitive impairment who are at risk.

Delirium is an acute disturbance of attention and arousal with a characteristic fluctuating pattern throughout the course of the day. It should be considered in any cancer patients in either an agitated or hypoactive state with altered behaviour or levels of consciousness. It is common in the elderly, particularly in those with dementia, advanced disease receiving chemotherapy and other medications, or who suffer from pain, sepsis, or cerebral metastases. Careful clinical assessment is important since hypoactive delirium is often mistaken for depression in clinical settings.

When cognitive impairment is present, it is mandatory to assess its impact on quality of life and on the capacity for self-management and to make informed decisions about treatment. However, the presence of cognitive impairment does not necessarily imply a lack of capacity, which must be assessed in relation to the specific decision or situation at hand. The four core features of capacity that must be elicited in a clinical assessment are: an understanding or appreciation of the treatment; awareness of its risks and benefits; the capacity for reasoning; and, a statement of choice from the patient regarding the treatment decision. Techniques that can be employed to improve and to demonstrate capacity include: disclosing information in small amounts, using vocabulary which is familiar to the patient, and asking for regular feedback from the patient about what has been discussed before ultimately asking if the patient feels able to decide.[10]

Assessment of depression

The clinical assessment of depression in cancer patients should take into account the varied manner in which it may present across the life cycle. Compared to their younger counterparts, depressed older individuals may be less likely to endorse affective symptoms, such as sadness, anhedonia and worthlessness, and more likely to express psychological distress in terms of physical symptoms. This symptom pattern, combined with the greater overall reluctance of the elderly to disclose emotional difficulties to health professionals, increases the likelihood that depression will not be detected in this age group. Weinberger and colleagues[11] suggest that attention to the typical symptom patterns of depression in the elderly and in cancer patients may increase detection of depression in individuals with this comorbidity. These include general malaise, diffuse somatic symptoms, late insomnia, diurnal mood variation, agitation, anxiety and loss of sexual interest.

Screening tools for depression

Routine distress screening has been widely recommended and is increasingly being implemented in cancer care. A depression scale specific for older cancer patients has not yet been developed, although many of the commonly used scales do not assess the depressive symptoms that are often reported by these patients. Nelson and colleagues concluded, in their recent review of self-report depression rating scales for elderly cancer patients, that the CES-D has been the most extensively validated in both geriatric and cancer populations.[12] However, they noted that it does not include a number of the common depressive symptoms in elderly cancer patients. There is clearly a pressing need for further research in this area.

Social support and attachment security

Supportive relationships are one of the most significant factors influencing the well-being of all cancer patients. Such relationships enhance psychological well-being, the sense of meaning and connectedness, buffer emotional distress, and facilitate access to medical and palliative care. However, social networks tend to shrink with advancing age, as a result of the death of family and friends, retirement from employment, and declining health and functional ability. This loss of meaningful relationships places the older adult at greater risk of depression, social isolation, and loss of meaning in life, although some are protected by long-term marital and family relationships and by greater attachment security. The latter, which is distinct from actual social support, refers to internalized expectations of support and the capacity to make use of relationships for this purpose.

Psychosocial interventions

During the past several decades, numerous psychosocial interventions to reduce and prevent distress in cancer patients have been tested (see Chapters 6 and 7). The majority of these interventions are structured, time-limited psychotherapies or educational programmes for individuals or groups. The impact of age has not been evaluated in most of these interventions or in reviews of their effectiveness, although some evidence suggests that older adults prefer interventions that include both education and support.

Holland and colleagues[13] have developed a novel theoretically grounded group psycho-educational intervention specifically for elderly individuals with cancer. It draws upon both Erickson's life stage developmental theory and on Folkman's cognitive coping paradigm in which life review discussions, sharing memories, and finding meaning and contributing to the good of others facilitates adaptation. Holland and her colleagues proposed that elderly cancer patients who are distressed, lonely or isolated may have failed to use such age-appropriate coping strategies. This intervention, currently being tested for its effectiveness, addresses the following domains: coping with cancer and ageing; loneliness; making peace with one's life; and generativity or the passing on of wisdom to others. Although outcome evaluations are not yet available, this approach holds promise as a tailored intervention for this population.

Supportive-expressive therapies also allow consideration of contextual and life-stage developmental challenges that contribute to distress in the cancer patient. Such therapies tend to be focused on emotion modulation, reflective functioning, and the promotion of psychological growth. They allow the processing of painful affect states associated with the trauma of diagnosis, recurrence and advancement of disease and with the multiple losses that have occurred and are anticipated. Three such therapies, which are outlined below, are Life Review Therapy, Dignity Therapy, and CALM (Managing Cancer and Living Meaningfully).

Life review therapy,[14] an individual or group-based therapy, may be particularly useful intervention for the elderly cancer population. In this intervention, time is spent reminiscing on past experiences throughout the patient's life cycle in order to enhance the sense of integration and meaning of self-experience and self-discovery. Research has demonstrated that it may have a positive impact on life satisfaction, mood, self esteem, and self-acceptance in the elderly, when used either in group or individual format. Within the oncology literature, there is some evidence that life review therapy can reduce suffering through an improvement in both depression and self-esteem.

Dignity therapy is a brief individual therapy designed to address psychosocial and existential distress in patients with advanced disease near the end of life.[15] It includes such themes as the maintenance of hope, the leaving of a legacy, sustaining a sense of meaning at the end of life, and alleviating concerns about burden to others and about the quality of care that is received. Younger patients may be more distressed because of the 'untimely' nature of the disease, and older patients may be more concerned about their legacy. In dignity therapy, the patient is helped to describe aspects of their lives which were most meaningful to them, what they want to be remembered for, and/or what they want to share with loved ones. The intent of the intervention is to facilitate greater acceptance of their existential dilemma and a sense of meaning to their past and current life experiences. This is a brief therapy of only 1 to 3 sessions, usually with a subsequent 'generativity document' returned to patients to leave to a family member or friend. Recent research found that dignity therapy was associated with improvement of depressive symptoms in patients with a life expectancy of less than six months. An international, multicentre randomized trial is currently underway to test this intervention in different palliative care settings.

CALM therapy (Managing Cancer and Living Meaningfully) is a brief, individual psychotherapeutic intervention that has been designed to address the practical and existential questions that face patients who are living with advanced disease. This intervention provides support for symptom management, navigation of the health care system and for the psychological, relational and existential problems that the disease has imposed. The therapy consists of 3–6 individual sessions delivered over 3 months, with 2 booster sessions offered in the subsequent 3 months. Based both on empirical research and on relational and attachment theory, this brief supportive-expressive intervention for patients with an expected survival of at least six months focuses on four main domains: (i) symptom management and communication with health care providers; (ii) changes in self and relations with close others; (iii) spirituality or sense of meaning; (iv) concerns for the future, hope and mortality. These domains provide a framework for the intervention, but the time devoted to each and the sequence in which they are addressed varies according to the individual patient's needs. Preliminary qualitative research[16] has identified benefit from CALM in terms of the reduction of distress, the experience of being understood as a whole person and in the capacity to tolerate mortality-related concerns and to communicate with significant others. Pilot quantitative research has found it to be associated with a reduction in death anxiety, depression, and attachment avoidance and with improved spiritual well-being.

Contextual factors

A variety of cultural and contextual factors may account for differences in the experience and communication of emotional distress between younger and older cancer patients. Culture influences how disease, disability and suffering are experienced, how concerns about them are expressed and how individuals relate to health care providers and to the health care system which serves them. Older individuals may have better support in traditional cultures in which there is greater respect for the elderly and obligation of the younger generations to care for them. Such collectivist cultures tend to be characterized by a wide network of relationships that extends across generations and have greater local community involvement in providing informal support to those in need. These familial traditions may protect against the social isolation which is common in the elderly in Western nations. In that regard, qualitative research on the experience of those living with advanced cancer in sub-Saharan Africa has demonstrated greater reliance on the local community than on formal services for care and support. This may help to engender in those who are ill or elderly a greater sense of value and support which helps to buffer against demoralization and despair, although it can sometimes be a barrier to timely engagement with formal care services or professional information or advice.

Increasing geographic mobility and emigration of younger generations have left older people in some cultures socially isolated and economically disadvantaged, thus diminishing their capacity to cope with declining health. It has also been suggested that there is an age cohort effect in Western cultures, such that older individuals may tend to have greater trust in health care systems, to value stoicism in the face of suffering and to be reluctant to advocate for themselves in medical settings. This age-related 'peer personality' may contribute to the reluctance of older cancer patients to utilize adequate analgesia or other available medical resources and supports. By contrast, those who grew up in the post-war generation may have a greater sense of legitimate entitlement than their older counterparts and may be more likely to advocate for themselves in modern health care settings.

Spiritual well-being

Spiritual well-being has been defined in the medical literatures as an outcome indicating the extent to which individuals are at peace with themselves, feel their lives have meaning and purpose, and derive comfort from their beliefs in the face of suffering.[17] The capacity to find meaning has been shown to grow with age and may be an important protection from distress in the elderly cancer patient.[2] Whereas spiritual well-being was formerly linked exclusively to religious faith, secular sources of spiritual well-being have increasingly been identified in Western cultures. In a recent study of spiritual well-being in a large sample of patients with metastatic cancer,[6] we have found it to be positively linked not only to religiosity but also to self-esteem and social relatedness, and to less physical suffering. Other research has highlighted the association between spirituality and the maintenance of dignity in older adults. Interventions which focus on meaning and self-reflection, leaving a legacy, and conducting a life review, may be of particular relevance for older individuals, although age-related differences in the acceptability and benefit of such interventions have not yet been established. The failure to adequately address spiritual needs can amplify the suffering experienced by many older adults with cancer, particularly those with advanced disease.

Caregiving

Research has demonstrated that family caregivers may experience even greater distress than cancer patients themselves.[18] This may occur because of the sense of loss and worry about the future and because of the disruptions to daily life, the role adjustments and lifestyle adaptations that are necessary to meet the needs of the cancer patient. The extent of such changes and demands differ according to the life stage of the patient and their caregivers. Studies have found that cancer causes greater financial disruption for middle-aged caregivers compared to their older counterparts. Additionally, younger caregivers report greater disruption to daily routines caused by the patient's illness and a greater impact on social networks. The families of younger patients may also face particular financial and social difficulties due to the needs of their children and due to less opportunity to acquire financial security. Culturally specific family beliefs regarding care-giving and care-receiving may also be important considerations. In particular, some older cancer patients, particularly in more individualistic cultures, may be greatly distressed by the role reversal that occurs when they become the recipient of care from their children.

Clinical case study

Mr K. was a 72-year-old married businessman who was referred for psychosocial assessment with his wife one year after the diagnosis of pancreatic cancer because of his and her distress. He had been married for the past 30 years to a woman who was 20 years younger and both described a satisfying and supportive marital relationship. They each had adult children from previous marriages and had remained close with these children and their grandchildren. Mr K. had remained active and continued to work despite his illness. Only recently, as his disease had progressed and his disability increased, had he begun to feel despondent about leaving his wife behind and worried about how she would manage without him. He said that his wife had 'got the worst' of the situation, because she was caring for him and her ailing parents and was required to face the future alone.

Mr K. and his wife benefited from a brief psychotherapeutic intervention. This included a life review and acknowledgement of his accomplishments and of the importance and value of their family and marital relationships. They were also able to discuss in the sessions planning for the end stages of his disease, a task that they had both avoided because it had felt too painful to face. Despite his sadness about leaving his wife behind, Mr K. said that he had come to feel 'at peace' with his illness and with his relatively short expected survival. He felt satisfied with his accomplishments, proud of his children and grandchildren, and confident that he and his wife would be able to manage the difficult journey ahead.

Mr K. is an example of the 'young-old', a man who had continued to work into his seventies and who became frail only with the progression of his cancer. Although he had become mildly depressed, his life stage and life experience allowed him to experience attachment security, to find meaning in his life and to accept the tragedy of his disease. His wife experienced more distress, a common experience for spouse caregivers, and her younger age and previous reliance on him as a confidante and mentor made the adjustment to his progressive disease more difficult for her than for him. The brief psychotherapeutic intervention facilitated the process of adjustment to this most difficult moment in both of their life trajectories.

Summary and conclusions

A life-stage approach in psychosocial oncology draws attention to the varying strengths, vulnerabilities and needs of individuals across the lifespan. Age is a rough proxy for life stage, although there may be large differences in the physical well-being, life tasks and life expectancy of individuals who are similar in age. Growing numbers of older individuals have been physically well prior to the onset of cancer and therefore may experience its onset as highly traumatic. However, most elderly patients are more psychologically prepared for the burden of disease than those who are much younger. Whereas emotional distress tends to be greater in younger cancer patients, older ones tend to be more frail and more sensitive to physical insults to the brain. Such individuals are more likely to develop cognitive impairment and delirium as a complication of cancer treatment and the frequent medical comorbidity, and are more likely to suffer from social isolation and suboptimal access to specialized psychosocial and medical care. However, there may be developmental growth in some capacities of older individuals, despite the more uniform decline in their physical functioning. In that regard, such individuals tend to have better spiritual well-being than those who are younger, and have a greater capacity to find meaning in the face of suffering and adversity.

There has been relatively little attention in the literature to the influence of life stage on the acceptability and benefit of psychosocial interventions. Older individuals may have greater potential to benefit from psychosocial interventions which focus on meaning, although such age-related treatment differences in the acceptability and benefit of specific interventions have not yet been empirically demonstrated. Much more research is needed to determine the appropriateness and effectiveness of psychosocial interventions at different life stages. However, from a clinical perspective, attention to life stage may be of value in that it draws attention to specific neurobiological vulnerabilities, age-related developmental tasks and appropriate interventions to alleviate the psychosocial complications of cancer.

Key points

- A life-stage approach in psychosocial oncology draws attention to the varying strengths, vulnerabilities and needs of individuals across the lifespan.
- Growing numbers of older individuals have been physically well prior to the onset of cancer and therefore may experience its onset as highly traumatic. However, most elderly patients are more psychologically prepared for the burden of disease than those who are much younger.
- There has been relatively little attention in the literature to the influence of life stage on the acceptability and benefit of psychosocial interventions.
- More research is needed to determine the appropriateness and effectiveness of psychosocial interventions at different life stages.

Suggested further reading

On a life-stage approach in psychosocial oncology:

Harden J. (2005) Developmental life stage and couples' experiences with prostate cancer. *Cancer Nursing*, 28, 85–98.

Rowland J. (1990) Developmental states and adaptation: Adult model, in *Handbook of Psycho-oncology: Psychological Care of the Patient with Cancer* (eds J. Holland, J. Rowland), Oxford University Press, New York, pp. 25–43.

On age, cancer, and culture:

Surbone A., Kawaga-Singer M., Terret C., Baider L. (2007) The illness trajectory of elderly cancer patients across cultures, SIOG position paper. *Annals of Oncology*, 18, 633–637.

On ageism in cancer care:

Kagan S.H. (2008) Ageism in cancer care. *Seminars in Oncology Nursing*, 24, 246–253.

References

1. Canadian Cancer Society/National Cancer Institute of Canada (2011) *Canadian Cancer Statistics 2011*, Toronto, Canada.
2. Lo C., Lin J., Gagliese L. *et al.* (2010) Age and depression in patients with metastatic cancer: The protective effects of attachment security and spiritual well-being. *Ageing and Society*, 3, 325–336.
3. Gagliese L., Jovellanos M., Zimmermann C. *et al.* (2009) Age-related patterns in adaptation to cancer pain: A mixed-method study. *Pain Medicine*, 10, 1050–1061.
4. Baltes, P.B. (1987) Theoretical propositions of life-span developmental psychology: On the dynamics between growth and decline. *Developmental Psychology*, 23, 611–626.
5. Bergman H., Ferrucci L., Guralnik J. *et al.* (2007) Frailty: An emerging research and clinical paradigm-issues and controversies. *Journals of Gerontology*, 64A, 731–737.
6. Lo C., Zimmermann C., Gagliese L. *et al.* Sources of spiritual well-being in patients with advanced cancer. *BMJ Supportive and Palliative Care* (in press).
7. Hall S., Gallagher R.M., Gracely E. *et al.* (2003) The terminal cancer patient: Effects of age, gender, and primary tumor site on opioid dose. *Pain Medicine*, 4, 125–134.
8. Ellis, J., Lin, J., Walsh, A., Lo, L. *et al.* (2009) Predictors of referral for specialized psychosocial oncology care in patients with metastatic cancer: The contributions of age, distress and relational need. *Journal of Clinical Oncology*, 27, 699–705.
9. Extermann M., Hurria A. (2007) Comprehensive Geriatric Assessment for older patients with cancer. *Journal of Clinical Oncology*, 25, 1824–1831.
10. Rodina M.B., Mohileb S.G. (2008) Assessing decisional capacity in the elderly. *Seminars in Oncology*, 35, 625–632.
11. Weinberger M.I., Roth A.J., Nelson C.J. (2009) Untangling the complexities of depression diagnosis in older cancer patients. *The Oncologist*, 14, 60–66.
12. Nelson C.J., Cho C., Berk A.R. *et al.* (2010) Are gold standard depression measures appropriate for use in geriatric cancer patients? A systematic evaluation of self-report depression instruments used with geriatric, cancer, and geriatric cancer samples. *Journal of Clinical Oncology*, 28, 348–356.
13. Holland J., Poppito S., Nelson C. *et al.* (2009) Reappraisal in the eighth life cycle stage: A theoretical psychoeducational intervention in elderly patients with cancer. *Palliative and Supportive Care*, 7, 271–279.
14. Ando M., Tsuda A., Moorey S. (2006) Preliminary study of reminiscence therapy on depression and self-esteem in cancer patients. *Psychological Reports*, 98, 339–346.
15. Chochinov H.M., Hack T., Hassard T. *et al.* (2005) Dignity Therapy: A novel psychotherapeutic intervention for patients near the end of life. *Journal of Clinical Oncology*, 23, 5520–5525.
16. Nissim R., Hales S., Zimmermann C. *et al.* Managing cancer and living meaningfully (CALM): A qualitative study of a brief individual psychotherapy for individuals with advanced cancer. *Palliative Medicine* (in press).
17. Canada A. L., Murphy P. E., Fitchett G. *et al.* (2008) A 3-factor model for the FACIT-Sp. *Psycho-Oncology*, 17, 908–916.
18. Braun M., Mikulincer M., Rydall A., Walsh A., Rodin G. (2007) The hidden morbidity in cancer: Spouse caregivers. *Journal of Clinical Oncology*, 25, 4829–4834.

CHAPTER 13

Psycho-oncology in Underserved and Minority Populations

Richard Fielding and Wendy W.T. Lam
Centre for Psycho-Oncology Research & Training, School of Public Health, The University of Hong Kong, Pokfulam, Hong Kong SAR, China

Introduction

Two major issues regarding cancers are considered: access to services and dealing with the consequences of that access. For many developed countries, access issues are less problematic for the majority, not so in developing countries, but as the growing trend towards withdrawing publicly funded health care accelerates these will become more pertinent for all. Even within countries that have extensive social medical systems there remain groups who face significant barriers to access and/or assistance with the consequences of the disease and treatment. This chapter examines these issues in the context of cancer.

Definitions

Underserved and minority populations comprise three main overlapping groupings (Figure 13.1): those facing social barriers, such as sexual minorities, prisoners, isolated community dwellers including many elderly and very elderly people; those facing financial or physical barriers, including low income groups, the physically disabled; and linguistic, racial and cultural minorities. These three groupings are underserved because in the first instance they tend to face discrimination on the basis of some characteristic, such as extreme age or sexual orientation, in the second instance cannot afford or access care, and in the third instance face language or cultural barriers to access. Several of these groups are at particular risk of being underserved because they belong to all three categories. Homeless groups are one example, illegal immigrants another, whilst prison populations face multiple barriers, with racial minorities, drug users and people with mental health problems making up a large fraction of prison and homeless populations. Inmates often face extreme difficulty in accessing care and only their most basic medical care needs are usually considered.

Psycho-oncology across cancer trajectories

Mostly, variation in psycho-oncology is by disease type and age group but except for including social impacts of cancer, psycho-oncology has tended to focus on clinical service provision. However, there is a strong argument for considering psycho-oncology from a much broader perspective. This is the perspective that we have taken in this chapter.

We consider psycho-oncology not just as clinical services, but as a discipline that can apply the tools and practices of psychological science to the whole spectrum of cancer. Hence, psychological inputs in cancer and morbidity prevention can then

Clinical Psycho-Oncology: An International Perspective, First Edition. Edited by Luigi Grassi and Michelle Riba.

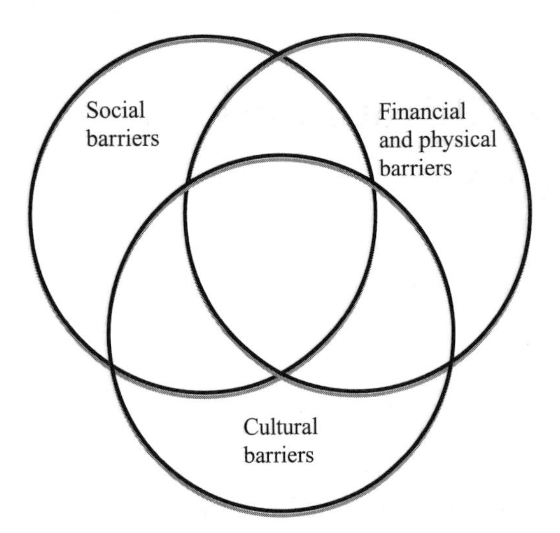

Figure 13.1 Main categories of underserved and minority populations

adopt the systemic orientation of public health thereby organizing efforts into primary, secondary and tertiary prevention. For primary prevention, behaviour change and health promotion efforts that reduce primary cancer risk, such as tobacco control efforts, dietary change, sun-smart practices and vaccinations where appropriate, fall under the rubric of psycho-oncology. General population cancer prevention, such as tobacco control, is not considered here for reasons of space. Secondary prevention would involve psychological inputs to prevent or minimize avoidable psychosocial morbidity during cancer, and involves traditional psycho-oncology and also facilitating prevention and detection among high-risk populations, optimizing clinic systems and surgeon/oncology practices to prevent avoidable psychological morbidity, screening for and treating distress, identifying unmet needs in cancer survivors, importantly including issues of access to appropriate care, and optimizing support services, particularly during later stages of disease trajectories. Tertiary prevention involves minimizing future occurrences of the problem and is particularly pertinent as numbers of cancer survivors inevitably increase.

Clearly the implementation of research findings plays a key role in this process and timely and relevant research is critical for underpinning the work of psycho-oncology, as it is for any other branch of health care.

Background

The magnitude of the problem of access to psychosocial care in cancer for underserved groups varies and for many disadvantaged groups there appears to be no published data, another way in which disadvantage raises problems for those affected – they are effectively invisible in the research arena. However, the existing literature indicates that several major issues are currently prominent and these are discussed below.

Major issues

Access to preventive and screening services

The best management for cancer is always to prevent the primary disease from ever developing in the first place. Once established, these diseases cause clinical and psychosocial consequences, which at best are usually only partially remediated. All treatments significantly impact patients, with usually life-long consequences, despite survival now being better than ever before. Hence a number of issues arise regarding prevention. These are: (i) the identification, informing, enrolment and appropriate screening of high-risk groups, and (ii) research and development of preventive and behaviour change strategies within such groups.

Identifying, informing and ensuring appropriate access to screening for high-risk groups

Many high-risk groups share the characteristic of being disadvantaged in some way. Those most emphasized are carriers of genes that have been associated with increased cancer risk. Perhaps the best known is the high prevalence of BRCA I & II variants among Ashkenazi Jewish communities. These and many other genetic variants have now been identified in a range of population subgroups, but most cancer genes remain apparently randomly scattered across the population and undetected. It is likely that as testing for genetic variation becomes more widespread patterns within this apparent randomness will emerge. In addition to genetic variants that increase cancer risk, numerous groups are known to be at high risk of specific cancers because of cultural or occupational practices.

High-risk groups include peoples from Southern China, Arctic communities, the Middle East and North Africa who are at high risk of nasopharyngeal cancer;[1] economically deprived groups in the United Kingdom who are at much higher risk for a whole range of cancers, including non-adenocarcinomas of the oesophagus;[2] whereas squamous cell carcinoma of the oesophagus, amongst other cancers such as those of the prostate, are much more prevalent in Black than White American males;[3] whilst peoples from the 'oesophageal cancer belt' which stretches from Turkey through Iran to China are at very high risk, primarily due to a mix of deprivation and dietary practices.[4] Liver and stomach cancer risk is high for first generation minorities living in the United States who originate from Korea, Northern Thailand, Laos and Vietnam (liver)[5,6] and Northern Asia (stomach). Tobacco smoking rates, the main risk factor for lung cancers, are often significantly higher in minority communities though minority smoking rates differ between countries,[7] in prisons,[8] and among persons with long-term severe mental health problems,[9] and in members of economically deprived communities.[10] Elderly adults are also at higher risk, with cancers being predominantly a set of diseases of the elderly. The list is lengthy and these few examples are illustrative.

Levels of knowledge about vulnerability to cancer and prevention are often low in minority and underserved groups.[11] For example Black, Hispanic and Asian Americans tend to view themselves, incorrectly, as not being vulnerable to melanoma. While melanoma prevalence tends to be lower than in fair-skinned groups, dark-skinned groups are vulnerable because perceptions of lower risk can lead to greater solar exposure.[12] Similarly, in the United Kingdom, ethnic minorities reported lower knowledge of cancer warning signs[13] and use of national cancer screening programmes than their White British counterparts.[14] Malay women showed high levels of misunderstanding of the purpose of Pap smear testing.[15] Notifying or educating these groups about their high risk is an important strategy. Men in particular tend to be less well informed of the benefits of screening than are women, as are African Americans compared to Whites.[16] Low educational achievement is also associated with less knowledge of screening benefits. In some jurisdictions prisoners may have access to cancer screening and for some screens, such as Pap smears uptake may be as high as 90%, while elsewhere they may be low. In a sample of US prisons, African-American male prisoners were the least likely to have had colonoscopy.[17]

Research and development of preventive and behaviour change strategies within such groups

Developing good models for preventive care in minority and underserved communities is an area that has been largely ignored in the literature. It is widely assumed that models developed on middle-class White Western urban populations are universally applicable[18] if translated into different languages. However, this is not the case. Because health care systems differ, from community attitudes to vulnerability, to service organization to personal values of clinical staff, requirements for different groups and times are likely to vary.[19] Moreover, any classification system is going to smooth out variation between subgroups. So, for example, among American Latinas, Mexican women more than other Spanish-speaking groups have the lowest uptake rates for mammography.[20] It is often the case that those minorities and underserved groups at the highest risk and with the lowest utilization of cancer services turn out to be also the most socioeconomically deprived,[20,21] irrespective of what ethnic or other grouping they belong to. Hence, the combination of minority status and low income can increase barriers to preventive services.

Most research on minority and underserved groups has focused on increasing screening uptake for these groups. Even between different minority and underserved groups screening rates differ for different cancer types. For example a survey of women living in homeless shelters in San Francisco found moderate rates of around 50% in screening for breast and cervical cancers.[22] Among Asian Americans, Korean women had the lowest screening rates for breast and cervical cancer, but while Japanese women had the highest breast cancer screening rates, they had low cervical cancer screening rates. Even so, rates were close to 80%[23] which is better than for many majority groups in other countries. For example in Switzerland Yugoslav, Italian and Portuguese women have lower mammography uptake than the majority Swiss population, but overall uptake rates in Switzerland are only around 33%.[24] In Spain, immigrant groups showed wide disparities in mammography utilization rates, with Eastern European (66%), Chinese (68%) and Filipino (69%) immigrant women having the lowest uptakes followed by Maghrebi (82%) women relative to native Spanish women (94%), with economic and social class differentiating uptake rates.[25] However, there are issues of appropriateness. For women amongst whom the prevalence of breast cancer is low, which is the case for some minority groups relative to the majority population, mammographic screening can result in increased harms but no reduction of breast cancer incidence.[26] The effectiveness of a screening programme is dependent on the population incidence of cancer and enrolment, and not simply enrolment alone. Thus, the incidence of breast cancer among Chinese women remains low relative to Caucasian women and Chinese female (particularly first generation) migrants to Western countries drawn into national mammography programmes based on the (higher) incidence among the native population may not always benefit as much as their Caucasian native counterparts. Eventually, after one or two generations migrant group incidence rates tend to converge on those of the majority population.

Most symptoms of cancer are self-detected, however, which can introduce disparities. Among 425 Hong Kong Chinese women, elderly women who tend to have less formal education, showed longer appraisal delay (time taken to decide on consultation) for self-detected breast symptoms than did middle-aged partnered women.[27] Similarly low education was a predictor for a sample of 664 Italian women who presented with delayed operable breast cancer,[28] among 190 Iranian women in Tehran[29] and in 565 Egyptian women.[30] Conversely, among a well-educated group of Cuban lung cancer patients in Havana, patient delays were on average low, with only 3% delaying more than 90 days.[31] Repeatedly, financial barriers to preventive uptake are reported,[21,32] particularly where co-payment or insurance is required, such as in the United States. The financial cost of screening may be compounded for minority women who are more likely to encounter job loss on diagnosis of cancers.[33] Within some minorities and lower educated groups, women may delay consultation for suspected symptoms of breast and gynaecological cancers because they wish to avoid examination by male doctors[27,34] and so limited access to female primary care physicians presents a further consultation barrier. This is one example where simply translating the language used to provide screening information may not increase uptake rates among minorities.

Interventions to improve prevention uptake

Attempts to improve preventive uptake among minorities and underserved groups have so far had mixed results. A community outreach colorectal cancer screening programme in Harlem, New York designed to increase uptake in African-American women encountered a refusal rate of 77% among 2616 eligible African-American women, and only 55% of the remainder actually received colonoscopy, a final rate of just 18%.[32] This is in contrast to a less-acculturated Chinese-American colorectal cancer (CRC) screening uptake rate in Seattle, Washington, of 'only' 40%,[35] while among 3953 British South Asian women, CRC screening uptake for the National Breast & Bowel Screening Programme was only 30% in contrast to 54% for non-Asians, and while more South Asian women who underwent mammography also received colon screening, rates were still lower (49% vs. 82%).[36] Moreover, screening in one programme was less likely to predict participation in the other among South Asian women, with

Muslim women in particular less likely to receive mammography compared to other Asian groups.[36]

Framing messages emphasizing disparities in ethnic groups may produce mixed results, depending on whether they generate a positive or negative emotional response in recipients.[37] Attempts have been made to operationalize the implications of theoretical work based on the Theory of Planned Behaviour[38] which suggests facilitating intention to action increases the probability of displaying a particular behaviour. So interventions to improve intention to adopt preventive practices among minorities and underserved groups are being evaluated.[39] While results are not yet available there is some reason to think that intention translates poorly into preventive behaviour in the absence of action planning, which might be a more important pre-determinant of preventive action.[40] Other studies have examined different outreach methods, including invitation and targeted phone calls, with disappointing results on mammography uptake.[41] Most studies, however, lack a robust theoretical basis.

Achieving a diagnosis and referral for treatment is a significant source of delay in many parts of the world, and once again lower educated groups seem to fare less well. Oncological pathology misdiagnosis rates range from 1–15% and can result in diagnostic delays in up to 50% of cases where they occur.[42] Pathology misdiagnosis is linked to poor specimen quality.[42] Inability to perform an adequate history, examination or specimen collection, because of language difficulties for example, are thus important contributing factors to misdiagnosis.[43] Lower availability of primary care physicians has also been linked to increased diagnostic delays in the United States,[44] and physician availability is inversely related to socioeconomic status of the community (the Inverse Care Law).[45]

Diagnosis, distress, adaptation, survivorship, families, interventions: secondary prevention

The primary focus of most psycho-oncology work in recent years has been on the prevention, detection and remediation of psychosocial distress as a consequence of the diagnosis and treatment of cancer. In the diagnostic, planning and treatment phases, there are a number of issues that disadvantage minority and underserved groups. These include difficulties in physical access to diagnostic facilities due to distance, transportation and, particularly for countries like the United States which are reliant on private medical insurance, cost, though cost can be an issue in the form of time off work and lost wages due to consultation and treatment everywhere.

Once diagnosed, minority and underserved groups are less likely to be offered aggressive treatment for cancer than are their majority population peers.[46] This has been demonstrated for prostate cancers in the United States, where poorer educated minorities receive less surgery than better educated Whites,[47] and for breast cancer where non-White women receive less aggressive treatment[48] and rural older women less breast-sparing surgery and radiotherapy.[49,50] Homeless people, the majority of whom come from disadvantaged and low-education groups are at particular risk due to low health care access, their itinerant nature and poor health habits[50] and may be less compliant with follow-up.[47] Such individuals are particularly vulnerable under all types of health care systems. Physicians may have more negative attitudes to minority groups and this might affect the choices they make.[52] Early reports of differences in terms of cancer treatment received by racial groups have not always been replicated in more recent studies, some reviews have concluded, though in some cancers, for example small-cell lung and prostate cancers, treatment differences by racial subgroups persist, even when staging and insurance differences are accounted for.[53] Patient refusal of cancer treatments is higher in minorities[54] which partially contributes toward the differences in treatment and survival rates seen in places like the United States[53] and other refusal rates may also be higher among ethnic minorities due to a greater fatalistic orientation.

Clinical communication

Communication within cancer-care-related clinical consultation has received considerable attention since being identified as a key influence on a range of psychosocial outcomes. Most of the content of diagnostic and treatment-planning consultations addresses biological and clinical aspects of the cancer and its management, as this is often the area that concerns most patients when first diagnosed: What is it? Why has it happened? Can it be cured? Survival is the predominant theme in many patients' minds.[34] Offset against this are the likely costs of that survival, in terms of physical and more subtly psychological and emotional impacts, which are often initially displaced by the physical focus surrounding diagnosis and primary treatment planning and implementation.[34] The negotiation of treatments remains problematic in most jurisdictions and for most patients, but people speaking different languages and from disadvantaged groups are often most vulnerable.[55]

Case study

Mrs Chan a 48-year-old Hong Kong Chinese woman recently arrived in Hong Kong from a rural part of China was referred to the oncology clinic for chemotherapy following surgery for primary colorectal carcinoma. During surgery she was found to have several lymph node metastases. The surgeon communicated this information to her and explained that she would be referred to the clinical oncology department for chemotherapy.

When Mrs Chan attended for her oncology outpatient appointment to assess her for chemotherapy, she was told by her oncologist that there are two chemotherapy regimes suitable to her condition. One is a standard regime that has been used for years, the cost of which is covered by the hospital. The other is a new regime recently introduced, but which is very expensive and patients therefore have to bear the treatment cost. Both options have similar survival benefits, but the new regime has reduced side-effects and toxicities. When asked, Mrs Chan stated that she could not afford the self-financed treatment so she opted for the standard treatment, despite worrying that the side-effects of chemotherapy might make her very sick and prevent her returning to work.

Several weeks later, Mrs Chan returned to the oncology clinic for her follow-up appointment. She complained to her oncologist that the surgical wound caused great discomfort. The oncologist told her to ask her surgeon as the oncologists only deal with the chemotherapy and its related concerns. Mrs Chan had mentioned the problem to the surgeon when she saw him, but he dismissed her concern and told her to check with her oncologist. Mrs Chan felt very frustrated as she felt that she was being passed around and no one was interested enough to listen to her concerns. Moreover, at each follow-up visit she was seen by a different physician none of whom knew her, but merely read about her from her case notes. When she requested to be seen by the same physician, she was told that such an arrangement is not possible in the publicly funded hospitals and only private hospitals can offer that kind of continuity of care.

Six months later, Mrs Chan had completed her chemotherapy and was told to come back every three months for surveillance purposes. Because of the chemotherapy side-effects Mrs Chan had lost her previous job as she was frequently absent from work. Mrs Chan recently found a new job, but she did not disclose her medical history to her new employer. She was afraid that she may not get hired. Therefore, Mrs Chan had not been able to adhere to her medical appointments as she is reluctant to take time off from her new job.

Evidence is now strong that, at least for some populations of breast cancer patients, difficulties in treatment decision-making are important markers or contributors for future psychological distress.[34,56–60] Our work shows that women with breast cancer who report difficulties in treatment decision-making for breast cancer surgery are significantly more likely to report being distressed at eight months post-surgery[59] and also at six years post-surgery.[60] Among minority and disadvantaged groups, such difficulties can include problems of understanding the relative merits and consequences of particular treatment options, or of not understanding the treatment plan.[61]

Even where there are no ethnic cultural barriers, use of jargon, task orientation and lack of continuity of care due to contemporary organization policies in clinics which allocate the next available doctor to see the next patient in the queue, mean that many of the needs that cancer patients may have for consistency and comprehensive information care[62] are lost, leading to communication and support deficits. When patients from the main sociocultural group express high levels of unmet need for improved communications in cancer care,[62] it is very likely that minorities and disadvantaged groups will experience these problems even more so.[63,64] Differences in unmet needs, either arising from majority cultural values or from differences in health service systems, or both, are seen between Caucasian German and Chinese women,[19] despite both groups having access to psycho-oncology services of some kind.

Whilst evaluations of training for physicians in communicating with cancer patients have shown improved communication skills,[65] the improved skills may not necessarily translate into lowered levels of anxiety or distress for patients or their relatives,[66,67] and again while there have been few evaluations of improved skills training targeted at minority and underserved groups, there is little reason to think that there would be any difference from the impacts faced by the majority of cancer patients.

Patient responses to cancer

How patients respond to a diagnosis of cancer is critical. The willingness to pursue treatment, to discuss and negotiate with surgeons and oncologists over treatment options, and to adhere to a course or courses of treatment can all determine treatment effectiveness and hence outcome. Distress, anxiety and depression are common negative affective states that are reported at high levels following a diagnosis of cancer. In many groups, pessimism/fatalism is also seen, and the belief that cancer is unavoidable and a death sentence is widespread in some groups. Fatalism is more likely to be present among groups who are less well educated and among whom cancer has a higher mortality rate, either through later presentation of symptoms and hence less successful treatment outcomes, or in groups who traditionally have faced barriers to treatment. As mentioned above, minority and disadvantaged groups often meet these criteria. Not surprisingly then we find that higher fatalism is associated with cancer information avoidance[68] and is also high in African-American groups,[69] particularly older African Americans who tend to be poorly educated.[70] This may in part reflect a sense of powerlessness.[70,71] Even where economic barriers may not exist, then, the kinds of treatments minority and disadvantaged patients receive may be suboptimal, and suboptimal treatments are often associated with more extensive physical and psychosocial impacts. For example Appalachian rural elderly women are more likely to undergo mastectomy than lumpectomy for breast cancer[48,49] (though in this particular example it may not translate into poorer psychosocial outcomes compared to younger women who, under some circumstances may suffer greater body image and related psychosocial decrements than older women),[72] a pattern that suggests that either older women are not offered a choice or are more willing to relinquish their breast.

Given the prevailing picture so far emerging that low socioeconomic status, low education and minority group membership are important predictors of poorer cancer outcomes, because of less knowledge, difficulties in accessing care and possibly fewer choices of care, and given that levels of distress among patients facing cancer are generally significant, we might therefore also expect to see higher levels of distress during cancer care and thereafter in such groups. Does the literature support this hypothesis? While there are very few studies looking at minority and disadvantaged group psychosocial reactions to the diagnosis and treatment of cancer, those studies do support this perspective. In Canada, a review of cancer distress among 2400 speakers of English as a second language found this accounted for a significant portion of explained variance in distress over and above gender, age and clinical features.[73] In the United States, rural Kentucky cancer survivors reported higher levels of distress than their non-rural counterparts.[74] A separate study of cancer pain found higher reported levels of pain and pain-related distress in African-American than Anglo-American cancer patients,[75] whilst elsewhere, African-American prostate cancer patients were reported to have significantly higher levels of traumatic stress,[76] and after adjustment for age and clinical status African-American cancer survivors reported lower self-rated health.[77] Similarly, at two months post-diagnosis British patients with lower socioeconomic status (SES) reported greater anxiety, depression, and more distress and social difficulties than higher SES counterparts.[78] It seems therefore that minority and disadvantaged groups also face greater struggles to cope with cancer. This is not surprising given that generally the less-well educated, people with different language or cultural orientation, and notably those with mental health difficulties, the homeless and similar groups may not cope well with excessive demands and therefore might manifest coping failure more often. Such groups also have less access to resources and are often less able to elicit help and assistance from formal and informal support services, lacking as they might, the skills or access to do so. Consequently, they form some of the most vulnerable groups during cancer. We will return to this point in the next section.

Finally, even in cancer survivorship, patients with lower socioeconomic status endure a poorer quality of life than their wealthier counterparts.[79] Members of these groups are less likely than their mainstream counterparts to hold professional or other jobs where they can take leave for treatment or leave of absence, for example to attend daily radiotherapy or for surgery, and be allowed a more gentle resumption of work on recovery. So not only does cancer present an existential threat but it also threatens financial security and family coherence. Any one of these is a major challenge to an individual; all together they represent a major coping load even for the strongest person.

The life-threatening traumatic nature of cancer and its treatment has been cited as a cause of post-traumatic stress disorder (PTSD). The USA National Institutes of Health National Cancer Institute web page states: 'People with histories of cancer are considered to be at risk for PTSD'. Around 16% of North American paediatric cancer survivors had symptoms of PTSD.[80] In bone marrow transplants patients' estimated PTSD rates have ranged from 5–35%[81,82] depending on when and how assessment is performed. Among 55 US women with breast cancer 5–10% were estimated to meet DSM-IV criteria for PTSD,[83] whilst in 155 other women, only 4% met PTSD criteria though 38% were distressed.[84] It is likely that there is symptomatic blurring between PTSD and generalized distress symptoms reflecting adjustment difficulties that confounds separating the distressed group from non-distressed patients.

This prevalence range for PTSD-like symptoms is much lower than the proportion of cancer patients in the United States who report being distressed.[85] A study of 9000 patients who completed the Brief Symptom Inventory found that around 1 patient in 3 overall was distressed (35%), ranging from 43% of lung cancer patients to 30% of gynaecological cancer patients. However, the BSI detects a range of symptoms (hostility, psychoticism, obsessive-compulsivity) some of which might have pre-dated the diagnosis of cancer or be otherwise unrelated, which would tend to inflate actual acute distress incidence. For breast cancer, 53% and 56% had depression and anxiety respectively. In contrast, rates of anxiety and depression in Canadian cancer patients were both 24%, with minority and lower income patients more likely to be distressed.[86] Elsewhere 'almost half' of all 'new' breast cancer patients showed 'high levels of distress' on the Distress Thermometer.[87] Among British cancer outpatients, levels of emotional distress were 'significant' in 22% (95% CI, 20–23%).[88] These different prevalence estimates are a function not only of how distress is defined, but when it is measured and how. Almost all studies of distress in different cancer groups report high levels of psychological distress.

As an example let us consider breast cancer. In Hong Kong Chinese women with breast cancer, rates of mild/severe distress one week and eight months following surgery were as high as 75% (95% CI, 73–83%), with around 39% of women achieving high/severe distress scores, and 64% (59–69%), with almost 50% (44–54%) of women remaining distressed over this period when a standard screening instrument based on the General Health Questionnaire was used.[56,57] However, it was apparent from this longitudinal study that women did not all follow the same pattern of high-to-low distress as time since diagnosis increased. When the same data were examined using more sophisticated modelling, the data revealed that four distinct trajectories of distress were apparent in this sample of over 300 women. Over 65% of women had persistent but very low levels of distress or no distress for the eight months of the study; 7% had low distress immediately post-surgery but by four months had high levels of distress, which gradually declined to baseline levels by eight months; 15%

of women had high levels of distress that remained high across the duration of the study, while only 12% of women showed the classic pattern of high-to-low distress over the eight-month period.[59] These data demonstrate that distress responses to cancer diagnosis and treatment vary among women with breast cancer in markedly different ways. When taken as one group, the overall rates of psychological distress imply a declining prevalence, but this was not the case for most women. What is surprising is that two thirds of women showed little or no distress across the disease trajectory, in other words a resilient response. This finding has quite profound implications for resourcing psycho-oncological services.

It is notable that despite being distressed, 44% of 3095 Canadian cancer patients felt that they did not need psychological help from a cancer support centre specifically providing psycho-oncology services, though other ethnicities than Canadian/European/British were more likely to make use of the services, as were women with breast cancer: 87% reported receiving support from family and 74% from friends.[86] Half a world away, 348 Hong Kong Chinese women with early-stage breast cancer rated continuity of care and better clinical information as their greatest unmet needs, in contrast to a comparable sample of 292 German women for whom psychological and physical/daily living needs and higher levels of depression and particularly anxiety predominated, and who reported more unmet psychosocial needs on average, though more Chinese than German women reported any unmet needs.[19] One possible explanation for these findings, taking into account the trajectory patterns experienced by Chinese women with breast cancer[59] is that, because greater psychological unmet need was associated with chemotherapy and greater health service and information needs were associated with physical symptoms, levels of distress are in many instances related to uncertainty in the context of high potential threat. Reported unmet needs reflect this uncertainty. Uncertainty in turn is prompted by several key triggers across the illness trajectory, including diagnosis, surgical treatment decision-making, physical symptom distress related to treatments, treatment cessation and novel bodily sensations. Numerous studies have identified these triggers to be strongly predictive of levels of distress in cancer patients.

However, in the Hong Kong–German study reported above,[19] distress did not equate with unmet needs, though women who were distressed tended to report more unmet psychological needs. This may help explain the findings of 44% of Canadian cancer patients not seeking support, while among 302 Dutch cancer patients, of those distressed (31–37%) in the two months following treatment 51% also refused help for their distress.[89] The presence of informal support networks is critical.[86] Younger and single people are more likely to seek and utilize formal psychosocial support services,[57] as are minorities,[86] presumably because their support networks are lacking or otherwise insufficient. Information needs are likely to be particularly acute among disadvantaged groups, though not necessarily always. Au *et al.* found that higher educational attainment was associated with greater unmet needs across all domains of the SCNS-SF34 except for activities of physical and daily living needs.[62] Perhaps more education confers more expectations, which are harder to meet.

Finally, the needs of caretakers or family members are largely neglected in the literature, with only a few studies considering this problem, mostly from the perspective of palliative or terminal care. A key determinant of distress for caregivers is the perceived burden of care they face.[90,91] A small Australian study of 57 advanced cancer patients found that caretaker unmet needs were greater than clinicians' unmet needs, with the patient's unmet needs being the least, but overall unmet need declined with time despite service provision remaining constant.[92] This final point is consistent with the idea that familiarity with both uncertainty and threats tends to be associated with adaptation to these and general decline in related distress, though background distress may remain high. Combining this with the insights from the trajectory studies of Lam *et al.* suggests that developing methods for the identification of people particularly at risk of persistent distress should be a priority. Because most patients and their relatives appear to experience only transitory distress which they seem to prefer to cope with on their own, resource use is optimized by identifying these high-risk individuals and those who want counselling or support services. Many minority groups have very strong family support ties and these may in part compensate for lack of access. For older and isolated individuals, coping with cancer is going to be a very lonely experience.

Implications for interventions

The studies reviewed above carry a number of implications for developing interventions that are particularly suited to benefit patients from minority and disadvantaged groups.

Improving access to preventive and screening services

Probably the most important preventive activities that are needed among underserved groups are appropriate advice on smoking cessation, exercise, control of infectious agents linked to cancer and improved diet.[93] These activities require targeted and culturally appropriate health promotion activities to be developed and operationalized. For some groups, barriers of time, opportunity and cost are significant and need to be overcome. We are a long way from the use of targeted culturally appropriate interventions, many of which struggle to achieve effects in the dominant cultural groups.

Education to recognize and respond to symptoms indicative of cancer is another area that needs to be emphasized. There are good arguments for primary care physicians to consider initiating discussions that can help to assess minority patient attendee knowledge of their cancer risk and symptom awareness needs. This may need to be done specifically by subgroups of clinicians, such as female doctors prompting these discussions with low response groups, such as Muslim women. For other groups, this is a task that can be done by practice nurses, particularly in more integrated community clinics which are now starting to be developed in some urban environments. However, language may remain a barrier in highly culturally diverse communities as it is unrealistic to expect multilingual staff in each clinic, but attendees usually bring a relative or friend who can translate, though this approach too has its own problems. The use of linguistically varied posters and print media detailing cancer risks is also potentially beneficial but low levels of health literacy – the ability to interpret health-related information even when presented in your own language – is widely problematic and urgently needs attention.[94] At a policy level, targeting of households in screening programmes with linguistically appropriate information and requests for screening is a minimum that needs to be done,[95] but again it faces the barrier of low health literacy in some underserved communities. Information on absolute as well as relative cancer reduction rates from screening programmes must be provided in an accessible and usable form to facilitate informed choice.

Identifying and triggering screening activities for low-uptake groups in clinics serving disadvantaged communities has been shown to be an effective way of increasing uptake for breast and CRC screening.[96]

Improving consultation and care options

The second major area in which interventions are needed is in the optimization of consultation and involvement in care decision-making for diagnosed cancer. In treatment decision-making (TDM), a study involving US women and their treatment decisions reported that greater numbers of women, including those from minority groups, choose mastectomy over breast-conserving treatment than women who allowed the doctor to make the decision on their behalf.[97] However, women who are involved in TDM evidence better mental health than those not involved,[98] provided that they want to be involved, do not encounter difficulties with, or do not receive insufficient information or support in making such decisions.[62] Women not offered involvement in TDM subsequently evidence higher levels of regret and reported lower quality of life.[98,99] Lam and colleagues studied Chinese women in Hong Kong and found that TDM difficulties, pessimism and physical symptom distress were important predictors of chronic distress trajectory membership in the eight months following primary surgery for early stage breast cancer.[59,62]

Very little research is available on participation involvement for other types of cancer, probably because the treatment options for other cancer types are more prescriptive based on disease characteristics, or no alternative treatments achieve comparable survival outcomes to mainstream treatments. One exception may be prostate cancers, but this is an area that does not seem to have been explored.

Improving clinical psycho-oncology support services

The literature on the benefits associated with psychological interventions for cancer patients is somewhat controversial. Whilst early studies reported significant and perhaps over-optimistic benefits, including survival benefits (e.g. Spiegel *et al.*),[100] as greater methodological rigor is applied to evaluate interventions, the benefits become less clear-cut. Reviews have been seriously compromised by the nature of the available studies, principally the lack of robust, blinded randomized controlled trials, but the better ones show more ambiguous intervention effects.[101] Meanwhile other reviews claim that cognitive-behavioural interventions are effective in reducing distress.[102] These discrepancies arise in part through lack of agreed definition of what constitutes 'psychological intervention'.[103] In relation to minority and disadvantaged groups, few studies have specifically examined interventions for these populations. In a group of 472 low income mostly Hispanic women with cancer who evidenced depression, more who were randomly allocated psychotherapeutic active intervention (63%) than enhanced usual-care control (50%) evidenced a greater than 50% decrease in depression and were more likely to receive treatment for depression which included antidepressant medication as well as psychotherapeutic intervention in a collaborative care programme. The problem-solving intervention was preferred to antidepressive medication.[104] Two years later, among the 44% of patients who were traced, around one third in both groups had recurrence of depression but intervention group patients were more likely to have received further intervention.[105] Similarly, a Scottish study of 200 depressed cancer patients began with ~4% already receiving antidepressant medication. Following an intervention comprising 10 sessions of problem-solving psychotherapy delivered by a trained oncology nurse, the proportion of patients on antidepressants increased substantially compared to usual-care group over the duration of the study, while lower anxiety and fatigue but not less pain or improved physical functioning was observed over the six-month follow-up.[106] However, almost 2 in 3 of these patients were disease-free and so the results may reflect difficulties in reintegration rather than difficulties in coping with the disease.[107]

Anxiety tends to co-occur with depression, though is more prevalent than depression and tends to be the major component of distress experienced by cancer patients, occurring in around 1 in 2 British cancer patients, around 1 in 5 of whom meet ICD-9 criteria for anxiety disorder,[108] while a German sample of breast cancer patients had slightly lower rates of 40% for anxiety and 6.3% for GAD.[109] In two small pilot studies that examined the effectiveness of a decision support tool, among the 95 (study 1) and 38 (study 2) Hong Kong Chinese breast cancer patients awaiting surgery who were involved, 11% in study 1 and 6% in study 2 reported anxiety exceeding the HADS-A cut-off for moderate/severe anxiety.[110]

Anxiety is closely related to uncertainty and management of information needs is important to help ameliorate uncertainty-related anxiety. Although information alone does not seem to be sufficient in reducing anxiety. Jones compared standardized versus personalized information booklets provided to UK cancer patients, but found no impact on anxiety level.[111] Au also found that their surgical decision support tool did not decrease anxiety before breast cancer surgery.[110] Other information seems beneficial, however, and is likely to be particularly so for minority and disadvantaged groups and those with low health literacy. An orientation education intervention that introduces patients to the clinical team, hospital setting and facilities, when evaluated showed a significant reduction in anxiety among new cancer patients.[112]

One area of work that holds promise is related to the concept of attentional bias. The literature on PTSD has shown that a persisting feature of this condition is attentional bias towards threat stimuli by the mechanism of trauma-related rumination. In cancer persisting PTSD may be maintained by or at least features negative cancer-related rumination.[113] Assisting patients to manage rumination using cognitive-behavioural approaches should help minimize PTSD-like symptoms.

A number of cognitive features have been identified as important influences on the coping process among patients. Anxiety tends to be a more common manifestation of distress in many cancer patients, and greater anxiety and depression are associated with more attentional and mnestic deficits when tests of neuropsychological function are considered, but subjective reports of poor cognitive function (so called 'chemo brain') do not correlate well with neuropsychological measures when affect and anxiety are controlled.[114] The effectiveness of attentional-control strategies to manage cancer-related pain are modulated by their affective-motivational significance suggesting that it is the degree of threat that the pain embodies which influences coping effectiveness for the patient.[115] Deploying attention away from threat-related information is generally acknowledged to hinder adaptive coping towards threat-related stimuli, such as cancer information, whilst active deployment of attention towards threat-related stimuli illustrates an adaptive strategy of engagement with the threat. Studies suggest that active engagement with cancer-related information is associated with less distress in breast cancer patients.[116] Reviews of anxiety/distress management in cancer indicate that social-cognitive problem-solving approaches confer the largest effect sizes,[117] though while a review of 56 articles identified effect sizes indicating benefits from individual and cognitive-behavioural therapies, the 95% confidence intervals of these effect sizes all include 0 and hence do not differ from chance.[118] The fact that different systematic reviews of the same literature reach different conclusions, with some being particularly unable to find clear evidence for benefit[119] indicates that there are significant outstanding issues to be addressed, not least methodological.[119,120] These include selective inclusion in studies of certain patient groups, such as North American and European Caucasian women with early stage breast cancer or Europeans with CRC leading to over-representation, and the under-representation of their late-stage disease and palliative care groups, minorities or disadvantaged groups (for the purpose of this chapter). An important problem identified by Jacobsen's review[120] is that there was a general assumption in many studies that all patients were anxious and therefore eligible for inclusion. As Lam *et al.*'s trajectory studies[59,60] show, this seems not to be the case and most cancer patients probably do not need psychological interventions to assist with managing distress; however, the ones that do need it require early identification and intervention.

A second key issue to address is the need to identify critical points in the cancer trajectory where interventions will be most effective in preventing problem amplification and chronicity from developing, and aspects of care provision that need to be changed to help prevent these. Evidence so far points to the provision of adequate tailored information to new patients, including orientation information, continuity of care over the duration of the cancer trajectory, assistance if desired with treatment decision-making where appropriate, problem-solving interventions and stress management for distressed patients, clear clinical information and good communication skills on the part of clinicians. These interventions are the best evidence-based options we currently have. They apply to all cancer patients, but are particularly pertinent to those who are already disadvantaged.

Recovery and rehabilitation

An issue very pertinent to many minority group cancer patients is the risk of facing discrimination and even ostracism following their diagnosis and treatment. Social responses within minority and subcultural communities are highly variable. For instance, in many parts of Asia, particularly in less-educated groups, superstition and misunderstandings about cancer abound. Beliefs that cancer is infectious remain, particularly among older members of such communities, the ones most likely to experience cancer. They may be unwilling to notify others of their diagnoses, and in turn there may be an unwillingness of adult children to agree to doctors telling their older parents if they have a diagnosis of cancer, for example for fear it will lead to fatalistic giving up of hope and quick death. This is a sure way to create massive tensions within the family which struggles to maintain the lie that the patient is not dying. Older patients still may believe that the way to find a good clinician is to rely on what is sometimes termed 'predestined medical affinity', whereby the patient and doctor are 'destined' to come together and because of this the doctor is to be trusted implicitly, and hence no patient involvement is required. Linked to this is the fact that, if the doctor is 'the right one' then s/he will know intuitively what the patient needs and there is no need for the patient to volunteer information. Many clinicians who trained and worked in Asia experience and may themselves become acculturated to such attitudes among their patients. The younger generation of clinicians is less affected because many have received specialist oncology training in Europe, North America and Australia.

In many non-European communities, disfigurement from cancer treatment brings with it a sense of shame within the community, fears are linked to discrimination and social isolation, and reticence to seek support from others. Suffering in silence remains a common attitude among older Asians for example, and social isolation, especially in the smaller expatriate communities that may exist in Western countries, may be severe, though family support systems are usually strong. Fatalistic views abound and influence willingness to seek help. These issues can overlay and compound the common wider difficulties of fear of diagnosis, uncertainty and low health literacy.

Finally, many ethnic minorities take recourse to traditional healing approaches when faced with cancer symptoms. Many may delay consulting allopathic clinicians seeking instead advice from traditional healers. It is important that these healers be very familiar with and willing to quickly refer to allopathic centres those patients who present with cancer symptoms. Even after surgery, many communities rely on traditional methods to maintain their health. For example Traditional Chinese Medicine (TCM) and dietary approaches are widely used by Chinese patients worldwide despite the primary management of cancer being based on surgery, chemotherapies and radiotherapy. Most often TCM is used to build health prior to treatment for example, or to help minimize the side-effects of chemotherapy. Clinicians therefore need to be aware of these traditional beliefs and accommodate them into care pathways for these groups of patients.

Key points

- Minority groups are usually underserved, remaining at the periphery of cancer prevention, detection, care and recovery.
- Several national oncology organizations have recommended guidelines to reduce disparities in survival and treatment of cancer as a result of minority status. In contrast to the growing amount of information on minorities regarding detection and prevention of cancer, there remains a clear lack of data on the latter parts of the cancer trajectory regarding these groups. In particular, such groups are seldom identified, let alone targeted for psychosocial interventions.
- On the question of psychosocial interventions, it is becoming apparent that a much more selective approach to the identification of patients who may benefit from support services is needed. Not all distressed patients want or need interventions and many who do have lower access to such services. More often, it will be peoples disadvantaged by income, education or ethnicity who are the ones that slip through the net. Such individuals tend to have fewer verbal and coping skills needed to negotiate treatment access and navigate the complexities of modern oncological care.
- Efforts need to be more inclusive of underserved groups in research and service provision, and to develop a more eclectic style of practice which more readily accommodates the educational, cultural and linguistic variation seen in contemporary communities.

Acknowledgements

We thank Ms Marie Kwok Nga Ting for her invaluable help in searching and compiling the literature that contributed to this chapter. We also thank the Hong Kong Cancer Fund for their longstanding and generous support of our work which is cited herein.

Suggested further reading

Holland J.C., Breitbart W.S., Jacobsen P.B. *et al.* (eds) (2010) *Psycho-Oncology*, 2nd edn, Oxford University Press, New York.

References

1. Chang E.T., Adami H.O. (2006) Nasopharyngeal carcinoma. *Cancer Epidemiology, Biomarkers & Prevention*, DOI: 10.1158/1055-9965.EPI-06-0353.
2. National Cancer Intelligence Network (2008) *Cancer Incidence by Deprivation, England 1995–2004*. Available at: http://www.ncin.org.uk/publications/reports/default.aspx (accessed January 2012).
3. Vizcaino A.P., Moreno V., Lambert R., Parkin D.M. (2002) Time trends incidence of both major histologic types of esophageal carcinomas in selected countries, 1973–1995. *International Journal of Cancer*, 99, 860–868.
4. Hormozdiari H., Day N.E., Aramesh B., Mahboubi E. (1975) Dietary factors and esophageal cancer in the Caspian Littoral of Iran. *Cancer Research*, 35, 3493–3498.
5. Alterkruse S.F., McGlynn K.A., Reichmann M.E. (2009) Hepatocellular incidence, mortality and survival trends in the United States from 1975–2005. *Journal of Clinical Oncology*, DOI: 10.1200/JCO.2008.20.7753.
6. Fielding R. (2010) Hepatobiliary cancer, in *Psycho-Oncology*, 2nd edn (eds J.C. Holland, W.S. Breitbart, P.B. Jacobsen *et al.*), Oxford University Press, New York, pp. 146–151.
7. Agyemang C., Stronks K., Tromp N. *et al.* (2010) A cross-national comparative study of smoking prevalence and cessation between English and Dutch South Asian and African origin populations: The role of national context. *Nicotine & Tobacco Research*, DOI: 10.1093/ntr/ntq044.
8. Belcher J., Butler T., Richmond R. *et al.* (2006) Smoking and its correlates in an Australian prisoner population. *Drug and Alcohol Review*, 25, 343–348.
9. Bremner J., Edmonds N. (2007) Supporting people with mental health problems to quit smoking. *A Life in the Day*, DOI:10.1108/13666282200700024.
10. Singh G.K., Miller B.A., Hankey B.E., Edwards B.K. (2003) *Area socioeconomic variations in U.S. cancer incidence, mortality, stage, treatment and survival 1975–1999*, National Cancer Institute, Bethesda, MD.
11. Macleod U., Mitchell E.D., Burgess C. *et al.* (2009) Risk factors for delayed presentation and referral of symptomatic cancer: Evidence for common cancers. *British Journal of Cancer*, DOI:10.1038/sj.bjc.6605398.
12. Robinson J.K., Joshi K.M., Ortiz S., Kundu R.V. (2011) Melanoma knowledge, perception, and awareness in ethnic minorities in Chicago: Recommendations regarding education. *Psycho-Oncology*, DOI: 10.1002/pon.1736.
13. Waller J., Robb K., Stubbings S. *et al.* (2009) Awareness of cancer symptoms and anticipated help seeking among ethnic minority groups in England. *British Journal of Cancer*, 101(Suppl 2), S24–30.
14. Robb K., Wardle J., Stubbings S. *et al.* (2010) Ethnic disparities in knowledge of cancer screening programmes in the UK. *Journal of Medical Screening*, 17, 125–131.
15. Wong L.P., Wong Y.L., Low W.Y. *et al.* (2009) Knowledge and awareness of cervical cancer and screening among Malaysian women who have never had a Pap smear: A qualitative study. *Singapore Medical Journal*, 50, 49–54.
16. Gourlay M.L., Lewis C.L., Preisser J.S. *et al.* (2010) Perceptions of informed decision making about cancer screening in a diverse primary care population. *Family Medicine*, 42, 421–427.
17. Binswanger I.A., White M.C., Perez-Stable E.J. *et al.* (2005) Cancer screening among jail inmates: Frequency, knowledge, and willingness. *American Journal of Public Health*, DOI: 10.2105/AJPH.2004.052498.
18. Marion M.S., Schover L.R. (2006) Behavioral science and the task of resolving health disparities in cancer. *Journal of Cancer Education*, 21, S80–86.
19. Lam W.W.T., Au A.H.Y., Wong J.H.F. *et al.* Unmet supportive care needs: A cross cultural comparison between Hong Kong Chinese and Caucasian German women with breast cancer. *Breast Cancer Research & Treatment*, DOI: 10.1007/s10549-011-1592-1. Epub ahead of print.

20. Miranda P.Y., Tarraf W., González H.M. (2011) Breast cancer screening and ethnicity in the United States: Implications for health disparities research. *Breast Cancer Research & Treatment*, Feb 6, Epub ahead of print.
21. Fernandes-Taylor S., Bloom J.R. (2010) Socioeconomic status and psycho-oncology, in *Psycho-Oncology*, 2nd edn (eds J.C. Holland, W.S. Breitbart, P.B. Jacobsen *et al.*), Oxford University Press, New York, pp. 47–55.
22. Long H.L., Tulsky J.P., Chambers D.B. *et al.* (1998) Cancer screening in homeless women: Attitudes and behavior. *Journal of Health Care for the Poor and Underserved*, 9, 276–292.
23. Lee H.Y., Ju E., Vang P.D., Lundquist M. (2010) Breast and cervical cancer screening among Asian American women and Latinas: Does race/ethnicity matter? *Journal of Women's Health*, 19, 1877–1884.
24. Fontana M., Bischoff A. (2008) Uptake of breast cancer screening methods among immigrant and Swiss women in Switzerland. *Swiss Medical Weekly*, 138, 752–758.
25. Pons-Vigues M., Puigpinos-Riera R., Serral G. *et al.* (2011) Knowledge, attitude and perceptions of breast cancer screening among native and immigrant women in Barcelona, Spain. *Psycho-Oncology*, DOI: 10.1002/pon.1940. Epub ahead of print.
26. Gray J.A.M., Patnick J., Blanks R.G. (2008) Maximising benefit and minimising harm of screening. *British Medical Journal*, DOI: 10.1136/bmj.39470.643218.94.
27. Li W.W.Y., Lam W.W.T., Wong J.H.F. *et al.* (2011) Waiting to see the doctor: Understanding appraisal and utilization components of consultation delay for new breast symptoms in Chinese women. *Psycho-Oncology*, Aug 26, DOI: 10.1002/pon.2038. Epub ahead of print.
28. Montella M., Crispo A., D'Aiuto G. *et al.* (2001) Determinant factors for diagnostic delay in operable breast cancer patients. *European Journal of Cancer Prevention*, 10, 53–59.
29. Montazeri A, Ebrahimi M, Mehrdad N, Ansari M, Sajadian A. (2003) Delayed presentation in breast cancer: A study in Iranian women. *BMC Women's Health*, 7, 3, 4.
30. Abdel-Fattah M.M., Anwar M.A., Mari E. *et al.* (1999) Patient and symptom related diagnostic delay in breast cancer: Evidence from Alexandria. *European Journal of Public Health*, 9, 15–19.
31. Valdes S., Garcia E., Perez H., Hernandez M. (2010) Length of diagnostic delay in patients with NSCLC. *MEDICC Review*, 12, 29–32. www.medicc.org/mediccreview/articles/mr_130.pdf (accessed January 2012).
32. Shike M., Schattner M., Genao A. *et al.* (2011) Expanding colorectal cancer screening among minority women. *Cancer*, DOI: 10.1002/cncr.25566.
33. Mujahid M.S., Janz N.K., Hawley S.T. *et al.* (2011) Racial/ethnic differences in job loss for women with breast cancer. *Journal of Cancer Survivorship*, 5, 102–111.
34. Lam W.W.T., Fielding R. (2003) The evolving experience of illness for Chinese women with breast cancer: A qualitative study. *Psycho-Oncology*, 12, 127–140.
35. Yip M.P., Tu S.P., Chun A. *et al.* (2006) Participation in colorectal cancer screening among Chinese Americans. *Asian Pacific Journal of Cancer Prevention*, 7, 645–650.
36. Price C.L., Szczepura A.K., Gumber A.K., Patnick J. (2010) Comparison of breast and bowel cancer screening uptake patterns in a common cohort of South Asian women in England. *BMC Health Services Research*, 10, 103.
37. Nicholson R.A., Kreuter M.W., Lapka C. *et al.* (2008) Unintended effects of emphasizing disparities in cancer communication to African Americans. *Cancer Epidemiology, Biomarkers & Prevention*, 17, 2946–2953.
38. Fishbein M., Ajzen I. (1974) Attitudes towards objects as predictors of single and multiple behavioral criteria. *Psychological Review*, 81, 59–74.
39. Engelman K.K., Cupertino A.P., Daley C.M. *et al.* (2011) Engaging diverse underserved communities to bridge the mammography divide. *BMC Public Health*, 11, 47.
40. Liao Q.Y., Cowling B.J., Lam W.W.T., Fielding R. (2011) Factors affecting intention to receive and self-reported receipt of 2009 pandemic (H1N1) vaccine in Hong Kong: A longitudinal study. *PLoS ONE*, DOI:10.1371/journal.pone.0017713.
41. Crane L.A., Leakey T.A., Rimer B.K. *et al.* (1998) Effectiveness of a telephone outcall intervention to promote screening mammography among low-income women. *Preventive Medicine*, 27, S39–49.
42. Raab S.S., Gryzibiki D.M. (*2010*) Quality in cancer diagnosis. *CA: A Cancer Journal for Clinicians*, DOI: 10.3322/caac.20068.
43. Singh H., Sethi S., Raber M., Peterson L.A. (2007) Errors in cancer diagnosis: Current understanding and future direction. *Journal of Clinical Oncology*, 25, 31, 5009–5018.

44. Roetzheim R.G., Pal N., Gonzalez E.C. *et al.* (1999) The effects of physician supply on the early detection of rectal cancer. *Family Practice*, 48, 850–858.
45. Hart J.T. (1971) The inverse care law. *Lancet*, 7696, 405–412.
46. Kahn K.L., Pearson M.L., Harrison E.R. *et al.* (1994) Health care for black and poor hospitalized Medicare patients. *Journal of the American Medical Association*, DOI:10.1001/jama.1994.03510390039027.
47. Krupski T.L., Kwan L., Afifi A.A., Litwin M.S. (2005) Geographic and socioeconomic variation in the treatment of prostate cancer *Journal of Clinical Oncology*, DOI: 10.1200/JCO.2005.08.755.
48. Haggstrom D.A., Quale C., Smith-Bindman R. (2005) Differences in the quality of breast cancer care among vulnerable populations. *Cancer*, 104, 2347–2358.
49. Freeman A.B., Huang B., Dragun A.E. (2011) Patterns of care with regard to surgical choice and application of adjuvant radiation therapy for preinvasive and early stage breast cancer in rural Appalachia. *American Journal of Clinical Oncology*, Mar 18, Epub ahead of print.
50. Dragun A.E., Huang B., Tucker T.C., Spanos W.J. (2010) Disparities in the application of adjuvant radiotherapy after breast-conserving surgery for early stage breast cancer: Impact on overall survival. *Cancer*, Dec 14, Epub ahead of print.
51. Moore C.E., Durden F. (2010) Head and neck cancer screening in homeless communities: HEAL (Health Education, Assessment, and Leadership). *Journal of the National Medical Association*, 102, 811–816.
52. van Ryn M., Burke J. (2000) The effect of patient race and socio-economic status on physician perceptions of patients. *Social Science in Medicine*, 50, 813–828.
53. Shavers V.L., Brown M.L. *(2002)* Racial and Ethnic Disparities in the Receipt of Cancer Treatment. *Journal of the National Cancer Institute*, DOI: 10.1093/jnci/94.5.334.
54. Merrill R.M., Merrill A.V., Mayer L.S. (2000) Factors associated with no surgery or radiation therapy for invasive cervical cancer in Black and White women. *Ethnicity & Disease*, 10, 248–256.
55. Kreps GL. (2006) Communication and racial inequities in health care. *American Behavioral Scientist*, DOI: 10.1177/0002764205283800.
56. Lam W.W.T., Fielding R., Ho E.Y.Y. (2005) Predicting psychological morbidity in Chinese women following surgery for breast cancer. *Cancer*, 103, 637–646.
57. Lam W.W.T., Chan M., Hung W.K., Fielding R. (2007) Treatment decision difficulties and post-operative distress predict persistence of psychological morbidity in Chinese women following breast cancer surgery. *Psycho-Oncology*, DOI: 10.1002/pon.1147.
58. Fielding R., Lam W.W.T. (2007) Surgical treatment decision-making in breast cancer among Chinese women: Predicting psychological morbidity. *Hong Kong Medical Journal*, 13, 19–22.
59. Lam W.W.T., Chan M., Hung W.K. *et al.* (2010) Resilience to distress among Chinese women diagnosed with breast cancer. *Psycho-Oncology*, 19, 1044–1051.
60. Lam W.W.T., Yee T.S., Bonnano G.A. *et al.* (2010) Distress trajectories at the first year following diagnosis of breast cancer in relation to 6-years survivorship. *Psycho-Oncology*, 2 Dec, DOI: 10.1002/pon.1875. Epub ahead of print.
61. Jean-Pierre P., Fiscella K., Griggs J. *et al.* (2010) Race/ethnicity-based concerns over understanding cancer diagnosis and treatment plan. *Journal of the National Medical Association*, 102, 184–189.
62. Au A., Lam W.W.T, Kwong A. *et al.* (2010) Validation of the Short-form Supportive Care Needs Survey Questionnaire (SCNS-SF34-C). *Psycho-Oncology*, Dec 12, DOI: 10.1002/pon.1851. Epub ahead of print.
63. Moody K., Mannix M.M., Furnari N. *et al.* (2010) Psychosocial needs of ethnic minority, inner-city, pediatric cancer patients. *Supportive Care in Cancer*, Sep 12, Epub ahead of print.
64. Ng R., Verkooijen H.M., Ooi L.L., Koh W.P. (2011) Unmet psychosocial needs among cancer patients undergoing ambulatory care in Singapore. *Supportive Care in Cancer*, May 10, Epub ahead of print.
65. Fallowfield L., Jenkins V., Farewell V., Solis-Trapala I. (2003) Enduring impact of communication skills training: Results of a 12-month follow-up. *British Journal of Cancer*, DOI:10.1038/sj.bjc.6601309.
66. Liénard A., Merckaert I., Libert Y. *et al.* (2006) Factors that influence cancer patients' anxiety following a medical consultation: Impact of a communication skills training programme for physicians. *Annals of Oncology*, DOI: 10.1093/annonc/mdl142.
67. Lienard A., Merckaert I., Libert Y. *et al.* (2008) Factors that influence cancer patients' and relatives' anxiety following a three-person medical consultation: Impact of a communication skills training program for physicians. *Psycho-Oncology*, 17, 488–496.

68. Miles A., Voorwinden S., Chapman S., Wardle J. (2008) Psychologic predictors of cancer information avoidance among older adults: The role of cancer fear and fatalism. *Cancer Epidemiology, Biomarkers & Prevention*, DOI: 10.1158/1055-9965.EPI-08-0074.
69. Morgan P.D., Fogel J., Tyler I.D., Jones J.R. (2010) Culturally targeted educational intervention to increase colorectal health awareness among African Americans. *Journal of Health Care for the Poor and Underserved*, 21, S132–147.
70. Powe B.D. (2001) Cancer fatalism among elderly African American women: Predictors of the intensity of the perceptions. *Journal of Psychosocial Oncology*, 19, 85–95.
71. Niederdeppe J., Gurmankin Levy A. (2007) Fatalistic beliefs about cancer prevention and three prevention behaviors. *Cancer Epidemiology, Biomarkers & Prevention*, 16, 998–1003.
72. Lam W.W.T., Chan M., Hung W.K. *et al.* (2009) Social adjustment among Chinese women following breast cancer surgery. *Psycho-Oncology*, 18, 1189–1198.
73. Thomas B.C., Carlson L.E., Bultz B.D. (2009) Cancer patient ethnicity and associations with emotional distress – the 6th Vital Sign: A new look at defining patient ethnicity in a multicultural context. *Journal of Immigrant & Minority Health*, 11, 237–248.
74. Burris J.L., Andrykowski M. (2010) Disparities in mental health between rural and nonrural cancer survivors: A preliminary study. *Psycho-Oncology*, 19, 637–645.
75. Vallerand A.H., Hasenau S., Templin T., Collins-Bohler D. (2005) Disparities between black and white patients with cancer pain: The effect of perception of control over pain. *Pain Medicine*, 6, 242–250.
76. Purnell J.Q., Palesh O.G., Heckler C.E. *et al.* (2010) Racial disparities in traumatic stress in prostate cancer patients: Secondary analysis of a National URCC CCOP Study of 317 men. *Supportive Care in Cancer*, Apr 23, Epub ahead of print.
77. Schootman M., Deshpande A.D., Pruitt S.L. *et al.* (2010) National estimates of racial disparities in health status and behavioral risk factors among long-term cancer survivors and non-cancer controls. *Cancer Causes & Control*, 21, 1387–1395.
78. Simon A.E., Wardle J. (2008) Socioeconomic disparities in psychosocial wellbeing in cancer patients. *European Journal of Cancer*, 44, 572–578.
79. Short P.F., Mallonee E.L. (2006) Income disparities in the quality of life of cancer survivors. *Medical Care*, 44, 16–23.
80. Rourke M.T., Hobbie W.L., Schwartz L., Kazak A.E. (2007) Post-traumatic stress disorder in young adult cancer survivors. *Pediatric & Blood Cancer*, 49, 177–182.
81. Widows M.R., Jacobsen P.B., Fields K.K. (2000) Relation of psychological vulnerability factors to posttraumatic stress disorder symptomatology in bone marrow transplant recipients. *Psychosomatic Medicine*, 62, 873–882.
82. Mundy E.A., Blanchard E.B., Cirenza E. *et al.* (2000) Posttraumatic stress disorder in breast cancer patients following autologous bone marrow transplantation or conventional cancer treatments. *Behaviour Research & Therapy*, 38, 1015–1027.
83. Cordova M.J., Andrykowski M.A., Kenady D.E. *et al.* (1995) Frequency and correlates of posttraumatic-stress-disorder-like symptoms after treatment for breast cancer. *Journal of Consulting and Clinical Psychology*, DOI: 10.1037/0022-006X.63.6.981.
84. Palmer S.C., Kagee A., Coyne J.C., DeMichele A. (2004) Experience of trauma, distress, and posttraumatic stress disorder among breast cancer patients. *Psychosomatic Medicine*, DOI: 10.1097/01.psy.0000116755.71033.10.
85. Zabora J., BrintzenhofeSzoc K., Curbow B. *et al.* (2001) The prevalence of psychological distress by cancer site. *Psycho-Oncology*, DOI: 10.1002/1099-1611(200101/02)10:1<19::AID-PON501>3.0.CO;2-6.
86. Carlson L.E., Angen M., Cullum J. *et al.* (2004) High levels of untreated distress and fatigue in cancer patients. *British Journal of Cancer*, 90, 2297–2304.
87. Carlson L.E., Grof S.L., Maciejewski O., Bultz B. (2010) Screening for Distress in lung and breast cancer outpatients: A randomized controlled trial. *Journal of Clinical Oncology*, 28, 4884–4891.
88. Strong V., Waters R., Hibberd C.J. *et al.* (2007) Emotional distress in cancer patients: The Edinburgh Cancer Centre symptom study. *British Journal of Cancer*, 96, 868–874.
89. van Scheppingen C., Schroevers M.J., Smink A. *et al.* (2011) Does screening for distress efficiently uncover meetable unmet needs in cancer patients? *Psycho-Oncology*, Mar 6, DOI: 10.1002/pon.1939. Epub ahead of print
90. Grunfeld E., Coyle D., Whelan T. *et al.* (2004) Family caregiver burden: Results of a longitudinal study of breast cancer patients and their principal caregivers. *Canadian Medical Association Journal*, DOI:10.1503/cmaj.1031205.

91. Hwang S.S., Chang V.T., Alejandro Y. *et al.* (2003) Caregiver unmet needs, burden, and satisfaction in symptomatic advanced cancer patients at a Veterans Affairs (VA) medical center. *Palliative and Supportive Care*, 1, 319–329.
92. Sharpe L., Butow P., Smith C. *et al.* (2005) The relationship between available support, unmet needs and caregiver burden in patients with advanced cancer and their carers. *Psycho-Oncology*, DOI: 10.1002/pon.825.
93. Denmark-Wahnefried W., Pinto B.M., Gritz E.R. (2006) Promoting health and physical function among cancer survivors: Potential for prevention and questions that remain. *Journal of Clinical Oncology*, DOI: 10.1200/JCO.2006.06.6175
94. Garbers S., Chiasson M.A. (2004) Inadequate functional health literacy in Spanish as a barrier to cervical cancer screening among immigrant Latinas in New York City. *Preventing Chronic Disease* [serial online]. Available from: http://www.cdc.gov/pcd/issues/2004/oct/03_0038.htm (accessed January 2012).
95. Beach M.C., Gary T.L., Price E.G. *et al.* (2006) Improving health care quality for racial/ethnic minorities: A systematic review of the best evidence regarding provider and organization interventions. *BMC Public Health*, DOI: 10.1186/1471-2458-6-104.
96. Roetzheim R.G., Christman L.K., Jacobsen P.B. *et al.* (*2004*) A randomized controlled trial to increase cancer screening among attendees of community health centers. *Annals of Family Medicine*, DOI: 10.1370/afm.101.
97. Hawley S.T., Griggs J.J., Hamilton A.S. *et al.* (2009) Decision involvement and receipt of mastectomy among racially and ethnically diverse breast cancer patients. *Journal of the National Cancer Institute*, DOI: 10.1093/jnci/djp271.
98. Anderson M.R., Bowen D.J., Morea J. *et al.* (2009) Involvement in decision-making and breast cancer survivor quality of life. *Health Psychology*, 28, 29–37.
99. Hack T.F., Degner L.F., Watson P., Sinha L. (2006) Do patients benefit from participating in medical decision making? Longitudinal follow-up of women with breast cancer. *Psycho-Oncology*, 15, 9–19.
100. Spiegel D., Bloom J.R., Kraemer H.C., Gottheil E. (1989) Effect of psychosocial treatment on survival of patients with metastatic breast cancer. *Lancet*, 8668, 888–891.
101. Lepore SJ, Coyne JC. (2006) Psychological interventions for distress in cancer patients: A review of reviews. *Annals of Behavioral Medicine*, DOI: 10.1207/s15324796abm3202_2.
102. Manne SL, Andryowski M. (2006) Are psychological interventions effective and accepted by cancer patients? II. Using empirically supported therapy guidelines to decide. *Annals of Behavioral Medicine*, DOI: 10.1207/s15324796abm3202_4.
103. Hodges L.J., Walker J., Klieboer A.M. *et al.* (2011) What is a psychological intervention? A meta-review and practical proposal. *Psycho-Oncology*, 20, 470–478.
104. Ell K., Xin B., Quon B. *et al.* (2008) Randomized controlled trial of collaborative care management of depression among low-income patients with cancer. *Journal of Clinical Oncology*, DOI: 10.1200/JCO.2008.16.6371.
105. Ell K., Xie B., Kapetanovic S. *et al.* (2011) One-year follow-up of collaborative depression care for low-income, predominantly Hispanic patients with cancer. *Psychiatric Services*, DOI: 10.1176/appi.ps.62.2.162.
106. Strong V., Waters R., Hibberd C. *et al.* (2008) Management of depression for people with cancer (SMaRT oncology 1): A randomised trial. *Lancet*, DOI:10.1016/S0140-6736(08)60991-5.
107. Rodin G. (2008) Treatment of depression in patients with cancer. *Lancet*, DOI: 10.1016/S0140-6736(08)60968-X.
108. Stark D., Kieley M., Smith A. *et al.* (2002) Anxiety disorders in cancer patients: Their nature, associations, and relation to quality of life. *Journal of Clinical Oncology*, DOI: 10.1200/JCO.2002.08.549.
109. Mehnert A., Koch U. (2007) Prevalence of acute and post-traumatic stress disorder and comorbid mental disorders in breast cancer patients during primary cancer care: A prospective study. *Psycho-Oncology*, DOI: 10.1002/pon.1057.
110. Au A.H.Y., Lam W.W.T., Chan M.C.M. *et al.* (2011) Development and pilot-testing of a Decision Aid for use among Chinese women facing breast cancer surgery. *Health Expectations*, DOI: 10.1111/j.1369-7625.2010.00655.x. Epub ahead of print.
111. Jones R.B., Pearson J., Cawsey A.J. *et al.* (2006) Effect of different forms of information produced for cancer patients on their use of the information, social support, and anxiety: Randomised trial. *British Medical Journal*, DOI: 10.1136/bmj.38807.571042.68.
112. McQuellon R.P., Wells M., Hoffman S. *et al.* (1998) Reducing distress in cancer patients with an orientation program. *Psycho-Oncology*, 7, 207–217.

113. Chan M.W., Ho S.M., Tedeschi R.D., Leung C.W. (2011) The valence of attentional bias and cancer-related rumination in posttraumatic stress and post-traumatic growth among women with breast cancer. *Psycho-Oncology,* DOI: 10.1002/pon.1761.
114. Poppelreuter M., Weis J., Kultz A.K. *et al.* (2004) Cognitive dysfunction and subjective complaints of cancer patients: A cross-sectional study in a cancer rehabilitation centre. *European Journal of Cancer,* DOI:10.1016/j.ejca.2003.08.001.
115. Buck R., Morley S. (2006) A daily process design study of attentional pain control strategies in the self-management of cancer pain. *European Journal of Pain,* 10, 385–398.
116. Glinder J.G., Beckjord E., Kaiser C.R., Compas B.E. (2007) Psychological adjustment to breast cancer: Automatic and controlled responses to stress. *Psychology & Health,* DOI: 10.1080/14768320600843168
117. Graves K.D. (2003) Social cognitive theory and cancer patients' quality of life: A meta-analysis of psychosocial intervention components. *Health Psychology,* DOI: 10.1037/0278-6133.22.2.210.
118. Osborne R.L., Demoncada A.C., Feuerstien M. (2006) Psychosocial interventions for depression, anxiety and quality of life in cancer survivors: Meta analyses. *The International Journal of Psychiatry in Medicine,* 36, 13–34.
119. Newell S.A., Sanson-Fisher R.W., Savolainen N.J. (2002) Systematic review of psychological therapies for cancer patients: Overview and recommendations for future research. *Journal of the National Cancer Institute,* 94, 558–584.
120. Jacobsen P.B., Jim H.S. (2008) Psychosocial interventions for anxiety and depression in adult cancer patients: Achievements and challenges. *CA: A Cancer Journal for Clinicians,* 58, 214–230.

PART 3
Other Topics

CHAPTER 14

Exploration of Family Care: A Multicultural Approach

Lea Baider[1] *and Gil Goldzweig*[2]
[1]Faculty of Medicine, Hebrew University Medical School, Hadassah University Hospital, Jerusalem; Psycho-Oncology Unit, Sharett Institute of Oncology, Department of Radiation and Clinical Oncology, Hadassah University Hospital, Jerusalem, Israel
[2]The Academic College of Tel-Aviv – Yaffo, Tel-Aviv, Israel

> We shall not cease from exploration, and the end of all our exploring will be to arrive where we started and know the place for the first time.
>
> T.S. Eliot[1]

Introduction

Cancer is not just a disease to be explained in terms of pathology in cells, tissues and organs. Cancer is an illness that should be described in terms of the social, cultural, religious and family responses to the underlying disease, including the ways in which the patient and family conceptualize and understand it. An individual's experience of illness cannot be considered in isolation from the family context in which it occurs. This is particularly true in the case of a life-threatening or life-chronic illness, such as cancer, where issues of meaning, appraisal and significance may assume great importance for the entire family.[2]

Cultural, social and religious factors are involved at every stage of the cancer journey from cancer prevention and screening, through to palliative care and end-of-life issues.[3] Definitions of what constitutes cancer, as an introspective appraisal, vary according to the normative family system as do explanatory models of the cancer trajectory. Understanding how and why cancer patients respond to their illness in the way they do will necessarily involve an appreciation of the role that the family culture plays in shaping all responses.[4]

In the Western world, individual autonomy, individual consent and patient approval are the core of the dominant bioethical framework.[5] This individual focus, while perceiving autonomy as empowering, tends to be blind to the fact that the knowledge base and the decision-making process of the individual shares a complex relationship with his/her social surrounding. Moreover, families may prefer to live with uncertainty about their fate rather than to be confronted with an accurate prediction of 'death threat'. There is an apparent incongruity in the 'right to know and the right not to know' debate. Can a fully autonomous individual make an informed choice with only partial knowledge? The right to know or not to know – whose right and to know what? – might have different theoretical and cultural bases. Who protects the patient's interests and the family as a unit of care and how are they protected?[6]

The total involvement of the family should be to discern as a reality and to recognize the long-standing values of respect for unconditional solidarity according to their normative cultural tradition. The existence of the family identifies it as a social entity whose being, integrity and cohesion are only understood within the family structure and not in its individualized members.[7]

Clinical Psycho-Oncology: An International Perspective, First Edition. Edited by Luigi Grassi and Michelle Riba.

As a system of interrelationships, another dimension is added to the images that the family has of illness, and that is the collision between the images of each family member and of the family as a collective identity. The family, as a normative system, influences each individual member; and each member influences the core of the family. In an autonomous system, events impinge on all members' actions, perceptions, fantasies and judgments. Moreover, each family member is perceived differently, assigned different roles and duties, is stimulated by different communication patterns and sees him/herself differently from any other system of individual care.

In contrast, a number of non-Western cultures de-emphasize autonomy, perceiving it as isolating rather than empowering. These cultures believe that communities and families – not individuals alone – are affected overtly by life-threatening illnesses of any of its members and the expected outcomes of the prognostic medical factors. The debate concerning knowledge, consent and approval revolves around the family. The family as the basic unit may be responsible for decisions about treatment and disclosure. Such cultures value non-maleficence (doing no harm) and protect patients from the emotional and physical harm caused by directly addressing illness and end-of-life care.[8]

Most societies recognize the significance of the interconnection between the individual and the family and the elaborate ways in which the illness and impending death of a member affect the family system. In most non-Western societies, it is accepted practice for families to contribute significantly to any decision-making process of cancer patients and to assume total caregiving responsibilities during the entire illness trajectory.[9] (Table 14.1)

Table 14.1 Cultural diversity

Cultural diversity
Emphasis on individualism versus collectivism
Definition of family (extended, nuclear, non-blood kinship)
Common views of gender roles, child-rearing practices, and care of older adults
Views of marriage and relationships
Communication patterns (direct versus indirect; relative emphasis on non-verbal communication; meanings of non-verbal gestures)
Common religious and spiritual-belief systems
Views of physicians
Views of suffering
Views of afterlife

Family illness: a private universe

The trajectory of chronic illness assimilates into a life course, contributing so intimately to the development of a particular life that illness becomes inseparable from the life history of the family.[10]

The life course of a family is manifest in its continuity over time. Each family arises from its particular history and is guided toward the future by sharing its basic values. These include the maintenance of health, personal development, education, work, community involvement, spiritual guidance and family cohesion.[11]

Is the family a universal institution of care and support?

The significance of the family, in regard to the society's value system, stems from the fact that the family is the basic social and ethical unit of care. Family groups have a diversity of illness narratives embedded within cultural, religious and historical contexts. Broader perspectives on the appraisal and value orientations towards the illness event are focused both between and within family cultures and traditional norms.

The meaning of cancer illness within the family culture is likely to be influenced not only by each individual's values and beliefs, but also by the family's convergence and diversity of meaning, their taboos and secrets. . . .[12]

Cancer poses the risk of separations and losses, which can best be contained within family relationships that are cohesive and mature. The threat of cancer to the family may be acknowledged by understanding the perception and appraisal within the social contexts in which it arises.[13]

Basic illness variables that lead to a diversity of family behavioural changes range from:

- disengagement, loneliness
- increased cohesiveness, spirituality
- stress and crises following recovery
- complaints, anger, withdrawal
- discovering new coping styles, strengths, autonomy, meaning.

Neither the patient nor his/her family can return to the pre-illness situation, and they neither remain the same people nor the same family system. Family memories and illusions of the past may become distorted in the face of the new reality of the illness. The family's expected emotional and/or instrumental support at this time is a crucial indicator of their cohesiveness, mutuality, flexibility and shared needs.[14]

The manner in which people manage illness and their terminal care is a particularly helpful window into the religious culture of a family. When focused on losses that are part of everyday life, we can learn a lot about a culture and about our shared humanity. As the management of grief and care are universal tasks confronting all families, a fuller understanding of Eastern and Western approaches to handling care and loss has the ability to stress our similarities without minimizing or overlooking our differences. Ultimately, we have an open space into the nexus of human relationships that comes by learning about a society's religious and cultural belief system regarding how to manage grief, illness and death.[15]

We will describe a variety of factors that constitute the experience of a traumatic life-threatening illness, both on the individual and collective dimensions of the family and the interplay between them. This orientation is applied from cultural and religious perspectives and affirms the link between clinical and conceptual viewpoints, using Israel as an example of a very diverse country.

Family culture: quandaries of care

Culture can be defined as the ideations, symbols, behaviours, values and beliefs that are shared by a human group. Culture, therefore, can be shaped by many factors including but not limited to religion, race, economic status, level of education and environmental factors.[16]

The culture of families 'is an ensemble of texts, themselves ensembles, which the anthropologist strains to read over the shoulders of those to whom they properly belong'.[17] This is an appealing image: like poems, narratives, myths or paintings, events can be imagined as texts, that, when properly interpreted, provide cracks of illumination upon an entire cultural system. The task is both challenging and complicated. The argument is not that a single event or set of behaviours provides the 'master text' for an entire culture.[18] Cultures are much too complex and contradictory to be properly reduced to a single stereotype. Nor is it claimed that there is a single correct interpretation or rendering of them. Yet, family illness events are so richly packed and glowing with meanings that unravelling them can provide new shades and levels of understanding.

Illness and loss provide an example of the continuous interplay between individuals and their religious and sociocultural contexts. The universal and particular elements of grief and mourning take place within a shifting and dynamic framework that evolves over time. The movement of the secular culture from emphasis on the collective to the families in society has major implications for how people respond privately and publicly to loss. Traditional family, community and religious values play a central role in determining people's attitudes toward life and death. Notably, these values are not held uniformly even within the same country and lead to conflicts in determining appropriate policy and universal practice standards regarding illness and death. Rituals remain a shared basis for the divergence into different meaning systems that are evolving to channel the illness and loss experience of differing subcultures within society.

Families in the Middle East: a protective fortress

As part of the Middle East, Israel's multicultural society has been affected over the years by the transition from a collective framework to a more individualistic one consisting of heterogeneous religious groups. This process has been taking place on an ongoing basis during the country's assimilation of successive waves of immigrants from around the world. At the same time, for important communal aspects of society, the significance of what it means to be a religious Jew, Muslim, Druze, etc. is shifting from an identity in dialogue within traditional religious society to an identity revolving around a more flexible system of family care. What is also being shed is the existing traditional religious society that provides a familiar approach to dealing with illness and death according to the norms of each historical system of traditions. Today's Israel encapsulates the multiplicity of cultural diversity; and as a living laboratory, it encounters illness, family-patient care and death.

Insofar as a community scheme tempers individual interests in favour of some collectively defined ideal such as family, ethnic group or religious community, it is sometimes assumed that autonomy is the first casualty of the communal revolution.[19] Israel is unusual in that it has tried to reconcile the utmost degree of autonomy, as characterized by the Western health care system, within the framework of a communitarian state – that is, within a society imbued with a high degree of collective consciousness, mutual concern, and family interdependence. The result, in the field of health care, is a unique blend of universal health insurance, compassion, presence and the highest levels of medical responsibility.

The ingathering to the land of Israel of people from so many scattered communities around the world has also exposed people to a multitude of varied religious and cultural rituals and practices that inevitably were influenced by the broader community around them. In effect, the reserved nature of families of northern European descent differ from families of North African, Russian, Arab and Druze descent in their emotional expression and behaviour, particularly when confronted with illness and death.[20]

Table 14.2 Population in Israel 2008.[21]

Total population: 7 552 000
Jews: 5 703 700 (75.5%) Among the Jewish population, 68% were born in Israel and the rest are foreign-born: 22% from Europe and North/South America, and 10% from Asia and Africa, including the Arab countries.
Arabs (including Muslim, Bedouin, Christians and Druze): 1 535 600 (20.3%) of total population) Muslim: 1 286 500 (17%) Christians: 151 700 (including non-Arabs) (2%) Druze: 125 300 (1.6%) The Arab population in Israel constitutes 20.3% of the general population (22.85% of whom are Arab women aged 20–60) and consists of several religious groups (Muslims 83.7%, Christians 8.9%, Druze 8.2%, and others). These groups speak the same language, share some likeness in historical background and in cultural norms and values; some of them live in mixed communities consisting of two or all three of the subgroups. Their society is more conservative and religious than the Jewish society in Israel.[22]
Others (non-Arab Christians or people who did not indicate religion): 312 700 (4.14%)
The total fertility rate among all populations in Israel remained unchanged over the past 10 years, except among the ultra-Orthodox and the Muslims. For more than 15 years, the average birthrate in the Muslim community has been 4.7 children per woman, Christian women an average of 2.5 children, and Druze women an average of 3 children.[23]

Israel population statistics (Table 14.2)

The attitudes of Orthodox Jewish and religious Muslim and Ethiopian families towards members affected by cancer will be examined and described. In addition, a glimpse will be provided into the cultural variations, religious orientations and differing socioethnic backgrounds – as they pertain to behavioural manifestations and narrative meanings – of these families as they experience illness and the trajectory of death. The purpose will be to illustrate the importance of the structure and function of culture, religion and social norms in offering and delivering care.

The ultra-Orthodox family

As of 2008, Israel is home to the largest ultra-Orthodox (*Haredi* in Hebrew meaning 'one who trembles') population, representing 10% of Israeli Jews.[24] The number is rising steeply. In 1992,

Table 14.3 Religiosity among Jews in Israel 2008.

Religiosity among Jews in Israel 2008 (%)				
	Not religious/ secular	Traditional	Religious	Ultra-Orthodox
Total	41.7	40.2	9.8	8.0
Males	43.2	37.1	10.0	9.1
Females	40.3	43.0	9.5	7.0

out of a total of 1 500 000 Orthodox Jews worldwide, about 550 000 were *Haredi* (half of them living in Israel).[25] An additional 10% as 'religious'; 14% as 'religious-traditionalists'; 22% as 'non-religious traditionalists' (not strictly adhering to Jewish law); and 44% as 'secular'. Among all Israeli Jews, 65% believe in God and 85% participate in traditional holidays. However, other sources indicate that between 15% and 37% of Israelis identify themselves as either agnostics or atheists.[21] (Table 14.3)

Ultra-Orthodox Jews are located at the strict end of the religious spectrum, living in tightly knit and highly integrated communities functioning in self-imposed cultural insularity. They believe that Jewish law is of divine origin and the observance of all biblical and rabbinic laws is obligatory. These laws comprise a sophisticated legal/religious framework guiding every aspect of life. Rabbinic authorities play a prominent role in establishing and maintaining guidelines for behaviour, issuing both public statements with general applicability and personal response to specific questions posed by individuals. Life is structured around comprehensive religious obligations and prescribed behaviour including strict observance of family values, modesty in behaviour and dress, separation of men and women in public domains and, for men, ongoing religious study and thrice-daily prayer.[26] Family, procreation and religious education – which is the basis for the moral and ethical system of family care – are the most fundamental pillars of Orthodox Judaism.[27]

This process goes yet further. Descendants of their own close communities also acquire a historical aura or depth after one knows a story or set of stories about one of the ancestors. When two people meet, there is a mutual awareness of each other's background – parents, grandparents, neighbourhood, religious places of study.

Perceptions of the community differ by gender. Traditionally, women's social space was confined to home, to shrines, baths and to caring for the children. Even today, women preserve a kind of closed section that is entirely their own, separating them from the men and establishing their own space and activities. While sitting together with their large extended families, they succeed in establishing their own private world. Men socialized in the communal town space and more often ventured outside the community. Men frequently, but not always, were the ones to occupy the mediating position between the home and the community and between the town and the rest of the world.[28]

Jewish beliefs regarding illness and the hour of death are founded in the Bible. It is written in Psalms 144:4 that 'Man is like a breath... His days are as a passing shadow....' According to Jewish lore, the patriarch Jacob approached the end of his life by imploring God to provide a transitional period between life and death that would give him time to take proper leave of his family. In response to Jacob's prayer, mortality was introduced into the world. Judaism's positions on care stem from its fundamental convictions that human beings are mortal, their body belongs to God, and they have both the permission and the obligation to heal themselves.[29]

Orthodox families are reluctant to disclose the diagnosis of an end-stage or terminal illness because of the belief that this may lead to emotional trauma for the patient or premature death – or both. This reticence is especially felt when it might involve informing patients who are on their deathbed. The reasoning is that a patient's hope for prolonged life may be undermined if he/she knows that the illness is terminal.[30] In fact, the word 'cancer' is often substituted for euphemisms such as 'the disease' or the 'known disease'. The duty and obligation to save and preserve life and non-disclosure or partial disclosure are often linked. Inevitably, this hinders the oncology professional's ability to communicate directly with the patient about illness matters, and decisions are made only by the family.[31] Judaism dictates that the sanctity of life, which is to be lived as fully as possible and valued above all else, and the imperative to preserve life supersede quality-of-life considerations. Compassion, hope and God are the basic pillars of family care for the dying patient.[32]

Clinical case

David: A family narrative

The following clinical case describes a man who serves as a rabbi of a large ultra-Orthodox community and is defined not only by his religious commandments and responsibilities, but also by the sociocultural environment and family system in which he lives and is expected to be a role model for all members.

Sociodemographic data

David was born in France in 1956 and immigrated to Israel with his parents in 1958. His parents were born in Algeria. He grew up in a religious family and studied in a religious school. He graduated and became a teacher and rabbi. David has 6 brothers and 4 sisters, all religious, living in Israel. David is married to Yaffa, 39 years old, and they have 5 daughters: a married daughter of 18 and a 16, 12, 7 and 3 year old. Besides being a full-time homemaker, Yaffa runs a private day care group for babies in their home. She was born in Tunis and came to Israel as a child with her extended family.

Medical history

In March 2009, David was diagnosed with metastatic prostate cancer. Treated with radiation and luteinizing hormone releasing hormone (LHRH). Despite clear, persistent symptoms, patient refused to see a physician for more than one year. Because of intense pain and urinary difficulties – and his desire for absolute secrecy – he finally consulted with a family doctor outside his community who sent him to the Institute of Oncology. There he received medical care from a senior oncologist.

Clinical data

Patient was referred to psycho-oncology services by the oncologist describing high psychological distress. David was suffering from high anxiety. He described himself as extremely embarrassed, ashamed and wishing for God's forgiveness. He thought that his wife could become pregnant again, if he discontinued all medical treatment (he may have been motivated by the biblical commandment to 'be fruitful and multiply'). His wife was young, very energetic and wanted to have many more children. According to David, she was totally unaware of his medical condition and just wanted to give him the honour of bringing him a son. She visited a very prestigious rabbi to receive his blessings for pregnancy. David and she had never discussed the possibility of any medical problems. It was clear to him that particular areas of life are only shared between God and his own soul. Yaffa blamed herself for not being able to conceive. David refused to communicate with her or any of his close family about the illness. Only an older brother knows about the present situation. David explained his absence from home by using the excuse that he had found a more suitable learning institution outside his religious community. The traditional separation of roles, time and space gave legitimacy to his behaviour. David regularly explained his illness by focusing on the attributes of a benevolent and wise God. He had been chosen by God to go through this test of his own devotion, fidelity and faith. David's sense of guilt was guided by his wish to succeed, his need to be recognized by his close community and his large family. He was the centre of his family and community who sought him constantly for advice and guidance. David maintained absolute privacy and confidentiality about disclosure, secrecy, ashamed of being ill, guilty that he cannot fulfil the commandment of giving his wife more children that she so much desires and expects, fear of being rejected socially by his community, and discredited by his family. He rejected any possibility of sharing his medical information with his wife and family for fear of shaming them and causing them to worry. He was certain that God is with him and will never abandon him. His faith emerges as a 'rock of Mt Sinai', waiting as Moses did for the miracle of health and fertility.

In our last meeting, he gave me a book of Psalms (*Tehilim*), which he inscribed with the following: 'Watch over me, God, for I seek refuge in You' (Psalms 16:1) [Translated from Hebrew, private material, Lea Baider].

Among ultra-Orthodox Jews, illness is described through invoking religious explanatory models and using coping behaviour based on faith in religious healing. Cancer is considered an embarrassing and deathly disease. God shared David's formidable preoccupation without inflicting any sorrow on his family or possible shame on his unwed children. His enduring faith allows David to hope for renewed health and balanced family harmony.

Whereas certain ultra-Orthodox male patients reportedly benefit from sharing their disease-related concerns with their families, others restrict communication to avoid upsetting conversations. Such concealment has also been found to be adopted for preventing social degradation.[33]

Patients live in constant tension between withholding personal anguish about their disease and sharing private struggles to sustain emotional closeness by hiding their asexuality.

Shame may be one of the most hidden human feelings. Ultra-Orthodox patients are reluctant to talk about their own shameful experiences and often do not even want to admit having this feeling. It is the nature of shame that patients hide feelings of inadequacy or inferiority either from themselves or from others. Shame 'generates concealment out of a fear of rendering the self unacceptable', in contrast to guilt which 'invites confession and forgiveness'.[34] It is often experienced as the inner, critical voice that judges whatever we do as wrong, inferior or worthless. Shame and humiliation are closely connected to social exclusion, making the individual feel deviant and an outsider. These feelings contribute to the understanding of the psychological and cultural aspects of being pegged as 'different'.[35]

In any case, family involvement can never be, a priori, described as good or bad. The important thing is to understand the role of the family for each individual under different circumstances. Above all, the relationship between patient/family and God must be part of any equation.

Muslim families

> He said: O Musa! Surely I have chosen you above all the people with My message and with My words... Therefore, take hold of what I give to you and obey every word I say....
>
> Shakir, *Qur'an*, 007:144

Although it is wise to avoid underestimating the role of various factors in defining culture, Islam is undoubtedly the main factor responsible for shaping the Muslim culture. Islam is a faith with more than 1.3 billion followers, comprising the largest religious minority in industrial Europe and the largest non-Christian religious group in the world. Islam is the fastest-growing religion globally.[36]

Islam literally means total submission to the will of Allah (The Almighty God) by conforming inwardly and outwardly to His law. Islam is based on five fundamental pillars, which are adhered to by Muslims who believe in a life after death where retribution will take place and people will be judged to Paradise or Hell based on their deeds. As a fundamental doctrine, people believe in pre-destination and attribute the occurrence of disease to the will of Allah.

Islamic teachings forbid unnecessary touch (including shaking hands) between unrelated adults of opposite sexes. The chastity of Muslim women is one of their most important values, and this is expressed by modesty in dress and behaviour.

Although power relationships in Muslim families vary from one family to another, generally, male members in descending order of age from father, older brothers and adult male children, and male spouses have greater decision-making power than other family members.[9] The family leader is often the breadwinner, protector, disciplinarian and spokesperson. He is usually the ultimate decision-maker, with female members unable to influence. Females enjoy familial social security, because male relatives are legally and culturally responsible for meeting their basic needs (food, clothing, habitation, health, etc.). The social norms generated by this system quash the tendency for independency and autonomy among females.

Belief in pre-destination and life after death helps Muslims to cope with the diagnosis of a terminal illness. Nevertheless, breaking bad news can be difficult and considerably impact the family. In the Islamic doctrine, no one but Allah knows the future. Families will usually be satisfied if reference to this doctrine is made during discussions about life expectancy.[37] However, the natural history of a terminal illness can be explained in general terms.[38] The underlying belief is that one should and can take comfort knowing that life and death are in accord with God's will, that the soul returns to God, and that the community is supportive of the bereaved. The nature of the private experience of family grief, and the extent to which it is expressed publicly, are related to an interpretation of the Islamic worldview of what is acceptable and desirable.[39]

In Muslim culture, the authority of the family overrules the individual's autonomy. Decisions taken by patients can often be altered according to the views of the family. The custom is for the family rather than the patient to know first about any medical information. The family then decides whether and how much to tell the patient.[40]

When patients are dying, their families might want them to face Mecca; and, therefore, the patient's bed might need to be moved to achieve the desired position. During this phase, the family usually recites chapters from the *Qur'an* at the bedside.

Visiting the sick is highly encouraged and hence considerably practised. Relatives often travel long distances to visit patients admitted for relatively minor ailments or operations. The number of relatives, friends and neighbours who visit at any single time can occasionally interfere with health care delivery. It is culturally unacceptable to ask the visitors to leave and can be embarrassing to the entire family.

Clinical case

Suriat: A family narrative

Ibrahim, 53-year-old patient; Suriat, his 46-year-old wife and caregiver; six children aged 7–23 years.

Medical condition in 2010: lung, small-cell undifferentiated carcinoma, hepatic metastases, hospitalized for the last three weeks with pneumonia.

Ibrahim has 4 brothers and 2 sisters, one of whom is single and living at home with their widowed father in a small village in the north of the country. The family has a clothing store business in which all the male members work together.

Suriat, the patient's wife, has spent the last three weeks – day and night – in the hospital with Ibrahim. She has not gone home once. Other family members are always available to care for the children. Most days, Ibrahim's room is filled with his sisters-in-law, who go home at night. Ibrahim's father and brothers spend three times a day during prayer time outside his room. At the family's request, his hospital bed faces Mecca.

Suriat does not request any help from the nurses. She washes him, attends to his needs and prepares some food every day, even though he cannot eat and receives nourishment only by infusion. Ibrahim is sedated and receiving oxygen. At times, he responds to Suriat's whispers and tender care.

Near the end of the three weeks, the physician discusses Ibrahim's imminent death with the male members of the family; and they request that he be sent home. The medical staff asks the brothers for permission to speak to Ibrahim and Suriat about the risks and consequences of leaving the hospital, but the family absolutely opposes our intervention.

Ibrahim was transferred home. We spoke with a nurse who lives near the family's village to ask that she be in contact with the family and to begin home hospice care. Ibrahim died the day after he arrived home, in his bed, surrounded by his brothers and the rest of the males in the family, his soul facing Mecca.

Suriat's narrative

During Ibrahim's hospitalization, I met with Suriat each evening at the entrance to his room. She seemed exhausted most of the time, sad, trying to control her tears and anguish. We shared – in silence – a cup of mint tea that Suriat brought for me.

Through our silence and scattered dialogue, there was an underlying theme that was pivotal to Suriat's strength. 'God decides our fate and observes our actions.' 'God's decision cannot be changed by any doctor.' 'I owe my husband everything . . . without him, I am worth nothing. . . .' 'I will always obey God and my husband's family. . . .' 'And I will wait for Ibrahim . . . always.'

Each time I departed, Suriat put some mint leaves in my hand as if to say 'thank you'.

The day Ibrahim left the hospital to return home, Suriat came to me, embraced me, and without a word, placed a piece of paper with something written in Arabic. She said, 'For later, not now'. On it was written:

Indeed, I am to die . . .
Just as death is certain,
So is the resurrection of the dead.

Qur'an, 2:153

I will wait for Ibrahim . . . always . . . God is also in your soul . . .

Suriat

Ethiopians: the mysterious tribe

After major airlifts, the Ethiopian population in Israel has risen to well over 70 000 representing more than 1% of the population. They arrived as consanguineous families, mainly illiterate peasant farmers from the Gondar and Tigray provinces. They preserved their cultural integrity, observing the rituals and traditions of their faith, especially the Sabbath and the rules of ritual purity, including detailed customs of mourning and burial rituals.[41]

According to this custom, when an Ethiopian does not die in his house, the message is delivered to one of the neighbouring families, who serves as a middleman. They first bring the bad news to the elders who then tell the close relatives, usually in the afternoon when people have returned from work or early in the morning before work. In no case is the tragic news to be delivered directly to the family, but always through the middleman who volunteers to take upon himself the difficult mission. This custom enables the family to begin the rituals and lamentations immediately and with the participation of many people. The process of mourning is not held in the deceased's home because of 'death impurity', but rather in a special tent (*das*). During the first seven days of mourning, many visitors are likely to come to comfort the bereaved. They enter the *das* in groups while singing mourning dirges (*likso*). The mourners stand up while the visitors file by, one by one, and while singing a dirge place hands upon the mourner's shoulders. Afterwards, they all sit down and talk particularly about the deceased's positive qualities. Visitors are offered a cup of coffee (*buna*). It is customary for the community to pray in the mourning tent during these seven days. At some point afterwards, the mourners organize a memorial service for the deceased to which they invite religious leaders, the extended family, friends and acquaintances. At this service, prayers are offered for the deceased, their life story is told, and a festive meal is served. This ritual is seen as a final parting gesture towards the departed one.[42]

Case study

Aniel: A family narrative

'... What makes us cause our rain to fall and smoke to evaporate?... What makes us ill?...'

Aniel is a 17-year-old patient with metastatic melanoma. Twelve family members were sitting near a circular formation of candles. The small room had a distinct odour of incense combined with an aroma of herbs and the strong smell of heat outside in a Negev-like desert village. Aniel was near the main room in a bed where three older women were spreading the air through straw blowers. Other family members were on their knees, outside in the entrance, singing prayers.

Aniel was diagnosed with metastatic melanoma more than one year ago. The extended family and the community did not move from their place. They believe that their prayers for Aniel go directly to angels like smoke and air... Aniel spent time at the hospital. She was treated with chemotherapy and a new vaccine. However, neither treatment produced any positive illness response.

The family took her home, very far from the hospital. Their silent thoughts were that chemicals had poisoned Aniel's blood and that she needed to be clean from the inside... Only two of her brothers and one cousin spoke Hebrew. Because one of the authors (LB) did not speak Amharic, the expression of eyes, body language and the silences filled with smells, songs and whispers became the bridge to mutual care and compassion.

LB spent two days with Aniel and her family. Smiles, crying, grief and suffering were embedded in a ritualistic form of mourning. No lights... only candles. Angels will search for the candles and give Aniel the paradise of God... white flowers surrounding her body. Their singing and prayers will endure the most beautiful dreams inside her eyes... And Aniel will dream within a sea of chants and golden rain.

A few days after returning to Jerusalem, I received an envelope containing dry white flowers and a note written in Amharic: 'From Aniel's angels...' [Translated from Hebrew, private material, Lea Baider].

Family care: an inconclusive exploration ...

In a world characterized by significant cultural, economic and social complexities, theoreticians and researchers have noted a fault line or sphere of incongruence that divides Western and Islamic cultures and civilizations.[43] Without a doubt, Western and Islamic societies have different normative meanings and value systems. They differ in their degree of emphasis upon individualist versus collectivist values, their championing of traditional versus 'modernist' appraisals of family care, and their degree of tolerance for diversity and pluralism.[44] In trying to understand a culture and its ways of structuring the world, much can be learned from addressing the manner in which intimate family relationships are ordered and the manner in which family crises are channelled toward care.

Studies on family culture suggest that those who have established strong religious beliefs are particularly likely to employ religious explanations that preserve their existing beliefs.[45] Additionally, validated experiences are more likely to attract religious explanations. Families who confront the 'boundary conditions of life', including life-threatening diseases, are more likely to find religious interpretations of their illness compelling.[46] Therefore, groups of religiously observant families facing life-threatening diseases tend to frame their experiences in religious terms that fit with their existing family beliefs.

In cultures across the world today, the process of secularization, urbanization and social mobility has resulted in a weakening of ritual, community and family buffers in the experience of loss. Cultures that place a higher value on beneficence and non-maleficence relative to autonomy have a long tradition of family-centred health care decisions. In this collective decision process, families receive information about the patient's diagnosis and prognosis and make treatment choices, without the patient's input.[47]

In a study by Pargament,[48] he reported that families reframed their assertions that although they were unable to discern a reason behind illness, they were certain that one did exist. In this way, the perceived meaninglessness of the situation remained at the level of human perception, and the inability to perceive the true and real meaning was due to a limited and inadequate capacity for comprehension. This admission of the inability to understand why a traumatic event has happened does not reflect negatively on God or on the situation; and the belief in a sacred design behind all events, including the traumatic, remains intact. What is changed is the belief about the human capacity to comprehend God's plans. Pargament notes that this is in some respects paradoxical, since 'we make sense of a life crisis by concluding that we cannot make sense of it; some things . . . are just beyond our comprehension'.

How much do we fully understand the psychological relevance of cultural, social and family factors in health, illness and death? Can illness behaviour be understood and reinterpreted in terms of normative family culture?[49]

As professionals, we have developed and held fast to our own culture, set of traditions and belief system, influenced and nurtured by our collegial 'family'. When we meet new patients, we must be willing to understand higher concepts of family, tradition and God. This will open the door wide to allow new kinds of debate regarding family, health and autonomy, and novel concepts of therapeutic processes. In so doing, controversy and quandaries will assume new qualities and new challenges. The ethos of openly sharing unresolved conflicts brought about by the illness may then find a different normative expression embedded in other societies and traditional systems of belief. We should strive for meaningful responses, interventions and compassionate acceptance of the multicultural diversity of norms regarding family care.

'They asked Rabbi Levi Yitzhak: "Why is the first page number missing in all the tractates of the Babylonian Talmud? Why does each begin with the second?" He replied: "However much a man may learn, he should always remember that he has not even gotten to the first page . . .".'[50]

Key points

- How much do we fully understand the psychological relevance of cultural, social and family factors in health, illness and death? Can illness behaviour be understood and reinterpreted in terms of normative family culture?
- Cancer is an illness that should be described in terms of the social, cultural, religious and family responses to the underlying disease, including the ways in which the patient and family conceptualize and understand it.
- The significance of the family, in regard to the society's value system, stems from the fact that the family is the basic social and ethical unit of care. Family groups have a diversity of illness narratives embedded within cultural, religious and historical contexts.
- Most societies recognize the significance of the interconnection between the individual and the family and the elaborate ways in which the illness and impending death of a member affect the family system.
- Ultimately, we have an open space into the nexus of human relationships that comes by learning about a society's religious and cultural belief system regarding how to manage grief, illness and death.

References

Key references: 2,3,6,7,12,14,18,19,20,30,33,34,40,47, 49. The remaining references are for recommended reading.

1. Eliot T.S. (1943) *The Four Quartets*, Harcourt, Brace and Co., New York.
2. Dein S. (2006) *Culture and Cancer Care Anthropological Insights in Oncology*, Open University Press, Maidenhead, UK.
3. Rolland J.S. (2005) Cancer and the family: An integrative model. *Cancer*, 104, 2584–2595.
4. Kirmayer L.J. (2004) The cultural diversity of healing: Meaning, metaphor and mechanism. *British Medical Bulletin*, 69, 33–48.
5. Fan R., Tao J. (Issue Editors) (2004) Informed consent and the family: A cross-cultural study. *The Journal of Medicine and Philosophy*, 29(2), Taylor & Francis, The Netherlands.
6. Kagawa-Singer M., Valdez D., Yu M. *et al.* (2010) Cancer, culture and health disparities: Time to chart a new course? *CA: A Cancer Journal for Clinicians*, 60, 12–39.
7. Baider L. (2007) Cancer in different cultural contexts: How is the family affected? *EONS Newsletter*, 17, 18–19.
8. Searight H.R., Gafford J. (2007) Cultural diversity at the end of life. *American Family Physicians*, 72, 515–522.
9. Sparling T.G. (2006) Caring for Fatima. *Journal of Clinical Oncology*, 24, 2589–2591.
10. Kleinman A. (1988) *The Illness Narratives*, Basic Books, New York.
11. Weihs K.L., Enright T., Simmens S. (2002) High quality spousal or long-term partner relationships predict time to recurrence of breast cancer, after control for disease severity. *Psychosomatic Medicine*, 64, 107.
12. Goldzweig G., Hubert A., Walach N. *et al.* (2009) Gender and psychological distress among middle- and older-aged colorectal cancer patients and their spouses: An unexpected outcome. *Critical Reviews in Oncology/Hematology*, 70, 71–82.
13. Manne S., Ostroff J., Sherman M. *et al.* (2004) Couples' support-related communication, psychological distress, and relationship satisfaction among women with early-stage breast cancer. *Journal of Consulting and Clinical Psychology*, 72, 660–670.
14. Hodges L.J., Humphris G.M., Macfarlane G. *et al.* (2005) A meta-analytic investigation of the relationship between the psychological distress of cancer patients and their carers. *Social Science and Medicine*, 60, 1–12.
15. Gomes B., Higginson I.J. (2006) Factors in influencing death at home in terminally ill patients. *British Medical Journal*, 332, 515–521.
16. Hallenbeck J.L. (2006) Intercultural differences and communication at the end of life. *Palliative Care*, 28, 1–8.
17. Geertz C. (1973) *The Interpretation of Cultures*, Basic Books, New York.
18. Kagawa-Singer M., Kassim-Lakha S. (2005) A strategy to reduce cross-cultural miscommunication. *Academic Medicine*, 78, 577–587.
19. Gross M.L. (2001) Autonomy and paternalism in communitarian society in Israel. *Hastings Center Report*, 29, 13–20.
20. Goldzweig G., Meirovitaz A., Hubert A. *et al.* (2010) Meeting cancer patients' expectations. *Journal of Clinical Oncology*, 28, 1560–1565.
21. Central Bureau of Statistics (2010) *Statistical Abstract of Israel No. 61*, Jerusalem, Israel.
22. Ben-Ari A., Lavee Y. (2004) Cultural orientation, ethnic affiliation and daily occurrences: A cross-cultural analysis. *American Journal of Orthopsychiatry*, 74, 102.
23. Lavee Y., Katz R. (2008) Division of labor and marital quality: The effect of gender ideology. *Journal of Marriage and Family*, 64, 27–36.
24. Erlanger S. (May 22, 2008) A modern marketplace for Israel's ultra-orthodox. Middle East. *The New York Times*.
25. Baumel S.D. (2005) *Sacred Speakers: Language and Culture among the Haredim in Israel*, Berghahn Books, New York.
26. Spitzer J. (2002) *A Guide to the Orthodox Jewish Way of Life for Healthcare Professionals*, 3rd edn, Sage, London.
27. Weinstein L.B. (2004) Orthodox Jewish families and their community. *Journal of Community Health Nursing*, 20, 233–243.
28. Wellen Levine S. (2003) *Mystics, Mavericks, and Merrymakers. An Intimate Journey among Hasidic Girls*, New York University Press, New York.
29. Daniels C.C. (1996) Crisis and comfort: The Halakhah and the moribund patient. *Le'ela*, 11–13.
30. Baider L., Surbone A. (2010) Cancer and the family: The silent words of truth. *Journal of Clinical Oncology*, 28, 1269–1272.
31. Dorff E.N. (2005) End-of-life: Jewish perspectives. *Lancet*, 366, 862–865.
32. Isaacs R.H. (1999) *Judaism, Medicine and Healing*, Jason Aronson, Inc., New Jersey.

33. Baider L. (2008) Communication about illness: A family narrative. *Supportive Care in Cancer*, 16, 607–611.
34. Baider L. (2010) My illness myself: On the secrecy of shame. *Asian Pacific Journal of Cancer Prevention*, 11(MECC Supplement), 59–62.
35. Navon L., Morag A. (2003) Advanced prostate cancer patients' way of coping with the hormonal therapy's effect on the body, sexuality, and spousal ties. *Qualitative Health Research*, 13, 1378–1392.
36. Breivik H., Cherny N., Collett B. *et al.* (2009) Cancer-related pain: A pan-European survey of prevalence, treatment and patient attitudes. *Annals of Oncology*, 20, 1420–1433.
37. Bener A., Alwash R., Miller C.J. *et al.* (2010) Knowledge, attitudes and practices related to palliative care among Arab women. *Journal of Cancer Education*, 16, 215–220.
38. Zafir Al-Shahri M. (2003) The future of palliative care in the Islamic world. *Western Journal of Medicine*, 176, 60–61.
39. Yasien-Esmael H., Rubin S.S. (2005) The meaning structures of Muslim bereavements in Israel: Religious traditions, mourning practices, and human experience. *Death Studies*, 29, 495–518.
40. Abyad A. (2009) Health care services for palliative care in the Middle East. *Middle East Journal*, 12, 1–4.
41. Hodes R.M. (2000) Cross-cultural medicine: Ethiopians abroad. *Western Journal of Medicine* 166, 29–36.
42. Witztum E., Malkinson R., Rubin S.S. (2001) Death, bereavement and traumatic loss in Israel: An historical cultural perspective. *Israeli Journal of Psychiatry*, 38, 157–170.
43. Lewis B. (2002) *What Went Wrong?: Western Impact and Middle Eastern Response*, Oxford University Press, New York.
44. Sacks J. (2002) *The Dignity of Difference*, Continuum, New York.
45. Bussing A., Ostermann T., Matthiessen P.F. (2005) Search for meaningful support and the meaning of illness in German cancer patients. *Anticancer Research*, 25, 1449–1455.
46. Rogers S.A., Poey E.L., Reger G.M. *et al.* (2002) Religious coping amongst those with persistent mental illness. *International Journal for the Psychology of Religion*, 12, 161–175.
47. Surbone A. (2004) Cultural competence. Why? *Annals of Oncology*, 15, 697–699.
48. Pargament K.I. (1997) *The Psychology of Religion and Coping: Theory, Research, Practice.* The Guilford Press, New York/London.
49. Biasco G., Surbone A. (2009) Cultural challenges in caring for our patients in advanced stages of cancer. *Journal of Clinical Oncology*, 27, 157–158.
50. Buber M. (1947) *Tales of the Hasidim*, Schoken Books, New York, p. 232.

CHAPTER 15

Bioethical Challenges: Understanding Cultural Differences and Reducing Health Disparities

Antonella Surbone
Department of Medicine, New York University Medical School, New York, NY, USA

Case study

Mrs A was a 60-year-old Hispanic woman who came to my office accompanied by her daughter and her 9-year-old grandson. She had a large fungating mass in her right breast due to locally advanced breast cancer. Although I knew Spanish well enough to speak to her without an interpreter, she asked that her daughter and grandson be present for both the physical examination and consultation to 'give her courage'. She had never seen a physician about her present problem. When I asked her why she had not, she told me that women in her country of origin are reluctant to expose parts of their bodies. I was concerned about the presence of her grandson, in front of whom she undressed, but it became clear that Mrs A was not. I later learned that he was the 'man' in the family, as both the patient and her daughter were widows.

I asked her what had made her decide to come to see an oncologist. Her daughter explained that they both heard an ad on the radio about the importance of regular check-ups for breast cancer in women after a certain age. She asked me if I thought her breast mass could be breast cancer and I replied affirmatively. She then asked me if we could do something to find out with absolute certainty and I proposed and ordered a biopsy that was performed by a surgeon colleague that day.

Mrs A came back with her daughter and grandson a few days later to receive the test results. She started by asking me to tell her the truth, When I completed my detailed explanation of the biopsy finding, which combined with her clinical presentation confirmed that she had locally advanced breast cancer, I told her about further tests we could perform to rule out metastatic disease, and about her treatment options, based on her cancer stage. She listened carefully, at times asking her daughter for help when my Spanish was not sufficient. She said she had understood everything her daughter and grandson had to. She told me that she had only wanted to know if she had breast cancer. Mrs A did not want any form of treatment, including local surgery, radiation therapy, or hormonal therapy. She explained that she believed in God and in letting nature take its course. She asked me to be her doctor and see her regularly.

I saw her once a month for several months, witnessing her slow progressive deterioration. Each time, I recommended treatment since, especially at the time of her early visits, there was still a chance of arresting the cancer growth and possibly even reducing it. I also suggested to her the option of second opinion. She always refused. She was always very sweet and grateful for my time, as were her daughter and grandson. When her breast cancer had spread beyond control, I offered her the opportunity/option to meet with a psycho-oncologist, who, while not interfering with her decision, could help her and family clarify their reasons for refusing treatment. She and her family agreed to see the psychoncologist on the same day. He met Mrs A and her family members an additional several times, and Mrs A started palliative radiation therapy. Her quality of life improved and she lived for more than a year following treatment.

The case of Mrs A illustrates the powerful role of culture and religion in patients' and families' attitudes toward prevention, diagnosis and treatment. It shows the ethical challenges inherent in cultural diversity and the importance of an ongoing trusting relationship

Clinical Psycho-Oncology: An International Perspective, First Edition. Edited by Luigi Grassi and Michelle Riba.

between patients, families and oncology professionals. Finally, it highlights the role of the psycho-oncologist in helping patients and families untangle the various threads of their cultural tapestry and understanding their own family dynamics. By clarifying their motivations for different attitudes and choices, as well as those of physicians, psycho-oncologists can help patients explore treatment options and, often, assist oncology teams in providing the best care and improving quality of life, while respecting patients' and family members' cultural and religious values and beliefs.

Introduction: culture as a bioethical challenge

This chapter will (1) briefly describe ethics of principles and ethics of care theories; (2) analyse the concept of culture and its influence on patients' and families' perceptions and beliefs with regard to cancer causation, prevention and treatment; (3) illustrate through a clinical case a bedside ethical dilemma related to cross-cultural differences between patient and family on one hand and oncology team on the other; (4) discuss the relevance of cultural competence to the ethical practice of psycho-oncology. The chapter aims at providing practical suggestions to help psycho-oncologists approach their cancer patients with cultural sensitivity in regard to attitudes, preferences and health values in order to achieve a common therapeutic goal.

Progress in oncology treatment, associated with technological advances and discoveries in genetics, has been paralleled by a growing number of ethical issues and dilemmas. Health care disparities that persist throughout the world, and among minorities within Western societies, add a layer of complexity to the field of bioethics.

As discussed in the 2007 Institute of Medicine (IOM) report *Care for the Whole Patient* (http://www.iom.edu/Reports/2007/Cancer-Care-for-the-Whole-Patient-Meeting-Psychosocial-Health-Needs.aspx) and declared in the 2010 International Society of Psycho-Oncology (IPOS) Statement on Standards and Clinical Practice Guidelines in Cancer Care (www.ipos-society.org), 'quality cancer care must integrate the psychosocial domain into routine cancer care'.

Global care of each cancer patient, including medical, rehabilitation and psychosocial care, should be provided to all patients by respecting their individual and cultural identity and taking into consideration the available community resources.

The American Cancer Society (ACS) established three major goals to be met by 2015: (1) to reduce cancer mortality by 50%, (2) to reduce cancer incidence by 25%, and (3) to improve the quality of life of cancer patients.

The word 'bioethics', or ethics of life, was coined in 1970 by the oncologist Van Rensselaer Potter.[1] While ethics has accompanied the development of medicine since ancient times, bioethics differs from earlier medical ethics in two ways: first, it was born in response to the sudden progress of science and technology that expanded tremendously the sphere of possible medical interventions, and second, it was developed in the United States where individual rights and personal autonomy are highly valued.

Bioethics is defined, argued, and practised on the basis of different theoretical frameworks and with different practical applications. While a systematic review of these is beyond the scope of this chapter, two – the ethics of principles and the ethics of care – should be noted because of their wide diffusion and application to the approach and solution of ethical dilemmas in oncology.

The ethics of principles in medicine is based on the four *prima facie* principles of autonomy, beneficence, non-maleficence and justice. *Prima facie* principles hold an absolute value and yet can enter into conflict with each other in specific clinical circumstances. In such cases, one principle may prevail in determining a particular ethical decision. *Prima facie* principles are thus extremely useful to orient clinicians in approaching and assessing ethical dilemmas in clinical care.[2]

The ethics of care is centred on the notions of trust and vulnerability as key to understanding and addressing ethical issues related to the asymmetry of the patient–doctor relationship. Care ethics, largely based on the contribution of women philosophers, nurses and clinicians, is built on the premise that asymmetrical relationships of help, such as parenting and caregiving, in which the partner needing help is more vulnerable than the one providing it, cannot be understood in terms of equal partnership. Hence, trust becomes the essential element upon which the involved partners can establish a reciprocity of care.[3]

The ethics of principles and care ethics are not mutually exclusive. Rather, they provide different perspectives to solve bedside dilemmas in an integrated way. Key to this integrated approach is taking into account the importance of fairness and justice in health care at individual and collective levels.

Regardless of different schools and perspective, the foundations of clinical bioethics lie within the patient–doctor relationship, and are based on reciprocal trust and on sharing a common therapeutic goal.[4] Such goal is possible only through effective ongoing communication among all involved partners. As cross-cultural communication can be especially difficult in increasingly multiethnic societies, some of the major bioethical challenges of contemporary medicine relate to dilemmas that arise in multicultural clinical encounters, as well as to those stemming from the profound health care disparities among different ethnic groups in Western countries and between developed and developing countries.

Culture and oncology

The coexistence of multiple cultures is both a source of enrichment and a potential cause of stress and conflicts, the latter including health care matters. Cultural perceptions and reactions to severe illnesses such as cancer, suffering and dying are different, and these differences influence the provision and effectiveness of cancer care.

Culture shapes patients' and communities' perceptions of cancer risk, their trust in oncology professionals and institutions, and their views of human experimentation. Sociocultural values are also linked to cancer outcomes through beliefs, attitudes and behaviours that influence adherence to medical treatments and recommendations.[5]

Along with biological and social factors, cultural variables contribute to racial/ethnic differences in cancer incidence, morbidity, mortality and quality of life. Cultural factors contribute to inequities in minority patients' access to cancer prevention, screening, optimal standard care, enrolment in clinical trials, effective pain control, adequate supportive and palliative care, end-of-life care, psychosocial care, research interventions and survivorship care.[5] Cultural factors influence the interpretation and expression of ethical norms with regard to health and illness. Patient's autonomy or beneficence may prevail in any given culture, according to the weight that is attributed to each sick person's right to self-determination versus the importance given to the duty to protect the sick person.[6]

A common example in oncology is non-Western families' efforts to shield the cancer patient from painful truths by asking oncologists to withhold information about a cancer diagnosis or prognosis, or by taking upon themselves the right and responsibility to make decisions about treatment or end-of-life choices without sharing them with the cancer patient.

Until the 1990s, non-disclosure to cancer patients was common practice in many countries. A comparable situation had been reported in the United States in the 1960s, with dramatic change by the end of the 1970s under the influence of many factors, including progress in cancer treatments, the law, and public and patient advocacy. Similarly, a major shift toward more open communication with cancer patients has occurred worldwide in the past two decades. Still, attitudes and practices of non-disclosure persist in many countries. These must be understood in the cultural context in which they occur.[6]

When a cancer patient is treated in the United States, oncology teams face a dilemma in responding to family requests not to tell the truth to the patient. Disagreements and conflicts concerning truth-telling often are resolved by expressing respect for values and norms of patients and families, while at the same time making clear that US oncology professionals are bound by the ethical and legal norms of their country of practice.[7] It is essential to explain to families the rationale for disclosure as a way to respect cancer patients and to foster their involvement in the decision-making process, so that cancer care can be provided according to the patient wishes and priorities. Finally, as a means of helping family members to be more open to including patients in treatment decision-making processes, oncology professionals can teach patients and families that cancer is becoming a curable illness.

In the Anglo-American context, each person is viewed as autonomous, rational, self-assertive and self-aware. All adult patients, with the exception of those deemed to be mentally incompetent, are considered able to make decisions about their health and health care on the basis of the information they receive, and full disclosure is viewed as a necessary step to empower patients to actively participate in their cancer care. By contrast, in more family and community-centred societies, where individual rights are not as valued and autonomy is often seen as synonymous with isolation or lack of support, there is often reluctance to disclose the truth to cancer patients.[6]

Western beliefs and values, however, are too often assumed to be universal and perceived as binding. As a consequence, health care professionals and institutions may lack sufficient respect for cultural differences in the clinics and display stereotyping or judgmental attitudes toward their patients and families that negatively impact the quality of health care provided. By contrast, culturally competent and sensitive cancer care involves the establishment of effective communication with patients and families of different cultures, improving both the quality and effectiveness of care and contributing to reduced disparities in cancer outcomes.[5]

Culture, health and illness

Culture is the sum of the integrated patterns of knowledge, values, beliefs and behaviours of different groups. Culture is the system of life designed to ensure the survival and well-being of its members by sharing meaning, purpose and means and manners of caring for each other throughout life. Different tools are used by every cultural group to survive and thrive, to make cognitive and emotional sense of external reality and life events, and to shape meaningful, structured and effective interpersonal and institutional social interactions.[5] Finally, culture provides a way to make sense of life events, especially during crises and trying times, such as when a person develops cancer.

Through specific beliefs, values and rituals, culture shapes people's emotional reactions and behavioural responses to cancer, as well as ways of caring, providing safety, and assuring social support. Cultural beliefs and values are not static. They change over time for individuals and groups, especially when interactions occur in multicultural settings.

With regard to health care matters, culture frames attitudes toward the concepts of illness and suffering, the meaning of body parts, and decisions about life, illness and death. The social structures of families, the decision-making pattern of the group, and the impact of characteristics such as gender, age and community status on decision-making in health care matters are in large part culturally determined. The notion of culture is therefore extremely complex and there is still limited consensus on the various terms employed to define sociocultural constructs of race, ethnicity and culture. This fact, along with a tendency to reduce cultural issues to socioeconomic issues, is an obstacle to research and scholarly study of the relationship between culture and medicine.[5]

In general, race refers to the genetic, while ethnicity to the social aspects of cultural groups. Ethnicity, as one's sense of identity as a member of a cultural group, is socially constructed, contextual and dynamic. For example, a non-White child adopted by a European family will likely grow identifying with the culture of the adoptive parents and may never have experienced his or her original culture, including some specific cancer risk factors associated with diet and lifestyle. By the mere fact of looking phenotypically different from other community members, however, a person diagnosed with cancer may be perceived as different by health professionals and may experience some degree of stereotyping or even discriminatory attitudes.[5] In oncology, cultural differences are magnified by the severity of the illness and of treatment-associated side-effects, by the the physical pain and the psychological and existential suffering experienced by many cancer patients, and by the negative metaphoric meaning of cancer itself and associated social stigmatization in many cultures.

There is no right or wrong way to cope with cancer. All individuals do so according to their personality, past experiences and social support systems. Culture also plays an important role in coping with cancer, as demonstrated by many studies and anecdotal reports. The emotional responses of Japanese Americans and European Americans to cancer have been found to be equally adaptive, yet focused on different goals and achieved through different coping strategies.[8] For Japanese Americans, strength was found to be synonymous with stoic endurance and the metaphor was that of strong, but pliant, bamboo growing in a group. For European Americans, strength is associated with fighting an external enemy and symbolized by the oak tree, resistant and singular.[5,8] Gender affects cancer patients' responses to cancer, as well. Japanese-American men and European-American women are more accepting of the limitations imposed by treatment side-effects and rely more on social support networks than Japanese-American women and European-American men, who are less accepting of dependence on others and less willing to rely on support systems.[5]

Cross-cultural communication and its impact on decision-making: a global challenge

Patients' and families' information needs and preferences are different and they change during the course of the illness, under the influence of many factors, including the evolution of the cancer and the quality of the patient–doctor–family relationship. When the latter is positive, oncologists can communicate in a culturally sensitive way the nature and development of the illness, explain the rationale behind different treatment options and guide the patient and family through the difficult transition from curative to palliative care without taking away hope.

Cultural differences affect communication expectations on the part of both patients and clinicians.[9] Physicians' personal assumptions and biases on race and their individual values concerning autonomy, gender, age and class affect the quality of communication with their patients. At the same time, patients and families react to medical information provided according to their culture, age, sex, gender, education, role expectations and degree of adherence to social and religious traditions. Because of these variations in what is considered 'respectful' communication in different cultures, the content of the patient–doctor communication may be the same, but verbal and non-verbal manners and etiquette may change both the message's meaning and its resonance and perception. In one study, Chinese-American and Japanese-American women, for example, tended to accept information from their doctors in silence, because in their culture asking questions would burden the doctors or make them lose face, as though the information provided was unclear or insufficient.[5]

Inadequate or poor cross-cultural communication can undermine patient and family trust in individual members of oncology teams, as well as in institutions and in health care systems, with a negative impact on the decision-making process and on the quality of overall cancer care. By contrast, culturally consonant communication fosters trust and, while not eliminating all conflicts, it provides a means to reduce their impact or resolve most of them.

The recent paradigm shift in Western countries toward early introduction of palliative care (PC) and end-of-life (EOL) care requires candid ongoing communication about PC and EOL care to be initiated early during the course of each patient's illness, especially when cancer patients are diagnosed at advanced stages.[10] This new communication paradigm is based on reciprocal trust and on those cross-cultural communication skills that are key to developing a trusting relationship with patients and their families at each stage of the illness trajectory.

In oncology, shared decision-making, which requires good communication, is an essential element in patients' assessment of the quality of care that they received. Several studies show that decision-making styles differ based on personal and cultural factors as well as on the constraints of structural and socioeconomic factors. For example, non-Hispanic White women and African-American women seem to be more likely to make decisions on their own than Hispanic women, for whom family involvement in decision-making is common. A population-based study showed that 58% of Asian-American women chose mastectomy over breast-conserving therapy compared to 42% of non-Hispanic White women.[11] Beyond demographic, medical and socioeconomic characteristics, choosing between equally effective treatments of mastectomy or breast-conserving surgery followed by radiation therapy is often related to the multiple caregiving obligations of minority women toward their young or elderly family members. Many women choose mastectomy because radiation therapy would necessitate longer periods of absence from home or transportation that is expensive or unavailable.

Oncology professionals also play a key role in differences found in patients' decisions: many inform minority patients of treatment options less often than they do their non-Hispanic White counterparts. Whether due to language or health literacy barriers, or to unconscious biases, inadequate information leads to limited or suboptimal treatment choices.

Another example of inequity in treatment options is minority under-representation in oncology trials. Among the many barriers to accrual to cancer-related trials, lack of culturally appropriate education materials and language barriers are potential sources of unequal enrolment. Inadequate or missing information provided by oncologists to minority or underprivileged patients has been reported as an additional contributing factor.

The ethical challenge of cultural differences in palliative and end-of-life care

The ethical challenges of palliative and end-of-life care (PC and EOL care) are many and the following paragraphs will address the influence of sociocultural differences on acceptance and provision of PC and EOL care, and the ethical implications of designing and implementing PC and EOL care programmes worldwide.

Major sociocultural differences exist regarding both acceptance and provision of PC and EOL care by patients, families and physicians. Physical and existential pain are interpreted and expressed differently, based on religious values and social mores. Some cancer patients refuse adequate pain control because of the value attributed in their cultures to suffering in silence. Others choose to bear pain as God's test of their faith, or as a form of divine punishment. Some may perceive cancer as a mark of shame and guilt, and do not admit to feeling intense pain. Others may fear becoming addicted to analgesics.

In Western societies, many cancer patients still suffer unnecessary pain due to socioeconomic and cultural factors. For example, studies have documented that cancer facilities and pharmacies in low income minority-populated areas in the US lack narcotics and other pain and supportive medications. Even if prescribed optimal palliative and supportive regimens, cancer patients often cannot obtain the necessary drugs to alleviate their suffering.

In most Anglo-American countries, hospice care is increasingly chosen as providing the highest quality EOL care when compared to hospital or home care. Yet, only a few hospice patients belong to minority groups. A study of predictors of Advance Care Planning (ACP) among African-American, Hispanic and non-Hispanic White patients showed that African Americans tend to request more intensive treatment than other cancer patients.[12] This is thought to result from African Americans' general tendency toward vitalism – a complex attitude related to religious, social and historic factors rooted in the African-American spirituality, as well as in their long history of abuses and discrimination – which has led many African Americans to mistrust medical institutions and fear being prematurely deprived of life.

Studies of EOL decisions in emergency rooms showed that African-American participants tended to value life prolongation and requested information on suffering and spiritual guidance to support the extended family in making decisions. Non-Hispanic White participants, on the other hand, tended to prefer to make EOL decisions on their own. Oncology professionals, including psycho-oncologists, must tailor the content and the structure of information that they convey to the cultural norms and expectations of different patients and their family members. Patients and families should be asked how they would want to hear and discuss serious medical information, and the different values and preferences of minority patients and families should be integrated into cancer care at all stages, but especially in palliative and EOL settings. Fostering patients' trust by way of culturally sensitive communication and care is even more important for minorities, who tend to have access to medical care only through acute care centres or teaching hospitals, where residents and sometimes attending physicians often rotate, leaving cancer patients with less opportunity to build a trusting relationship with the oncology team.[5]

A limited use of palliative and EOL services, especially hospices, has been reported in non-Western countries, especially in communities with strong religious values and traditions. This paucity of hospice care is related to social, economical, political and cultural factors, as well. Professional societies such as IPOS, ASCO, MASCC, UICC and WHO are actively involved in promoting the diffusion of PC and EOL care standards as affordable and feasible also in low- and medium-income countries (LMCs). Four out of five patients diagnosed with cancer in LMCs have incurable disease at presentation due to lack of prevention, screening and general medical care, and this contributes to the higher cancer mortality in LMCs compared to higher income countries.[13] The ethical challenge is to find solutions not by exporting or imposing Western models, which may be culturally inadequate, but by working with local communities to educate people and health professionals and find applicable strategies based on existing facilities and resources.

The ethical challenge to understand cultural differences in survivorship care

As of 2008 there were 12 million cancer survivors in the United States. The first published review on cancer survivorship among ethnic groups of colour found that between 1966 and 2002, only 65 articles had been published, compared with more than 50 000 studies on primarily non-Hispanic Whites. These studies indicate that the needs of these diverse populations are as significant as those non-Hispanic White cancer survivors, but that the ability of clinicians or community groups to provide adequate services is compromised by lack of sufficient information, support and education for minority cancer patients and their families.

A few studies, along with the accounts of many ethnic-specific community leaders, indicate that mainstream survivorship programmes in the United States have not been found helpful by minority groups because they did not integrate cultural differences in communication styles or modes of providing social support. Some community organizations have now implemented programmes tailored to the needs and culture of their members. Survivors and their families require medical and psychosocial support to manage the long-term sequelae of cancer treatment, along with information on how to maintain physical, emotional, social and spiritual well-being. This should be provided through a culturally based integrated approach.

The ethical challenge of cultural differences includes family caregiving

Cancer is always a disease of the entire family, as the illness of one member alters the family dynamics and roles, requiring a readjustment of family relationships. While most research and interventions on coping with cancer continue to focus on the individual in the doctor/patient dyad, we should consider the triad of doctor, patient and family as the focus of our efforts to provide optimal cancer care.

The importance of family and communities in relation to oncology care is increasing as cancer care moves from inpatient to outpatient facilities, with a consequent increase in informal caregiving provided at home by family and friends. Of the many ethical aspects related to informal caregiving, this chapter will focus on two. First, caregiving is associated with high levels of stress and with different forms and degrees of physical and psychological morbidity, as well as with high financial costs. As a consequence, medical and psychosocial support to caregivers should become an integral part of oncology care and psycho-oncologists should take the lead as experts in this field.

Second, the modalities of providing caregiving, as well as the meaning and values associated with it, are strongly related to sociocultural factors and appear to differ by ethnic group. Caring for a loved one may be perceived as a burden, a duty, a privilege, or an opportunity to reciprocate the love and caring received in one's life. The quality of life of all involved in the provision of care is clearly affected by such differences, and psycho-oncologists are in a position to elicit and understand different caregivers' perspectives in order to maximize the efficacy of psychosocial support and interventions that both patients and caregivers may require.

The ethical challenge includes overcoming language and cultural barriers

Language and cultural barriers can become a major source of stress for patients, families and physicians. In such cases, the communication process tends to be confined to an exchange of basic information about medical, technical or bureaucratic aspects of the patient's cancer treatment. Effective communication requires a deeper knowledge of the patient by the treating oncology team, built upon conversations and exchanges that go beyond the strict medical sphere. This allows the team to familiarize with the patient as a whole person with values, preferences, wishes and priorities. Inadequate communication, whether verbal or non-verbal, engenders frustration and reciprocal mistrust. Errors may occur, and their seriousness may be enhanced, if patient safety rules cannot be adequately communicated and comprehended. Patients may feel less understood and accepted by their oncologists, especially when they have been subjected to prior discrimination by society or by the health care system. Unless clinicians are skilled in cultural competence, language barriers may easily lead to patient dissatisfaction and engender bedside misunderstanding and conflicts. These may reduce patients' adherence to treatments or preventive measures, or limit their participation in screening programmes or clinical trials, resulting in lower quality of care.[14]

To overcome language barriers in the clinic, the help of medical interpreters, considered as professionals who can mediate among different languages and cultures, is essential. Interpreters must be introduced to patients and family members, at the outset, to enhance the latter's acceptance of them as members of the medical team. The interpreter's role goes well beyond providing an accurate translation; it makes possible effective reciprocal communication between patients and cancer care professionals, even in the absence of shared language and meanings, and helps them establish trusting relationships.

In all cases of patient–doctor relationships mediated by a translator, it is necessary to elicit direct patient feedback about his or her understanding of what has been interpreted. Oncologists and psycho-oncologists must learn how to communicate with patients and families through professional interpreters and to consult with them during the course of the patient's illness and treatment, especially at times of difficult decision-making or of transition from curative to palliative or EOL care.

Providing language services to cancer patients and families requires 'cultural' and social commitment, along with adequate funding. Not all cancer facilities, however, can afford to have on-site professional interpreters or phone services offering medical translation, and not all patients and families feel comfortable with the presence of professional interpreters. Not all communication models can be exported from one culture to another. For example, phone or e-mail counselling, interviews or follow-up, or the use of written or audio material may not be considered appropriate means of communication in some cultures and may fail if patients or family members perceive them as disrespectful. As a result, we often need to rely on the patient's relatives or friends as translators. Non-professional translators, however, may not convey all information the oncologist gives, either for lack of health literacy or to protect the cancer patient from painful truths.

It can happen that minors are placed in the very difficult position of translating information about cancer to a non-English-speaking relative, because family members oppose the oncology team's suggestion to involve a professional translator. Conveying difficult, and distressing, medical information through a minor would raise ethical concerns in western cultures, yet it is considered appropriate in some cultures, especially when the minor is a male. Involving a psycho-oncologist can prove helpful over time in resolving such delicate situations.

The ethical duty to acquire cultural competence in oncology

Cultural competence is the set of knowledge and practical skills needed to understand and respond to different health beliefs and values in medical encounters and to reduce communication misunderstandings and ethical conflicts that may arise from cultural differences among patients, families and health care professionals.[15] Cultural competence is an important individual and system factor in our efforts to eliminate health care disparities and reduce the burden of unequal cancer treatment, along with bringing attention to disparities and fostering work force diversity. Patient-centred care includes cultural competence and sensitivity toward the patient and family, considered as a unity of care.[14] Teaching and training programmes in cultural competence have been developed and implemented and have been made mandatory for medical students and health care workers in some countries, such as the United States. Outcome evaluation of its impact is ongoing. Guidelines for the acquisition of individuals' and institutional cultural competence have been published in oncology and continuing medical education and online courses are available.[16]

A key element of cultural competence in medicine is to understand that cultures are dynamic and evolve with time and through mixing with other cultures. Individual members of the same community may have various degrees of acculturation or adherence to traditional customs. At times, these differences may lead to underlying conflicts within families about matters of illness and care, which psycho-oncologists may help to reveal and resolve.[5]

Finally, cultural competence requires awareness of one's own culture and biases, including their impact on one's response to the cultural attitudes and norms of others. With such awareness, oncology professionals become less judgmental and more accepting of others and of themselves. For example, it may be easier to discuss difficult life-and-death medical decisions with patients who share one's cultural background. By contrast, providers may become annoyed, and react judgmentally, when family members answer personal questions or make important EOL decisions while the patient remains silent or is not even in the room. Acknowledging differences and potential biases helps to reduce the risk of stereotyping patients and families or a lapse into discriminatory attitudes.

Biases can escalate into racism in the practice of medicine. Most often, racism is not an attitude of individual health care workers, but the product of an institutional and systemic 'culture of discrimination' that influences the behaviour of professionals. Subconscious racial biases among individual physicians who displayed discriminatory attitudes toward minority cancer patients have also been observed in clinical oncology practice.[5] Overcoming prejudices and racism in medicine and oncology is thus another major ethical challenge to be faced, given the rapid demographic shifts of contemporary times.

Practical suggestions are needed for an ethical psycho-oncology practice in a global perspective

As previously stated, all professionals, including psycho-oncologists, can now benefit from intensive interactive courses, whether residential or online, and continuing medical education courses, as well as from guidelines and publication of practically oriented research tailored to students and communication teachers. Recent publications include useful and simple clinical tips on how to approach patients and families of different cultures. Published material is available on making best use of individual and institutional resources to meet the needs of culturally diverse patients and their communities.[16]

Information regarding a patient's culture is generally obtained through the social history as part of the basic information required in any medical encounter. Such information should be augmented with questions about the patient's lifestyle, beliefs and values that will enable oncology professionals to consider the cultural, social and family context of each patient in its complexity and uniqueness.

As studies show that spirituality and religiosity are important dimensions in the lives of all cancer patients, and that their expression varies in different cultural groups, it is necessary to be open to addressing the spiritual concerns and needs of our patients, without imposing our own spiritual beliefs. Instruments to assess cancer patients' spiritual and religious needs have been developed and validated, and should be integrated into the patient's history.

Finally, as all cultures have developed healing strategies to maintain health and contrast illness, different patients may use these practices alone or in parallel with traditional Western medicine. Although complementary and alternative medical practices are increasingly used by many Western cancer patients, the majority of whom are well-educated and of middle to upper class backgrounds, oncology professionals tend to underestimate the fact that for patients of different cultures such practices often are seen as forms of traditional healing rather than an alternative practice. When healing practices are neutral or beneficial and do not have negative interactions with cancer therapies they may benefit cancer patients and their families by helping them to draw upon their natural resources to maintain and promote health.

It takes time to gather a comprehensive sociocultural history, including spiritual aspects as well as information about non-Western healing practices, but the time invested upfront can prove to be treatment- and cost-effective by facilitating development of a trusting relationship and reducing the risk of misunderstandings and conflicts due to cross-cultural differences.

Conclusion

The practice of oncology involves many ethical issues, both in clinical care and in research. In this chapter I have focused on the ethical challenges posed by cultural differences, both due to the growing multiethnicity of most countries and to the rapid increase of cancer diagnoses and deaths in developing countries, with their own sociocultural contexts and resources. Cultural differences enrich our lives and societies, but can also give raise to profound moral and social conflicts and to ethical quandaries. They can be the source of misunderstandings among patients, families and health care providers, and of ethical dilemmas for oncologists. For this reason, acquiring cultural competence is now necessary to the ethical practice of oncology and psycho-oncology.

Through understanding culture, cancer care providers, including psycho-oncologists, will be in a better position to establish meaningful and trustworthy therapeutic relationships with patients of diverse cultural backgrounds and to contribute to reducing cancer care disparities in Western countries. Furthermore, by acquiring cultural competence, leading oncology professionals will enhance their abilities to communicate with policymakers and other stakeholders involved in integrating psychosocial care into global cancer care worldwide.

Key points

- The main ethical goal of optimal cancer care is to foster excellence in the medical and technical aspects of oncology, including palliative and end-of-life care, as well as survivorship care, integrated with psychosocial care for cancer patients and their families.
- Cultural differences with regard to health care matters and serious illness, such as cancer, are increasingly common in progressively more multiethnic Western societies. It is important to understand and respect them in order to reduce the burden of unequal cancer treatment of minorities in both Western and developing countries.
- Culture has an impact on cancer at every stage of the cancer continuum from prevention, screening and early detection, to access and response to treatment, enrolment in clinical trials, rehabilitation and survivorship/palliative care, and end-of-life care.
- Cultural competence is a set of knowledge, skills and professional values necessary to effective cross-cultural communication in order to overcome linguistic, health literacy and cultural differences that tend to prevent or limit mutual understanding.
- Effective communication in medical encounters is a bidirectional process that enables health care professionals to know their patients as whole persons living with a specific illness in specific family and sociocultural contexts. Cancer patients can and should be actively involved in decision-making and receive the best medical care in the context of individual and cultural values, wishes and priorities.
- Proper cross-cultural communication facilitates the reciprocal trust between patients, families and oncology professionals that is necessary to negotiate and reach a common therapeutic goal for the patient's good.
- The patient–doctor relationship has an inherent therapeutic value, based on relational and spiritual dimensions: specific cross-cultural communication skills are needed to communicate effectively with cancer patients and families in the context of cross-cultural differences.
- From the perspective of patient/family-centred care, cultural competence is key to oncology practice, as it improves the quality and effectiveness of the global cancer care provided to cancer patients in developed and developing countries.

Suggested further reading

Crawley L, Kagawa-Singer M. (2007) Racial, Cultural, and Ethnic Factors Affecting the Quality of End-of-Life Care in California: Findings and Recommendations) California Health Care Foundation. Available at http://ehealth.chcf.org/documents/chronicdisease/Cultural FactorsEOL.pdf

Goss E, Lopez AM, Brown CL, *et al.* (2009) American Society of Clinical Oncology policy statement: Disparities in cancer care. *Journal of Clinical Oncology*, 27:2881–2885.

Association of American Medical Colleges. (2005) Cultural competence education for medical studies. Academic Medicine. Available at http://www.aamc.org.ezproxy.med.nyu.edu/meded/tacct/start.htm

Sabin J., Nosek B.A., Greenwald A., Rivara F.P. (2009) Physicians' implicit and explicit attitudes about race by MD race, ethnicity, and gender. *Journal of Health Care for the Poor and Underserved*, 20, 896–913.

Searight HR, Gafford J. (2005) Cultural diversity at the end of life: Issues and guidelines for family physicians. *American Family Physician*, 71:515–52

Sherwin S. (1998) A relational approach to autonomy in health care, in *The Politics of Women's' Health: Exploring Agency and Autonomy* (The Feminist Health Care Ethics Network, S. Sherwin, Co-ordinator), Temple University Press, Philadelphia, PA, pp. 19–44.

Surbone A., Baider L., Weitzman T.S. *et al.* on behalf of the MASCC Psychosocial Study Group Psychosocial Study Group at www.massc.org (2010) Psychosocial care for patients and their families is integral to supportive care in cancer: MASCC Position Statement. *Supportive Care in Cancer*, 18, 255–263.

References

1. Potter, Van Rensselaer (1971) *Bioethics: Bridge to the Future*, Prentice-Hall, Englewood Cliffs, NJ.
2. Beauchamp T., Childress J.F. (1994) *Principles of Biomedical Ethics*, 4th edn, Oxford University Press, New York.
3. Surbone A. (2010) Care ethics: An approach to the ethical dilemmas of psycho-oncology practice, in *Psycho-Oncology*, 2nd edn (eds J. Holland, W.S. Breitbart, P.B. Jacobsen *et al.*), Oxford University Press, New York, pp. 619–624.
4. Pellegrino E.D., Thomasma D.C. (1988) *For the Patient's Good. The Restoration of Beneficence in Health Care*, Oxford University Press, New York/London.

5. Kagawa-Singer M., Valdez A., Yu M.C., Surbone A. (2010) Cancer, culture and health disparities: Time to chart a new course? *CA: A Cancer Journal for Clinicians*, 60, 12–39.
6. Surbone A. (2006) Telling the truth to patients with cancer: What is the truth? *The Lancet Oncology*, 7, 944–950.
7. Anderlik M., Pentz R.D., Hess K.R. (2000) Revisiting the truth telling debate: A study of disclosure practices at a major cancer center. *Journal of Clinical Ethics*, 11, 251–259.
8. Kagawa-Singer M. (2001) From genes to social science: Impact of the simplistic interpretation of race, ethnicity, and culture on cancer outcome. *Cancer*, 91(suppl 1), 226–232.
9. Surbone A. (2006) Cultural aspects of communication in cancer care. *Recent Results Cancer Research*, 168, 91–104.
10. Peppercorn J.M., Smith T.J., Helft P.R. *et al.* (2011) American Society of Clinical Oncology Statement: Toward individualized care for patients with advanced cancer. *Journal of Clinical Oncology*, 28, 1–6.
11. Prehn A.W., Topol B., Stewart S. *et al.* (2002) Differences in treatment patterns for localized breast carcinoma among Asian/Pacific islander women. *Cancer*, 95, 2268–2275.
12. Smith A., McCarthy E.P., Paulk E. (2008) Racial and ethnic differences in advance care planning among patients with cancer: Impact of terminal illness acknowledgment, religiousness, and treatment preferences. *Journal of Clinical Oncology*, 26, 4131–4137.
13. Patel J.D.P., Galsky M.D., Chagpar A.B. *et al.* (2011) Role of American society of clinical oncology in low- and middle-income countries. *Journal of Clinical Oncology*, 29, 3097–3102.
14. Surbone A. (2010) Cultural competence in oncology: Where do we stand? [Editorial] *Annals of Oncology*, 21, 3–5.
15. Betancourt J.R. (2006) Cultural competency: Providing quality care to diverse populations. *The Consultant Pharmacist*, 21, 988–995.
16. Surbone A., Baile W.F. (2010) *Pocket Guide of Culturally Competent Communication*, The University of Texas MD Anderson Cancer Center, Houston, TX. Available at http://www.mdanderson.org/education-and-research/resources-for-professionals/professional-educational-resources/i-care/ICARE_Guide8pg_final.pdf.

CHAPTER 16

Post-traumatic Growth in Cancer Patients Across Cultures

Michael Diaz[1], *Matthew Cordova*[2] *and David Spiegel*[3]
[1]Stanford University, Stanford, CA, USA
[2]Palo Alto University, Palo Alto, CA, USA
[3]Department of Psychiatry & Behavioral Sciences, Stanford University School of Medicine, Stanford, CA, USA

Introduction

WHAT CANCER CANNOT DO
Cancer is so limited that:
It cannot cripple love
It cannot shatter hope
It cannot corrode faith
It cannot destroy peace
It cannot kill friendship
It cannot suppress memories
It cannot silence courage
It cannot invade the soul
It cannot steal eternal life
It cannot conquer the spirit.

—By an anonymous cancer survivor
Source: http://www.cancernet.co.uk/poems.htm

Having cancer is an extremely stressful experience for most people and an extensive literature has documented the negative emotional sequelae of cancer diagnosis and treatment. Since the mid 1990s, the idea that cancer can be experienced as a traumatic stressor has received considerable research attention, including investigation of post-traumatic stress disorder (PTSD) symptoms and diagnoses in cancer patients.[1] At the same time, there has been increasing recognition that those with cancer may experience positive personal changes, or post-traumatic growth (PTG), in a number of life domains. PTG, which has alternately been referred to as stress-related growth, benefit-finding, perceived benefits, growth through adversity, and existential growth, has been studied in a broad range of cancer patient populations to date.

Despite this burgeoning area of interest, most research on PTG following cancer has come from the United States. While some studies of cancer-related PTG have been conducted in Europe, Asia, Australia and elsewhere, there are still limited data from non-Western cultures. Although recent studies demonstrate that positive changes are reported by cancer patients from a wide range of countries, the extent to which this phenomenon differs across cultures is unclear. This chapter seeks to review what is known about cancer-related PTG across cultures and to draw conclusions that will inform clinical care and research.

Background

Growth after trauma: historical overview and theoretical underpinnings

The idea that an individual can grow after suffering is neither new nor culture-specific. Ancient

Clinical Psycho-Oncology: An International Perspective, First Edition. Edited by Luigi Grassi and Michelle Riba.

texts from many of the world's religions, including Judaism, Christianity, Islam and Buddhism, stress the connection between pain and growth. The crucifixion of Jesus has been used for thousands of years to teach Christians about the healing power of suffering. Buddha's concept of *dukkha* demonstrates the ubiquity of suffering and disquietude in ordinary life.[2] Islam teaches that suffering is used by Allah to test one's faith. Hinduism emphasizes the cycle of birth, death, and rebirth, and the idea of meaning-making may be related to the culture-related constructs of *dharma* and *karma*. Existential philosophers have emphasized that authentic living only comes from a true confrontation with non-being.[3–5] However, only recently has growth through suffering been explained as a psychological construct that reflects explicit and adaptive changes in an individual who has experienced trauma.

Theories that explain the phenomenon of PTG have been put forward. American psychologists Tedeschi and Calhoun (1995) coined the term post-traumatic growth in their book, *Trauma and Transformation: Growth in the Aftermath of Suffering*, and described cognitive, emotional, social and spiritual contextual factors that may lead to personal growth after trauma.[6] United Kingdom psychologists Joseph and Linley (2005) described a similar model of PTG, termed the 'Organismic Valuing Theory of Growth through Adversity'.[7] While there are some differences, these models share the idea that traumatic experiences can shatter previously held assumptions about the self (e.g. regarding goodness, control, invincibility) and the world (e.g. regarding safety, predictability), and can challenge or block pre-trauma life goals. While this disruption may lead to sadness, anger, fear and the constellation of symptoms known as PTSD, the process of reconstructing more flexible and accurate beliefs and revising goals through cognitive-emotional rumination and accommodation, though painful, may lead to perceptions of positive change in a number of life domains. According to these theories, only experiences of a significant magnitude, 'seismic events', can lead to the disruption that ultimately gives rise to PTG.

Through struggling with adversity, trauma survivors may experience positive changes in several areas of living.[6,8,9] This approach does not seek to dismiss the many adverse consequences of cancer, including existential threat, treatment side-effects, loss of function and pain.[10] However, in relation to these major stressors, cancer patients may experience a renewed appreciation of life, including a shift in priorities regarding what is important and recognizing the value of each day in their own lives. They may develop new interests or pursue a more meaningful path in life. They may feel closer to loved ones, value relationships differently, and have more compassion toward others. Those who face trauma may realize that they are stronger than they previously thought and may develop a greater sense of self-reliance. Many trauma survivors identify a better understanding of spiritual matters or a stronger religious faith.

The construct of PTG differs from resilience. Rather than a return to baseline following extreme stress, the hallmark of resilience, the individual experiencing PTG is thought to function at a higher or improved level than prior to the trauma. Wortman's quote from Lance Armstrong, world-renowned cyclist and cancer survivor, reflects this idea, 'Looking back, I wouldn't change anything . . . I learned a lot and grew tremendously the last two years' (p. 81).[11]

Clinical case

Ramon, a married 63-year-old Filipino father of 3, presented with newly diagnosed colorectal cancer. In addition to fatigue, pain and functional limitations, he reported severe anxiety regarding his uncertain prognosis, and sadness, guilt and anger at not being able to continue working. As the leader of his family and household, he felt 'worthless ... like a burden', and withdrew from his wife and adult children to protect them from his distress. While struggling to recover from surgery and chemotherapy, Ramon came to view his role in the family differently. He talked about being a model to his children for how to overcome difficult challenges. He became more disclosing and demonstrative to his wife and experienced an increased sense of closeness with his family and friends. He elected to retire and increase his time spent volunteering at his church and exercising. He stated, 'Everyday is precious – I want to spend my time with the people and causes that matter.'

The post-traumatic growth inventory: finding good in the bad

Although several instruments have been developed, the most widely used measure of PTG is the Post-traumatic Growth Inventory (PTGI).[9] Originally developed using a sample of American university students who had experienced a significant negative life event within the past five years, this 21-item self-report measure asks respondents to indicate the degree to which they have experienced positive life changes due to a given traumatic experience. Items are rated on a 0 ('I did not experience this change as a result of the event') to 5 ('I experienced this change to a very great degree as a result of the event') Likert-type scale. The PTGI yields a total score and five subscale scores: new possibilities (5 items), relating to others (7 items), personal strength (4 items), spiritual change (2 items), and appreciation of life (3 items). Tedeschi and Calhoun stress that the five factors can be reduced to three subdomains of growth: changes in self, in relationships, and in philosophy of life.[9]

Critiques of the PTG construct

Questions have been raised regarding the validity and accuracy of reports of positive change following trauma in general, and cancer specifically.[12] It has been argued that PTG may reflect a self-illusory process that allows an individual to maintain his/her identity in the face of catastrophe.[13] Further, emerging data suggest that cross-sectional reports of PTG may differ from actual changes reported over time from pre- to post-trauma.[14] Some have questioned whether the 'shattering of assumptions' is needed or even beneficial to the process of PTG.[11] Others have questioned whether cancer should be considered a 'trauma', akin to recognized discrete traumatic stressors, such as rape, disaster, or severe accidents. Maerker and Zoellner (2004) suggest that PTG may be best conceptualized through a two-part model that includes both adaptive and illusory components.[15] Despite this skepticism, it is common for those who have faced malignant disease to identify positive changes as a result of their experience.

Major issues relative to the theme of the chapter

Prevalence of cancer-related PTG

Some degree of post-traumatic growth is endorsed by a majority of cancer patients. In qualitative studies, 60–90% of breast cancer patients, 76% of testicular cancer patients, and 60–95% of survivors of childhood/adolescent cancers report some beneficial impact of their disease.[16] Qualitative methodologies for assessing PTG vary widely, from open-ended questions about the 'impact of cancer' to more directive questions regarding 'positive changes' as a result of cancer, making interpretation of these reports complex.

Because PTG is not a dichotomous construct, it is more common to use scores on the PTGI or other quantitative instruments as a measure of the extent to which PTG is endorsed in a given sample. Studies of cancer-related PTG using the PTGI[17] tend to yield total scores ranging from the mid 50s to upper 60s, suggesting mean item ratings around 3 on the 0–5 scale, reflecting a 'moderate' amount of positive change, on average.

Correlates of cancer-related PTG

Attempts have been made to identify correlates and predictors of PTG in cancer patients, with variable results. Sociodemographic factors have been one focus of investigation. At least some studies have found that higher socioeconomic status, as reflected by greater income[18] and education,[19] is associated with greater PTG after cancer. Others have found that younger age,[20] being married and employed,[19] and being of minority ethnicity[21] are linked with greater perception of positive change in cancer patients. Positive relationships have been found between cancer-related PTG and social support,[22] optimism[23] and coping through positive reframing.[24] While theory holds that greater threat posed by cancer would be more likely to elicit PTG, results have been mixed. Some studies have found greater disease severity to be associated with greater PTG,[25] whereas others have found earlier[26] or intermediate[27] disease stage to be associated with greater reports of growth. Other studies have found that greater subjective perceived threat and stressfulness of cancer is associated with greater PTG.[18,24]

Cancer-related PTG and distress

The relationship between reports of positive and negative adjustment to cancer is not clear. A number of studies have examined the relationship between PTG and indices of distress, including measures of depression, anxiety, PTSD and emotional well-being. Results have been mixed.[17] In cross-sectional studies, positive change has been linked to better adjustment in some cases (e.g.[28]) but has been unrelated to adjustment in others (e.g.[29]). Similarly, longitudinal studies of cancer patients have found perception of growth and distress to be positively related (e.g.[30]), negatively related (e.g.[21]), unrelated (e.g.[18,24,31]), and related in a curvilinear fashion.[32] These inconsistent findings are consistent with multidimensional views of well-being, which hold that negative and positive aspects of adjustment may vary independently of one another.

Reasons that cancer-related PTG may differ across cultures

The majority of the previously reviewed studies of cancer-related PTG were conducted in the United States. While this literature has provided some insight into the phenomenon, the extent to which it is representative of the experience of cancer patients from other cultures is unclear. Extending this line of research to non-Western countries would enhance our understanding of the phenomenon of cancer-related PTG, highlight possible cross-cultural differences, and inform clinical care and research.

There are several reasons that PTG following trauma in general, and cancer specifically, may differ across cultures. First, cultural differences in worldview and assumptions may affect perceptions of and attitudes towards growth after a crisis. Stereotypically, Western cultures more strongly emphasize independence and individualism, whereas Eastern cultures stress interdependence and collectivism.[33,34] American culture's emphasis on individuality and enhancement of the self may affect processes and norms that support the experience of growth through adversity. Several domains of the PTGI, such as 'personal strength', 'spiritual change', and 'new possibilities', are consistent with a more individualistic worldview, and therefore might not accurately reflect growth processes in collectivistic cultures. Indeed, it has been argued that PTG exemplifies the American ideal of overcoming strife through personal strength.[35]

Evidence from studies of PTG in non-cancer populations suggests such differences. Taku and colleagues (2007) found relatively low PTG in Japanese university students who had experienced various traumatic events.[36] Japanese culture emphasizes harmony and suppression of individual needs in the service of the good of the group; this may foster self-criticism and deflection, and may make perception of positive change after trauma less likely.

Second, cultural differences in religion and spirituality may impact the experience and measurement of PTG. For example, the 'spiritual change' items on the PTGI (i.e. 'better understanding of spiritual matters'; 'stronger religious faith') may perform differently across religious groups. Certain religions, such as Buddhism and Shintoism, do not stress strict professions or demonstrations of faith; thus, the impact of trauma on spirituality in these groups may not be adequately assessed by existing measures of growth. At the same time, some cultural and spiritual traditions view trauma as a possible transition with the potential for positive and negative outcomes; for example, the Chinese character for crisis combines symbols for danger and opportunity. Such views may create a context for greater perception of PTG.

Together, cultural differences in collectivism and spirituality may impact the pattern of reported PTG as well. Powell and colleagues studied PTG in Bosnian refugees using a translation of the PTGI.[37] Factor analysis failed to replicate the five-factor model of the original PTGI. Results yielded factors for 'relating to others' and 'changes in self/positive life attitude'; separate factors for 'spiritual change' and 'appreciation of life' did not emerge. While the low number of items in the original spiritual change and appreciation of life factors (2 and 3 items, respectively) may have accounted for this finding, Powell *et al.* suggested that the integral role of religion in Bosnian culture may have made it difficult to separate spirituality from other adjustment domains. The authors also suggested that the failure to detect an 'appreciation of life' factor may have been attributable to the Bosnian emphasis on collectivism over individualism, and the value of multigenerational patterns as opposed to individual outcomes.

Maercker and Herrle (2003) examined PTG in victims of the Dresden bombing 50 years post-trauma using a German translation of the PTGI. Factor analysis yield a four-factor model; only the 'personal strength' factor from the original PTGI was not replicated. These findings were attributed to differing concepts of the self between Germans and Americans.[38]

Similarly, Weiss and Berger used a Spanish translation of the PTGI to evaluate growth in Latina immigrants. Factor analysis yielded a five-factor model, but one factor labelled 'philosophy of life' combined items measuring 'spiritual change' and 'appreciation of life'. The authors suggested that the findings might have reflected the central role of religion and the emphasis on collectivism in Latino culture.[39]

Third, cultural variation in views of cancer may influence reports of PTG following malignant disease. The Western perspective of cancer as a biological condition differs from some other cultures. For instance, some Asian cultures view health in terms of role fulfilment, as opposed to physical status. Such differences may impact threat perception and subsequent adaptation.

Navon noted cultural differences in patient and health care professional responses to cancer. For instance, in India, cancer patients typically do not report pain until it becomes unbearable, as pain is considered a normal and natural part of life; this high threshold for stress may influence what is and is not considered to be traumatic. Physician disclosure of health threats differs across cultures. For example, it is considered cruel and untactful in nations as diverse as Italy, Egypt and Japan to fully disclose information regarding prognosis to a patient, whereas in the United States it would be considered dishonest to withhold such information.[40] Thus, cross-cultural differences in flow and appraisal of threat information may influence PTG outcomes.

Within culture, socioeconomic status may play a role in perception of illness. Low-income African-American women may minimize the severity of early stage, non-fatal cancer diagnoses.[40] Low-income Latinos and African Americans in the United States may hold more fatalistic and pessimistic perspectives on cancer than Caucasians.[41] Such views may influence treatment-seeking and coping responses, which may impact both distress and perception of positive change due to cancer.

Evidence of cancer-related PTG in non-Western countries

A growing number of studies of cancer-related PTG are being conducted in non-Western countries. Thombre and colleagues studied PTG in a sample of male and female breast, head/neck, and lung cancer patients ($n = 59$) from western India. Pilot testing of the PTGI for understanding in Indian patients led the researchers to change the metric to a 3-point rating scale ('did not experience this change', 'not sure', 'did experience this change'). PTG was positively associated with meaning-focused coping and with re-evaluation of worldviews, but was unrelated to uncertainty or fear of recurrence. Re-evaluation of worldviews having to do with social roles and relationships, religious beliefs and meaning in life were more common than those having to do with fairness or control, consistent with the 'collectivist and spiritual values of Indian culture' (p. 20).[42]

Jaarsma *et al.* evaluated the psychometric properties of a Dutch translation of the PTGI in a sample ($n = 294$) of male and female patients with diverse malignant diseases (e.g. breast, gynaecological, prostate, head/neck). Findings suggested that the original five-factor structure of the PTGI was maintained. Female gender and younger age were associated with greater PTG. PTGI scores were positively related to intrusive ideation and to emotional expression about the illness, openness to experience, and 'innerness', but were unrelated to avoidance, depression, anxiety, or neuroticism.[43]

Mystakidou and colleagues evaluated PTG in a Greek sample ($n = 58$) of advanced cancer patients with diverse diseases on a palliative care unit. They found that greater PTSD-related distress involving intrusive ideation, avoidance and hyperarousal was associated with greater PTG in a number of domains. They concluded that among these Greek cancer patients, greater disruption caused by cancer set the stage for greater opportunities for growth.[44]

Morris and Shakespeare-Finch investigated whether PTG differed across disease site in a sample ($n = 235$) of male and female cancer patients in Australia. Breast, prostate, haematological and colorectal malignancies were the most frequently occurring diagnoses. Younger age and female gender were associated with greater PTG. Greater PTG was related to greater perception of threat from cancer and to greater cancer-related distress. Patients with breast cancer reported greater PTG than those with haematological and colorectal cancer, but did not significantly differ from those with prostate cancer, even after controlling for gender.[45]

Mols *et al.* examined PTG in a sample ($n = 183$) of Dutch long-term (i.e. ~10 years post-diagnosis) breast cancer survivors. Both PTG and benefit finding (on a scale that asked participants to rate various life domains from negatively to positively impacted by cancer) were assessed. Life-satisfaction was higher in the cancer survivor sample than in a group of healthy matched controls. Almost 80% of the sample found benefits in their cancer experience, including in relationships with family and friends, community and civic involvement, diet, recreation, self-expression/self-improvement, outlook on life, mental health, character and trust in one's own body. PTG was particularly evident in domains of relating to others, personal strength and appreciation of life. Greater satisfaction with life was associated with greater PTG. Receipt of radiotherapy was negatively associated with PTG on some subscales, and higher tumour staging was associated with less benefit finding.[46]

Lelorain and colleagues studied PTG in a sample ($n = 307$) of French long-term (i.e. 5–15 years post-diagnosis) survivors of breast cancer. Notably, factor analysis of the French translation of the PTGI did not replicate the original five-factor structure, but because Cronbach's alphas were acceptable, the five subscales were still used in the analyses. PTG was positively associated with overall mental health, happiness and vitality. Positive affectivity, and active, positive, relational and religious coping were all positively associated with PTG. Interestingly, there was a curvilinear relationship between negative sequelae of breast cancer and PTG, such that an intermediate degree of difficulties was associated with greater perceived growth.[47]

Ho and colleagues conducted a series of studies of PTG in Chinese cancer patients. One study[48] evaluated PTG in ethnic Chinese male and female patients ($n = 188$) with various malignant diseases. Factor analysis of a Chinese translation of the PTGI did not replicate the five-factor structure of the English measure. Rather, a four-factor model, with factors labelled self, spiritual, life-orientation, and interpersonal, emerged. A second-order factor structure, with two factors labelled interpersonal and intrapersonal (consisting of self, spiritual and life-orientation items) was ultimately used in analyses. Both interpersonal and intrapersonal dimensions of PTG were negatively associated with depression, anxiety and negative coping, and were positively associated with positive attitude.

Ho *et al.*[49] conducted a study of the impact of explanatory style on PTG and PTSD in a sample ($n = 90$) of Chinese breast cancer patients. Women who made internal, global, and stable causal attributions for good events reported greater cancer-related PTG. In a separate study of PTG in Chinese oral cavity cancer patients ($n = 50$), being married and having greater optimism and hope were associated with greater PTG.[50]

Schroevers and Teo studied PTG in a sample ($n = 113$) of male and female Malaysian cancer survivors who were heterogeneous with respect to diagnosis.[51] Reports of PTG were common, particularly with regard to appreciation of life. PTG was unrelated to indices of cancer-related distress but was positively associated with coping through instrumental support, positive reframing and humour.

In sum, a number of recent non-US studies have investigated cancer-related PTG. These efforts have necessitated translation of the PTGI into several different languages and introduction of the concept of PTG into new cultural contexts. However, it is not immediately clear that the pattern of findings regarding PTG in these samples differs significantly from prior studies conducted in the United States.

Analysis of the evidence

Similarities and differences in cancer-related PTG across cultures

While cross-cultural comparisons of cancer-related PTG are made difficult by methodological differences between studies, several notable similarities and differences emerge. Some findings from the previously reviewed non-US studies of positive changes following cancer parallel results of US studies. First, reports of PTG in cancer patients across cultures are common. Across studies, mean item ratings (calculated by dividing the mean total PTGI score by 21 items) range from 2 to 3, reflecting small to moderate positive changes, on average. Thus, across cultures, most cancer patients derive at least some degree of PTG from their illness experience.

Second, there is some cross-cultural consistency with regard to correlates of PTG. In both US and non-US studies, female gender is associated with greater reports of cancer-related PTG. Gender differences in emotional expression, elicitation of social support, and meaning-making may underlie these findings. In addition, across countries, age is inversely associated with perception of positive change due to cancer, such that younger patients report greater PTG. Older patients' life perspectives and sense of personal stability may make perception of growth from cancer less likely. US and non-US studies have yielded parallel findings with regard to coping and PTG; several investigations suggest that active engagement and positive reframing are linked with greater perception of positive change. Greater perception of threat, stress and disruption due to cancer has been linked to greater cancer-related PTG in studies across various cultural samples. These cross-cultural patterns are consistent with both Tedeschi and Calhoun's and Joseph and Linley's prediction that active processing in the face of great threat may promote PTG.[6,7]

Variability in results of cancer-related PTG studies across cultures is also apparent. The process of translating the PTGI to other languages has led to some important observations regarding scaling and interpretability of the construct. Thombre *et al.*[42] revised the response options (from the original 6-point scale to a 3-point scale) in their adaptation of the PTGI for patients in India; this change was made to increase understandability and acceptability of the measure for their sample. With regard to the structure of PTG, factor analytic studies attempting to replicate the five-factor model based on the original English version of the PTGI have yielded mixed results. A five-factor structure was found in Jaarsma *et al.*'s[43] Dutch sample but not in Lelorain *et al.*'s French sample[47] or in Ho *et al.*'s Chinese sample.[48] Attempts to explicate these differences could include the proposition that PTG is understood and experienced differently across cultures, in part due to differences in collectivism and individualism.

However, drawing definitive conclusions regarding differing findings of cancer-related PTG studies across cultures is difficult due to limitations of the PTGI and to methodological variability across studies. The fact that the original English version of the 21-item PTGI has relatively few items (ranging from 2 to 7) per subscale has resulted in questions about the stability of its factor structure, regardless of language or culture. In fact, Tedeschi and Calhoun suggest that the PTGI may be appropriately reduced to three subdomains of growth: changes in self, in relationships, and in philosophy of life.[9]

In addition, variations in findings may be attributable to differences in study samples and methods. Most US studies of cancer-related PTG have focused on female patients, predominantly breast cancer survivors, relatively early in their disease or survivorship trajectory. As reflected in this review, non-US studies have been more likely to include samples that are heterogeneous with respect to gender and disease site, and have tended to include more long-term survivors. Given that female gender has been associated with greater reports of PTG and that time since diagnosis may influence adjustment, differences in results across studies may be confounded with sampling differences and are difficult to interpret.

Cultural implications

Convergent findings suggest that cancer patients across cultures report positive changes due to their illness. While there is reason to suspect that the phenomenology and specific kinds of growth patients experience may vary based on cultural differences in religion or in emphasis of individualism versus collectivism, evidence to date does not support clear distinctions in PTG across culture. Although differences may exist, methodological variability across studies has posed an obstacle to detecting and fully understanding them. Thus, it may be important to augment theory-driven hypothesis and model testing with more culture-based, 'bottom-up' approaches.[45]

In this light, moving from an *etic* to an *emic* approach to cancer-related PTG may be warranted.[35] An etic approach views a culture from an observer's perspective; this has been the stance of most research conducted on PTG in different cultures.[39] An emic approach, on the other hand, takes the perspective of a member of a certain culture to gain subjective, culturally relevant information. This important distinction can be used to create better, more culturally sensitive methods of measuring and observing PTG. By beginning with knowledge based on cultural values and assumptions, and using this information to design new and innovative measures of growth, researchers can move away from an etic approach and more towards an emic approach that develops assessments that are culturally pertinent and useful.

As inspiring and attractive as the construct of PTG is, caution and sensitivity are warranted in approaching this topic with cancer patients and other trauma survivors. Those who experience PTG appear to do so through a natural and unfolding process. While there is evidence that some intervention approaches may facilitate this kind of positive change,[23,52–55] it is important to avoid being prescriptive with regard to advocating growth to patients. Pushing or pulling patients toward PTG is likely to be experienced as invalidating and constricting and ultimately may result in alienation and increased distress.

Conclusions

The idea of having positive experiences in the face of trauma is not new or culture-bound. As Nietzsche said, 'That which does not kill us makes us stronger'. People report beneficial changes in the aftermath of trauma. While trauma can foment extreme stress in victims, they can also emerge stronger, with transformed relationships, new life priorities, increased appreciation of life, increased self-confidence, and an enhanced sense of spirituality.[52,53,55] Cancer confronts people with their mortality, undermining beliefs about control and predictability and apparently blocking valued goals; however, it is apparent that across cultures, patients' active confrontation with this threat can lead to enhanced functioning and well-being. As noted by Weiss and Berger, 'ordinary humans from diverse cultures and subcultures view their traumatic experience as "a supreme ordeal" by which they are transformed and from which they receive certain gifts'.[56]

Summary

There is growing evidence that most cancer patients perceive positive life changes as a result of their experience. This post-traumatic growth may coexist with emotional distress and appears to have some reliable correlates. Although most research on cancer-related PTG has been conducted in the United States, recent studies from other countries suggest that perception of growth after trauma in general, and cancer specifically, is a cross-cultural phenomenon. While there are reasons to suspect that patterns of cancer-related PTG may differ across cultures, methodological differences across studies make it difficult to draw firm conclusions. It is recommended that health care professionals approach the topic of PTG with great sensitivity and in the context of the patient's culture and worldview.

Key points

- Post-traumatic growth is defined as: positive experiences gained from struggling with and overcoming significant adversity.
- Many individuals diagnosed with and treated for cancer experience post-traumatic growth.
- The Post-traumatic Growth Inventory is the most commonly used self-report measure of post-traumatic growth.
- Post-traumatic growth following cancer is more likely in patients who are female, younger, and actively processing their experience.
- Post-traumatic growth following cancer appears common across cultures but patterns may differ.
- Methodological variability in cross-cultural studies of cancer-related post-traumatic growth make drawing conclusions about cultural differences difficult.
- Researchers should practice cultural sensitivity when discussing post-traumatic growth with patients, and should try to utilize more qualitative measures of growth through a 'bottom-up' rather than 'top-down' approach.
- More research is needed on non-Western cancer survivors to make better generalizations about post-traumatic growth across cultures.

Suggested further reading

Butler L.D., Blasey C.M. *et al.* (2005) Posttraumatic growth following the terrorist attacks of September 11, 2001: Cognitive, coping, and trauma symptom predictors in an internet convenience sample. *Traumatology,* 11, 247–267.

Cadell S., Regehr C. *et al.* (2003) Factors contributing to posttraumatic growth: A proposed structural equation model. *American Journal of Orthopsychiatry,* 73, 279–287.

Calhoun L.G., Tedeschi R.G. (2004) The foundations of posttraumatic growth: New considerations. *Psychological Inquiry,* 15, 93–102.

Carboon I., Anderson V.A. *et al.* (2005) Posttraumatic growth following a cancer diagnosis: Do world assumptions contribute? *Traumatology,* 11, 269–283.

Classen C.C., Kraemer H.C. *et al.* (2008) Supportive-expressive group therapy for primary breast cancer patients: A randomized prospective multicenter trial. *Psycho-Oncology,* 17, 438–447.

Cohen M., Numa M. (2011) Posttraumatic growth in breast cancer survivors: A comparison of volunteers and non-volunteers. *Psycho-Oncology,* 20, 69–76.

Cordova M.J., Andrykowski M.A. (2003) Responses to cancer diagnosis and treatment: Posttraumatic stress and posttraumatic growth. *Seminars in Clinical Neuropsychiatry,* 8, 286–96.

Cordova M.J., Cunningham L.L.C. *et al.* (2001) Posttraumatic growth following breast cancer: A controlled comparison study. *Health Psychology,* 20, 176–185.

Cordova M., Giese-Davis J. *et al.* (2007) Breast cancer as trauma: Posttraumatic stress and posttraumatic growth. *Journal of Clinical Psychology in Medical Settings* 14, 308–319.

Goodwin P.J., Leszcz M. *et al.* (2001) The effect of group psychosocial support on survival in metastatic breast cancer. *New England Journal of Medicine,* 345, 1719–1726.

Mystakidou K., Tsilika E. *et al.* (2008) Post-traumatic growth in advanced cancer patients receiving palliative care. *British Journal of Health Psychology,* 13, 633–646.

Sawyer A., Ayers S. *et al.* (2010) Posttraumatic growth and adjustment among individuals with cancer or HIV/AIDS: A meta-analysis. *Clinical Psychology Review,* 30, 436–447.

Schroevers M., Ranchor A.V. *et al.* (2006) Adjustment to cancer in the 8 years following diagnosis: A longitudinal study comparing cancer survivors with healthy individuals. *Social Science & Medicine,* 63, 598–610.

Shakespeare-Finch J., Copping A. (2006) A grounded theory approach to understanding cultural differences in posttraumatic growth. *Journal of Loss and Trauma,* 11, 355–371.

Spiegel D., Kraemer H. *et al.* (1989) Effect of psychosocial treatment on survival of patients with metastatic breast cancer. *Lancet,* 334, 888–891.

Thornton A.A., Perez M.A. (2006) Posttraumatic growth in prostate cancer survivors and their partners. *Psycho-Oncology,* 15, 285–296.

References

1. Kangas M., Henry J.L., Bryant R.A. (2002) Posttraumatic stress disorder following cancer: A conceptual and empirical review. *Clinical Psychology Review,* 22, 499–524.

2. The First Noble Truth: The Noble Truth of *dukkha* [Access to Insight] (c.2010) Available from: http://www.accesstoinsight.org/ptf/dhamma/sacca/sacca1/index.html (accessed January 2012).
3. Kierkegaard S. (1954) *Fear and Trembling and the Sickness unto Death*, Double Day, Garden City, New York.
4. Sartre J.P. (1943) *Being and Nothingness* [*L'Être et le Néant*], Gallimard, Paris.
5. Yalom I.D. (1980) *Existential Psychotherapy*, Basic Books, New York.
6. Tedeschi R.G., Calhoun L.G. (1995) *Trauma and Transformation: Growing in the Aftermath of Suffering*, Sage Publications, Thousand Oaks, CA.
7. Joseph S., Linley P.A. (2005) Positive adjustment to threatening events: An organismic valuing theory of growth through adversity. *Review of General Psychology*, 9, 262–280.
8. Tedeschi R.G., Calhoun L.G. (2004) Posttraumatic growth: Conceptual foundations and empirical evidence. *Psychological Inquiry*, 15, 1–18.
9. Tedeschi R.G., Calhoun L.G. (1996) The Posttraumatic Growth Inventory: Measuring the positive legacy of trauma. *Journal of Traumatic Stress*, 9, 455–471.
10. Spiegel D. (1999) A 43-year-old woman coping with cancer. *Journal of the American Medical Association*, 282, 371–378.
11. Wortman C.B. (2004) Posttraumatic growth: Progress and problems. *Psychological Inquiry*, 15, 81–90.
12. Sumalla E.C., Ochoa C., Blanco I. (2009) Posttraumatic growth in cancer: Reality or illusion? *Clinical Psychology Review*, 29, 24–33.
13. Zoellner T., Maercker A. (2006) Posttraumatic growth in clinical psychology: A critical review and introduction of a two component model. *Clinical Psychology Review*, 26, 626–653.
14. Frazier P, Tennen H *et al.* (2009) Does self-reported posttraumatic growth reflect genuine positive change? *Psychological Science*, 20, 912–919.
15. Maercker A., Zoellner T. (2004) The Janus face of self-perceived growth: Toward a two-component model of posttraumatic growth. *Psychological Inquiry*, 15, 41–48.
16. Cordova M.J. (2008) Facilitating posttraumatic growth following cancer, in *Trauma, Recovery, and Growth: Positive Psychological Perspectives on Posttraumatic Stress* (eds S. Joseph, P.A. Linley), John Wiley & Sons, Inc., Hoboken, NJ, pp. 185–206.
17. Stanton A.L., Bower J.E., Low C.A. (2006) Posttraumatic growth after cancer, in *Handbook of Posttraumatic Growth: Research and Practice* (eds L.G. Calhoun, R.G. Tedeschi), Lawrence Erlbaum Associates, Mahwah, NJ, pp. 138–175.
18. Widows M.R., Jacobsen P.B. *et al.* (2005) Predictors of posttraumatic growth following bone marrow transplantation for cancer. *Health Psychology*, 24, 266–273.
19. Bellizzi K.M, Blank T.O. (2006) Predicting posttraumatic growth in breast cancer survivors. *Health Psychology*, 25, 47–56.
20. Bellizzi KM. (2004) Expressions of generativity and posttraumatic growth in adult cancer survivors. *International Journal of Aging and Human Development*, 58, 267–287.
21. Tomich P.L., Helgeson V.S. (2004) Is finding something good in the bad always good? Benefit-finding among women with breast cancer. *Health Psychology*, 23, 16–23.
22. Weiss T. (2004) Correlates of posttraumatic growth in married breast cancer survivors. *Journal of Social and Clinical Psychology*, 23, 733–746.
23. Antoni M.H., Lehman J.M., Kilbourn K.M. *et al.* (2001) Cognitive-behavioral stress-management intervention decreases the prevalence of depression and enhances benefit-finding among women under treatment for early-stage breast cancer. *Health Psychology*, 20, 20–32.
24. Sears S.R., Stanton A.L. *et al.* (2003) The yellow brick road and the emerald city: Benefit finding, positive reappraisal coping and posttraumatic growth in women with early-stage breast cancer. *Health Psychology*, 22, 487–497.
25. Andrykowksi M.A., Curran S.L., Studts J.L. *et al.* (1996) Psychosocial adjustment and quality of life in women with breast cancer and benign breast problems: A controlled comparision. *Journal of Clinical Epidemiology*, 49, 827–834.
26. Smith B.W., Dalen J. *et al.* (2008) Posttraumatic growth in non-Hispanic white and Hispanic women with cervical cancer. *Journal of Psychosocial Oncology*, 26, 91–109.
27. Lechner S.C., Zakowski S.G., Antoni M.H. *et al.* (2003). Do sociodemographic and disease-related variables influence benefit-finding in cancer patients? *Psycho-Oncology*, 12, 491–499.
28. Urcuyo K.R., Boyers A.E., Carver C.S. *et al.* (2005) Finding benefit in breast cancer: Relations with personality, coping, and concurrent well-being. *Psychology and Health*, 20, 175–192.

29. Andrykowski M.A., Brady M.J., Hunt J.W. (1993) Positive psychosocial adjustment in potential bone marrow transplant recipients: Cancer as a psychosocial transition. *Psycho-Oncology*, 2, 261–276.
30. Carver C.S., Antoni M.H. (2004) Finding benefit in breast cancer during the year after diagnosis predicts better adjustment 5 to 8 years after diagnosis. *Health Psychology*, 23, 595–598.
31. Salsman J.M., Segerstrom S.C. *et al.* (2009) Post-traumatic growth and PTSD symptomatology among colorectal cancer survivors: A 3-month longitudinal examination of cognitive processing. *Psycho-Oncology*, 18, 30–41.
32. Lechner S.C., Carver C.S., Antoni M.H. *et al.* (2006) Curvilinear associations between benefit finding and psychosocial adjustment to breast cancer. *Journal of Consulting and Clinical Psychology*, 74, 828–840.
33. Kitayama S., Markus H.R. *et al.* (1997) Individual and collective processes in the construction of the self: Self-enhancement in the United States and self-criticism in Japan. *Journal of Personality and Social Psychology*, 72, 1245–1267.
34. Markus H.R., Kitayama S. (1991) Culture and the self: Implications for cognition, emotion, and motivation. *Psychological Review*, 98, 224–253.
35. Splevins K., Cohen K. *et al.* (2010) Theories of post-traumatic growth: Cross-cultural perspectives. *Journal of Loss and Trauma*, 15, 259–277.
36. Taku K., Calhoun L.G. *et al.* (2007) Examining post-traumatic growth among Japanese university students. *Anxiety Stress Coping*, 20, 353–367.
37. Powell S.R., Rosner R., Butollo W. *et al.* (2003) Posttraumatic growth after war: A study with former refugees and displaced people in Sarajevo. *Journal of Clinical Psychology*, 59, 71–83.
38. Maercker, A., J. Herrle, J. (2003). Long-term effects of the Dresden bombing: Relationships to control beliefs, religious belief, and personal growth. *Journal of Traumatic Stress*, 16, 579–587.
39. Weiss T., Berger R. (2006) Reliability and validity of a Spanish version of the posttraumatic growth inventory. *Research on Social Work Practice*, 16, 191–199.
40. Navon L. (1999) Cultural views of cancer around the world. *Cancer Nursing*, 22, 39–45.
41. Dein S. (2004) Explanatory models of and attitudes towards cancer in different cultures. *The Lancet Oncology*, 5, 119–124.
42. Thombre A., Sherman A. *et al.* (2010) Posttraumatic growth among cancer patients in India. *Journal of Behavioral Medicine*, 33, 15–23.
43. Jaarsma T.A., Pool G. *et al.* (2006) Psychometric properties of the Dutch version of the posttraumatic growth inventory among cancer patients. *Psycho-Oncology*, 15, 911–920.
44. Mystakidou K., Parpa E. *et al.* (2007) Traumatic distress and positive changes in advanced cancer patients. *American Journal of Hospice and Palliative Care*, 4, 270–276.
45. Morris B.A., Shakespeare-Finch J. (2010) Rumination, post-traumatic growth, and distress: Structural equation modelling with cancer survivors. *Psycho-Oncology*, 16, 229–242.
46. Mols F., Vingerhoets A.J.J.M. *et al.* (2009) Well-being, posttraumatic growth and benefit finding in long-term breast cancer survivors. *Psychology & Health*, 5, 583–595.
47. Lelorain S., Bonnaud-Antignac A. *et al.* (2010) Long term posttraumatic growth after breast cancer: Prevalence, predictors, and relationships with psychological health. *Journal of Clinical Psychology in Medical Settings*, 17, 14–22.
48. Ho S.M.Y., Chan C.L.W. *et al.* (2004) Posttraumatic growth in Chinese cancer survivors. *Psycho-Oncology*, 13, 377–389.
49. Ho S.M.Y., Chan M.W.Y., Yau T.K. *et al.* (2011) Relationships between explanatory style, posttraumatic growth and posttraumatic stress disorder symptoms among Chinese breast cancer patients. *Psychology & Health*, 26, 269–285.
50. Ho S., Rajandram R.K., Chan N. *et al.* (2011) The roles of hope and optimism on posttraumatic growth in oral cavity cancer patients. *Oral Oncology*, 47, 121–124.
51. Schroevers M.J., Teo I. (2008) The report of posttraumatic growth in Malaysian cancer patients: Relationships with psychological distress and coping strategies. *Psycho-Oncology*, 17, 1239–1246.
52. Classen C., Butler L.D. *et al.* (2001) Supportive-expressive group therapy reduces distress in metastatic breast cancer patients: A randomized clinical intervention trial. *Archives of General Psychiatry*, 58, 494–501.
53. Spiegel D., Bloom J.R. *et al.* (1981) Group support for patients with metastatic cancer: A randomized outcome study. *Archives of General Psychiatry*, 38, 527–533.
54. Spiegel D., Classen C. (2000) *Group Therapy for Cancer Patients: A Research-Based Handbook of Psychosocial Care*, Basic Books, New York, NY.

55. Spiegel D., Yalom I.D. (1978) A support group for dying patients. *International Journal of Group Psychotherapy*, 28, 233–245.
56. Weiss T., Berger R. (2010) Posttraumatic growth around the globe: Research findings and practice implications, in *Posttraumatic Growth and Culturally Competent Practice: Lessons Learned from Around the Globe* (eds T. Weiss, R. Berger), John Wiley & Sons Inc., Hoboken, NJ, pp. 189–195.

Additional resources

Poems, Philosophy, and Cancer [Cancernet-UK] (c.2011) Available from: http://www.cancernet.co.uk/poems.htm (accessed 18 August 2011).

Post-traumatic Growth [Positive Psychology UK] (c.2011) Available from: http://www.positivepsychology.org.uk/pp-theory/post-traumatic-growth/105-post-traumatic-growth.html (accessed January 2012).

CHAPTER 17

The Need for Psychosocial Support in Genetic Counselling and Genetic Testing

Mary Jane Esplen[1], *Jonathan Hunter*[2] *and Kathryn M. Kash*[3]

[1]Department of Psychiatry, Faculty of Medicine, University of Toronto; Program of Psychosocial & Psychotherapy Research in Cancer Genetics, University Health Network, Toronto, ON, Canada

[2]Consultation/Liaison Division, University of Toronto Department of Psychiatry; Mount Sinai Hospital, Toronto, ON, Canada

[3]Jefferson School of Population Health, Thomas Jefferson University, Philadelphia, PA, USA

Background

Approximately 5–10% of cancers are hereditary.[1] Identifying people at risk for cancer allows for more targeted screening than general population-based programmes and thus the optimal use of resources. Genetic testing can assist in identifying those at substantially increased risk for cancer and can help individuals prepare both medically and psychologically. However, difficult emotional reactions can occur as a result of counselling and testing procedures. This chapter will describe the process of genetic susceptibility testing, associated emotions, and the current state of knowledge about supporting individuals psychologically through this process. Case examples are presented to illuminate the issues that can arise, and suggestions for their management. Given the psychosocial challenges that can occur during genetic testing, there is a need to incorporate psychological care into genetics services.

Genetic testing and counselling

Once a concern about a family history of cancer is identified, individuals are referred to specialty genetic clinics to see a genetic counsellor and/or geneticist. At least one counselling session is provided, usually by a genetic counsellor, geneticist or genetics nurse before a genetic test is performed. During this first session, genetic (and non-genetic) risk factors for the cancer are identified to determine eligibility for genetic testing. The genetic counsellor outlines benefits of genetic testing, its process and the potential results, along with the implications of the potential test results. For example, individuals are informed that they may test 'positive' (indicating the presence of a susceptibility mutation), 'negative' (indicating the absence of such a mutation), or 'uninformative', (a result that does not permit a definite risk to be assigned). Family implications are addressed in this session, as the cancer susceptibility genes are autosomal dominant, with each offspring of a gene carrier having a 50% chance of carrying the same genetic mutation. This means that other members of the family, for instance the siblings of the individual who has presented for testing, may well be affected by the result.

In this first session it would be important to assess the person's perception of their risk and the likelihood of developing cancer. This information is extremely helpful in the post-testing session as

Clinical Psycho-Oncology: An International Perspective, First Edition. Edited by Luigi Grassi and Michelle Riba.

it helps prepare the counsellor to address active risk as compared with perceptions of risk from the pre-testing (or first) session. Specific benefits are also discussed, for example, the opportunity to participate in surveillance programmes with close monitoring, or risk-reducing surgery. The potential for harm is also discussed, for example, issues around insurance (health, life, unemployment or disability – depending on the country), the potential that some family members may not wish to be informed, or have increased worry about their risk.

If testing goes forward there is a waiting period while laboratory DNA analysis occurs. When the result is available a post-test counselling session is then provided, wherein the test result and its impact are fully explored. This includes an assessment of the individual's understanding of their risk for disease, their assimilation of this new information, and how it compares with their previous expectations. Specific surveillance and prevention recommendations are discussed, and follow-up appointments for screening tests or consultations with specialists who can address such options as risk-reducing surgery are scheduled. The implications of the test for family members are also discussed, including an exploration of potential issues around communicating this new genetic information to relatives. Typically a follow-up appointment is booked, either in person or via telephone, within one to four weeks. This follow-up allows further exploration of the individual's ongoing adjustment and decisions about surveillance and prevention, or family communication problems.

The genetic counselling sessions are highly focused on risk, genetics and probabilities but are often highly emotional. Standard clinic processes, such as constructing a family tree depicting the cancer diagnoses or deaths of loved ones across generations can result in profound emotional reactions. Receiving information about the presence of a genetic mutation is, in fact, life-altering, as revealed by one patient's comment – 'Everything changed for me – now I have so many medical appointments and I wonder if I will have a long life ... I'm likely to develop cancer ... I never had to see doctors so much before'.

Psychosocial issues in genetic testing

Genetic testing precipitates awareness of a state of increased health risk, often with accompanying fears about developing cancer, feelings of anger (towards those who transmitted the disease) or guilt (about the potential transmission of the genes to offspring), as well as triggers of past emotional experiences with loved ones who dealt with or died from cancer in the past. Such emotional reactions affect the person's quality of life and can also interfere with family relationships or the communication of genetic information to at-risk family members. Even before testing occurs there are psychological issues that influence who comes forward for the testing. For example, those with higher perceived risk for cancer are most interested in genetic testing.[2,3] Individuals who feel vulnerable due to their family experience with illness, or those with anxious, preoccupied or monitoring coping styles are often interested in attending a genetics centre.[4–6] These individuals frequently have personal beliefs and associated emotions regarding their destiny.[7] For instance, women with a first-degree relative with breast cancer frequently profoundly overestimate their risk for cancer,[8,9] believing that the disease will inevitably strike. It is not uncommon for those feeling at high risk to report a perceived risk of a '100% chance' of developing the disease. These overestimations of risk can be persistent and challenging to modify when providing 'objective' risk information in the absence of psychological intervention aimed at addressing issues that may be contributing to a sense of an inflated personal risk.[6,10–12] Factors associated with elevated risk perception include: (1) having a family history of disease; (2) beliefs about the disease and risks; (3) previous loss of a family member from the disease; and (4) over-identification with a family member who has had the disease.[6] At times the person who is the most emotional about risk for cancer is someone whose perception is based on misunderstandings about their real risk. Frequently these are the people who have one elderly family member with a cancer and they inappropriately request genetic testing. Offering psychological counselling may help determine what is driving their fear and offer information and support about the use of genetic testing.

Testing positive – notification of the presence of a genetic mutation

Increased worry or concern about developing cancer is a common reaction and a person may wrongly assume that the illness is inevitable and not treatable. Responses after testing positively (and at times even prior to confirmation of a high risk for cancer) often result in a belief that 'it is just a matter of when, not if, the disease occurs'. Having younger children and a history of previous losses to cancer are associated with greater emotional distress.[13,14] While individuals typically understand that they did not intentionally pass along a gene mutation, they may still feel guilt or strong concern about the risk for offspring.[15,16] Having an expectation of receiving a negative test result, low social support and a monitoring coping style are associated with greater distress.[17] Following the provision of the test result, individuals are given medical risk-reducing options that pose challenges in decision-making, such as the choice to adopt close surveillance and monitoring, such as regular MRIs, or to opt for risk-reducing surgery or chemoprevention. Even personal decisions around marriage and childbearing are impacted by the test result.[13,16] In addition, the person receiving a positive test result also is typically given the responsibility to notify family members and offspring about potential cancer risk. In general, these decisions and tasks pose an additional psychological burden and a person may be psychologically unprepared for these often unanticipated consequences of genetic testing. For example, a woman at increased risk for ovarian cancer due to a BRCA1 mutation is highly recommended to have risk-reducing oophorectomy to reduce her risk for ovarian cancer.[16] For pre-menopausal women the removal of ovaries will lead to menopause and the end of child-bearing, an obviously profound consequence for many.

Case study

The story of Anne (not her real name)

Anne is a 39-year-old woman recently diagnosed with a BRCA1 mutation. She is unmarried and felt going into the genetic testing process that given her mother's history of breast cancer she was likely to be at increased risk for breast cancer. Although she was already engaging in routine screening, she now learned that she would be adding routine MRIs and additional clinical breast exams to her mammograms. She also was informed that she was eligible to have her breasts removed and reconstructive plastic surgery, and that it is also highly recommended to have her ovaries removed prior to her mid-forties.

'I was completely shocked. I knew I was at risk for breast cancer, but to remove my breasts that are healthy? Seems so drastic. I'm not sure whether to have just the screening or to do the surgery ... I had no idea that would come up. I'm kind of young for menopause. And, what about children? ... although I am not married, I still hope to meet someone and have a child ... but now, who would even want to marry me ... especially with all this surgery ... and when do I take work off to do all this?'

Following a positive test result individuals must weigh the potential costs of an intervention against its benefits. For example, those that undergo risk-reducing procedures do report a decreased sense of fear and anxiety about cancer risk;[13,18] however, there have also been reports of negative impacts on psychological functioning, body image, sexual functioning and self-concept.[13,19] As well, genetic information does not always lead to positive health behaviours or change. One study of female carriers in BRCA 1/2 families failed to demonstrate an optimal level of adherence to screening recommendations one year post-disclosure of a positive test result.[20]

For some individuals, ongoing family and personal reactions and distress can persist.[16,21] In reports using standardized measures approximately 10–25% of risk-counselled individuals demonstrate scores consistent with a clinical diagnosis of depression or anxiety.[17,22–24] However, most carriers of genetic mutations do not become more distressed over time.[25] One year post-test psychological functioning among the majority of individuals who were informed that they carry a genetic mutation is similar to those receiving a negative test result,[21,25–27] suggesting the effectiveness of genetic counselling.

Most individuals do identify specific benefits to testing,[28] which are important in buffering the impacts of the emotional costs. For example, the increased certainty around one's risk and the opportunity to have close surveillance contribute to relief. To illustrate, one young woman stated, 'My mother never had the chance to be closely watched like me. I feel lucky that now I do know and I can prepare. It is great to be watched by my clinic nurses and doctors. If I do get cancer, I have a much better chance to catch it early and have it treated . . . Mom didn't have that chance and we lost her too young.'

Additional quality of life benefits to genetic testing include the opportunity for an individual to examine his/her current life situation. A positive genetic test result has an existential impact through the gained awareness of being at increased risk for a serious disease. The existential threat can be a powerful motivator for the adoption of a healthier lifestyle and can contribute to a feeling that 'life is precious', motivating a person to reflect on his/her life and to make other positive changes, such as spending more time in desired activities or with valued others.[16] Genetic information can also be used to make career choices, plans for retirement or to obtain life insurance. Opportunities to support others or to participate in research that may assist future generations (including one's own relatives) have direct benefit in buffering the impact of a stress response and facilitating active coping.[16] Such outcomes can occur spontaneously, but for others psychological and behavioural interventions provide forums that can encourage these positive perspectives.

Receiving a negative test result

The news that one does not carry a genetic mutation is generally associated with relief and improved psychological functioning.[29] However, testing negatively can result in some individuals experiencing surprising challenges in adjusting to their new risk information. For example, most individuals with a strong family history of cancer have integrated a sense of being at increased risk into their self-concept.[13] They have a sense of 'merger' or a strong identification with the relative(s) affected by the disease. The negative test is unexpected and they have the task of integrating this new information into their sense of self. This task is challenged by a feeling that one is giving up a sense of belonging to a 'group', and it can be experienced as a distressing separation from the loved ones.[16] Alternatively, an individual can test negatively while other family members are notified that they are carriers, resulting in feelings of guilt about being spared the legacy of the familial disease. This response is consistent with 'survivor guilt'[24] and conflicts with the relief that usually accompanies a favourable test result.

Inconclusive test results

Another possible outcome of genetic testing is that of the 'inconclusive' test result. In these situations there may be a family history of a particular cancer but no affected individual is available to be tested. In this instance the person is tested for the most common genes that are carried by those with a similar family history. If no mutation is detected the result comes back as 'inconclusive' as it is still possible for the individual to carry rare gene mutations or those not yet detectable through sequencing. Such a result causes concern to clinicians who fear that the individual is falsely reassured. The individual's comprehension of an inconclusive test result must be examined during follow-up, particularly in relation to adherence with surveillance and preventive options.[30,31] In addition, an individual who misunderstands his/her inconclusive test result may communicate inaccurate information to family members.[30,31]

Family impacts

Genetic testing may start with an individual but it quickly becomes a family affair.[32] Some individuals describe feeling closer to family members who carry the same genetic mutation. But, as noted above, relationships among siblings, parents and offspring can be complicated by individuals receiving different test results. Other family relationships are also affected. Spouses can have difficulty adjusting and have demonstrated high levels of concern for their partner.[33] For example, spouses may feel unsure about how to support a partner through medical decision-making or in coping with his/her risk. A parent who carries a genetic mutation needs to decide when and how to inform adolescent or adult offspring.

Women with gene mutations related to breast and ovarian cancers (BRCA1/2) in a group support programme reported that a particular challenge was informing an adult daughter of the mutation. The mothers expressed wishes that their adult daughters were enrolled in the appropriate surveillance programmes that would be recommended following a genetic test, but also felt a strong need to protect them from the potential worry and psychological burden.[16] For parents with younger children there is the challenge of explaining absences or changes due to medical appointments or procedures,[34] such as in the case of a woman with the BRCA1 mutation who undergoes risk-reducing surgery and must find a way to communicate to her children the need for surgery, while reinforcing her current state of good health.

Other challenges occur around the responsibility of notifying extended family. Individuals can be burdened with trying to find ways to notify a cousin they may have never met or who does not live close by, and have concerns of causing emotional upset.[15] In addition, individuals with genetic knowledge may also feel a strong pressure to encourage family members to be tested, even when these individuals may not be interested, precipitating conflict. These family communication challenges can be addressed through guidance from health care professionals. Some clinics, for example, provide templates of letters that can offer a first step in communicating genetic information for further follow-up, including genetic clinic locations within their geographic areas.

Case study

Story of a family with an APC gene mutation

John is a 42-year-old man who carries an adenomatous polyposis coli (APC) gene mutation for Familial Adenomatous Polyposis (FAP) and is therefore at 100% risk for developing colorectal cancer. The gene is autosomal dominant with each of his children having a 50% chance of carrying the same gene mutation. He has one son age 20 (Tom), who is also a carrier, and two daughters, Sue and Barbara, who have not yet been tested. John complies with regular colorectal cancer screening and feels that by doing so he will prevent cancer. Their son, Tom, has refused to have colorectal cancer screening as he feels he is too busy graduating from college and applying to medical school. John's 47-year-old cousin, who also carried the APC gene mutation, recently died of colorectal cancer and this prompted John and Jane to bring their daughters for genetic counselling and testing. Both girls gave assent and consent to genetic testing during the counselling session.

The results at a follow-up session indicated that Sue, who is 18 years old, is not an APC carrier; however, Barbara, who is 13 years old, is a carrier. Prior to counselling and testing Barbara was very close to her mother while Sue was very close to her father. During this session however, Jane distanced herself physically from her daughter, Barbara, and told her she should '... never have children so this gene mutation will stop here'. Jane has also told her son, Tom, the same thing. Jane goes on to say that if she had known this would happen she would never have had children herself. Barbara was quite stunned and upset that she is a carrier and expressed feelings regarding being a teen and having to now start colorectal cancer screening. However, she was optimistic because her father does not have colorectal cancer. She was also surprised and very upset about her mother's shift in attitude towards her. Jane's reactions were experienced as hurtful and had a profound impact on the family, as did the APC genetic test result status for Barbara.

Sue, the non-gene mutation carrier had a different kind of impact, expressing feelings of 'survivor guilt'; feeling badly that, in contrast to her sister, she was spared the cancer risk. As they left the session, Jane avoided interacting with Barbara and chose to walk next to Sue. Six months later John developed colon cancer and had surgery. He became more concerned about his survival. His daughter, Barbara, began to wonder if the screening was really a 'waste of time', given that her father developed cancer, demonstrating a misunderstanding of the purpose of 'screening', which is to provide early detection and not primary prevention. Tom still had not gone for cancer screening.

This vignette highlights the challenging dynamics that can spontaneously emerge associated with genetic test results that vary within a family, and the changing issues that arise as a result of the evolution of illness over time.

Socio-cultural issues

Individuals and their families can face a number of societal and ethical challenges which may impact on quality of life and lead to potential distress.[6,35] These include the following: (1) the need to maintain confidentiality and privacy (e.g. Who will have access to genetic test results?); (2) the potential for discrimination (health, medical or life insurance, employment opportunities, the linkage of specific cultural groups to a genetic mutation); (3) disclosure issues associated with familial information (e.g. disclosing information concerning a genetic mutation to family members versus the right of relatives 'not to know'); and (4) interest in prenatal testing (which is currently discouraged for adult-onset disorders).

Cultural factors are also relevant in the provision of genetic testing,[36,37] as cultures may vary in specific beliefs and attitudes concerning genetic testing, affecting interest or uptake.[36] African-American women have been shown to have lower levels of knowledge about breast cancer genetics.[38,39] African Americans and older generations of Asian populations have expressed concern about how genetic information will be managed and utilized.[37,40,41] Differences among cultures have also been found in relation to the communication of genetic information, particularly around the role of consent.[42]

Culture can also play a role in preventive treatments. For example, in a support group for women with BRCA 1 and 2 mutations[16] a participant from an ethnic and religious community described her challenges around risk-reducing surgery. As she listened in the group to other women expressing personal views and choices, she became aware that such discussions were enhancing her feelings of fear and decisional conflict. She wished to follow the recommendation of her physician to remove her ovaries to minimize her ovarian cancer risk, given that she had completed childbearing. However, her husband did not agree as he believed it went against religious values and that they would require the permission of their male spiritual leader to proceed with the surgery. According to her, this passive position was typical of the female role within her culture, and it contributed strongly to her conflict around surgical decision-making. Further investigations are clearly needed on the impact of specific cultures in this arena. However, given the role that culture plays in health outcome[36] the literature to date indicates the need for the genetic counsellor and psychosocial personnel to be culturally sensitive during the assessment phase when genetic testing is being described and offered, in order to fully appreciate the person's context. Culturally sensitive approaches may be required to provide outreach to specific cultures which may not fully understand or see the benefit of genetic testing, and to address specific barriers to providing information or care in the management of risk.

Psychological approaches that support the impact of genetic testing

Psychological care is best integrated into the standard genetic testing process to facilitate optimal adjustment and support to individuals and their families.[7,43] A full appreciation of the personal and cultural context, including the prior history of cancer experiences in the family is needed. For those individuals who may have specific psychological risk factors as noted above, or who experience challenges around family communication or medical decision-making, ongoing support and referral to a mental health professional is important. Psychosocial screening instruments are useful and have recently been designed and tested specifically for cancer risk populations.[44,45] They identify empirically derived psychological risk markers related to the heritable cancer experience and genetic testing. Relevant risk factors for emotional distress detected by these measures are detailed in Box 17.1.[46–49]

Once the background and the level of distress are identified, it is helpful to apply the appropriate level of intervention (see Box 17.2). The empirical evidence to date has been focused on psycho-educational approaches or decisional aids to facilitate genetic counselling and decision-making about medical interventions, with research

Box 17.1 Factors associated with psychological risk or adjustment difficulties with a positive test

Socio-demographic
- Age/developmental level/ proximity to age of affected family member
- Gender
- Culture/ Ethnicity
- Socioeconomic status
- Having young children

Medical
- Penetrance
- Severity/ Nature of disease
- Prevention options and risk-reducing procedures

Psychosocial
- Loss of relative to disease (especially parent)
- Care-giving of family member with disease
- Prior history of additional life losses/trauma
- Pre-morbid psychological history/condition
- Current level of psychological functioning (e.g. presence of depression, anxiety, disease-specific worry)
- Current life stressors (e.g. job stress, divorce)
- Expectation of receiving a negative test result
- Coping style (e.g. anxious preoccupied, health monitoring)
- Social support level (low level)

Reproduced from Esplen M.J. (2006) Psychological aspects of genetic testing for adult-onset hereditary disorders, in *Genetic Testing: Care, Consent, and Liability* (eds N. Sharpe, R. Carter), John Wiley & Sons. Inc., Hoboken, NJ (pp. 61–77), with permission from John Wiley & Sons, Inc.

Box 17.2 Psychosocial and psychotherapeutic interventions recommended for distress levels

Low level of distress →	*Moderate level of distress →*	*High level of distress*
Educational pamphlets, CDs, Internet information Peer support	Cognitive-behavioural (e.g. stress management, coping strategies for living with uncertainty) Interactive CD ROMS Manual and computer-based decisional aids Telephone counselling and follow-up counselling Couple or family counselling Peer support (1:1; Group)	Individual psychotherapy/ Supportive counselling Professionally led support groups Family counselling Psychotropic medication

Reproduced from Esplen M.J. (2006) Psychological aspects of genetic testing for adult-onset hereditary disorders, in *Genetic Testing: Care, Consent, and Liability* (eds N. Sharpe, R. Carter), John Wiley & Sons. Inc., Hoboken, NJ (pp. 61–77), with permission from John Wiley & Sons, Inc.

on other psychotherapeutic approaches still at an early stage. Interventions can be considered along a continuum by level of distress as depicted in Box 17.2. For example, for individuals who experience low levels of worry straightforward educational materials are indicated. Interventions, such as in-person or telephone-based counselling 1:1 approaches,[11,12,50–53] and decisional aids[52,54–57] have demonstrated improvements in knowledge and coping.

Individuals with moderate levels of anxiety or communication challenges within their family that interrupt sleep, or interfere with optimal coping and decision-making will benefit from additional 1:1 sessions with a genetic counsellor or mental health professional. Individual or group peer supports and/or cognitive-behavioural strategies can be employed to promote stress management and to facilitate the tolerance of ongoing uncertainty.[58] When depressive symptoms or anxiety interferes with daily functioning or self-care, or when a person demonstrates feelings of hopelessness or suicidal expressions, more specialized services offered by a skilled mental health professional are necessary. For these highly distressed people, individual psychotherapy to address unresolved grief issues, psychotropic medication directed at a current psychiatric syndrome, professionally led support groups, and longer follow-up are warranted.

The use of social support, such as ongoing connections with the genetic clinic or a peer support group[16,58] can augment any of these levels of interventions. Groups have shown improvements by decreasing cancer worry or general anxiety, or by improving coping strategies.[16,58] They also facilitate decision-making around genetic testing or prevention, as well as assisting communication with family.[16,54]

Cognitive and behavioural strategies (CBT)

Behavioural interventions are frequently utilized in general settings to reduce anxiety and facilitate stress management. Relaxation or distraction[59] techniques can assist in addressing the lifelong stress associated with repeated medical and screening appointments. Specific programmes, such as mindfulness-based stress reduction training has been widely tested and is effective in improving quality of life and decreasing anxiety in various populations, including cancer patients.[60] Health promotion or wellness programmes can be used to promote the adoption of positive lifestyle behaviours, which often foster a sense of increased control over one's own health. These include as regular physical exercise, eating healthy foods and avoiding tobacco products, and excessive alcohol intake. Cognitively oriented strategies used routinely in CBT to manage anxiety or to facilitate medical decision-making are helpful and can be employed through individual or group formats.[54,59] To address an over-inflated personal cancer risk estimate, structured exercises that teach patients to identify and monitor 'catastrophic' thinking or 'dysfunctional' thoughts can be utilized. Exercises, such as logging of thoughts and patterns, role play, and journal-keeping allow individuals to gain insight on specific self-beliefs or rigid thoughts and learn about the connections amongst their thoughts, moods and behaviours.[61] Homework assignments and thought records are typically used and reviewed in sessions to help identify the person's inaccurate cognitions and to encourage more realistic interpretations of their circumstances. Self-beliefs are entrenched, often as a result of past traumatic experiences, such as the loss of a parent to serious illness in the family. Wellisch and colleagues,[12,23] have highlighted the unique issues that are highly relevant in young women who lost a mother to cancer, particularly during their adolescence. Women who have lost mothers to breast cancer can develop a sense that it is inevitable that they will suffer and die from cancer, just as their mothers did. This 'catastrophic' belief about the self can be identified and compared to a more realistic 'objective risk' in order to help facilitate adaption to the current day and improve functioning. CBT sessions can also lead to increased insight into one's cultural values, their role in adopting preventative health care or screening programmes, with the goal of addressing potential barriers to the uptake of recommended surveillance or procedures. Exercises can also focus on the future, for example, mental constructions of future health can be used to motivate a person to adopt screening or resolve challenging medical decisions.

Psychodynamic approaches

While little empirical research has been conducted to date in this clinical area, a psychodynamic approach may also be suitable. Psychodynamic therapies emphasize emotions more than cognition and utilize the alliance between the therapist and the individual as a means of understanding the individual and creating change. Insight is gained by appreciating how early life experience, such as previous relationships and bereavements – particularly those related to cancer in the family – relate to current distress. For example, for individuals who have lost a parent to cancer at a young age, the therapy would explore not only the loss of the parent and what occurred around the time of the event, but how such a loss and the subsequent events (such as having a grief-stricken remaining parent who was less available) led to great effort being spent on maintaining self-reliance and avoidance of close bonds, in an effort to avoid such a painful experience again. Once this self-awareness is established, these recognized established patterns can be explored and challenged through the understanding of how they evolved. New informed approaches about being in relationships can be adopted and tried out including within the relationship with the psychotherapist. The reflection upon distressing past events within the context of a trusted therapeutic relationship can inform an appreciation of how the consequences of the early experience impact on the current emotional reaction to genetic risk, or recommended procedures and family communication.

In other populations, a current dynamic approach utilized focuses on identifying the *attachment style* of people. Attachment style refers to the fundamental beliefs and behaviours that were formed in childhood about relationships, and which persist into adulthood for most people.[62,63] This approach has the benefit of being easy to understand and apply, and can be very helpful in gaining an understanding of an individual's motivations and behaviours. For instance, knowledge of attachment style allows one, with some certainty, to predict the person's capacity to trust others, regulate anxiety, process fearful information, and tolerate uncertainty, all functions that pertain to the genetic risk counselling circumstance.[62,64]

Principles of supportive-expressive group therapy (SEGT)[65,66] have been applied to the genetic counselling context.[9,67] This group approach involves bringing together 5–10 individuals with common challenges and issues, for example carrying a gene mutation or having a strong family history of cancer. The SEGT model for cancer risk populations involves a dose of 8 weekly, 90-minute sessions, followed by 4 monthly 'boosters'. Sometimes a family session is included where individuals are invited to bring a family member to the group to explore and discuss family impacts. The SEGT has the goals of using the existential impact of the risk/genetic situation as an opportunity to explore its relevance in relation to perceptions of cancer risk, and through the here and now of the group experience encourages individuals to live authentically and fully.[9,16,67] The foci are explorations of past events concerning the familial experience of cancer and its influence on current risk processing, viewpoints and emotional impacts and how they are impacting on current medical decision-making and adjustment. Mutual understanding and providing an opportunity for emotional expression within a safe culture of sharing and trust create a forum for the processing of unresolved grief or exploring adjustment challenges. Role modelling of others in the group and the vicarious learning that occurs through the sharing of various perspectives and coping strategies are helpful in facilitating coping. A key emphasis is on the legitimacy of a full range of emotion and the centrality of relationships in giving value to life, a perspective taken from existential psychotherapy.[65,66] Topics include medical decision-making, grief and loss, feeling vulnerable to cancer, impact on self, and family impacts.[16] SEGT has been tested with women at risk for cancer and those who carry mutations, demonstrating improvement in coping, grief and quality of life.[9,16,65] An interesting feature has included the inclusion of women who have survived cancer with those 'at risk' who have not had a diagnosis of cancer. This provides an opportunity for direct exchange and testing of assumptions between these two subgroups of women. For some young women the inclusion of older women who have survived cancer allows them to see for the first time that someone can survive cancer, directly challenging a strong belief that if diagnosed, death is inevitable.

Case study

The story of Betty (not her real name)

Betty is a 37-year-old woman whose mother died at the age of 38 from breast cancer, when Betty was 12 years old. Cancer was never discussed in her family and Betty's father became emotionally detached from Betty and her two younger siblings. Thus Betty never had the opportunity to grieve her mother's loss or discuss her own risk for developing breast cancer. Betty's assumption was that she too would develop breast cancer and die at age 38. For almost 20 years (since age 18), Betty lived with this fear and postponed thinking or trying to achieve any goal that involved living past this age (including marriage, children, future career opportunities, or other long-range plans). The group sessions had a powerful impact on her knowledge, current thinking, ability to connect with others, and support mechanisms.

At the one-year follow-up session, when she was past her 38th birthday and cancer-free, she realized that she had wasted her 20s and 30s and was not making plans for the future. 'If this support group, which gave me an opportunity to actually talk about what happened to my Mom, would have been available to me when I was in my 20s, my life would be so different now.' She then went on to state that her '... fear was no longer keeping her from dating and marriage and maybe even having children'.

The opportunity for Betty to participate in a support group, meet others with similar histories and to share her concerns and perspectives, provided her with a forum to hear of others' perspectives (often similar) and to gain insight into how her history and the loss of her mother was impacting on her own life and her choices. While she felt she had missed some opportunities she also realized it 'wasn't too late' to enjoy life and for the first time to give herself permission to believe that life could be longer. She began to take risks and allow herself to become emotionally closer to people, regardless of her cancer risk. She felt more open to 'taking a chance' and began to develop a sense of hope that she might not develop cancer.

This new perspective was described by Betty as 'freeing' and 'a whole new way of being' in relation to her future goals and hopes for herself. She no longer believed that she should opt not to have children and even hoped that this might occur as she began to believe that if she did meet someone she would consider having her own family. Betty ascribed these changes to the specific mechanisms of the group support programme – the sharing and forming of bonds with other women in the group, her new insight and her sense of trust that a future could evolve differently from what she had previously believed to be her only path in life. These changes provided her with greater confidence to take risks and to maintain a sense of hope for her future.

Summary

Genetic knowledge of disease predisposition resulting from this new and constantly evolving field has the potential to provide many benefits. However, genetic information can also pose challenges to individuals and their families that can result in emotional distress or decisional conflict around medical preventive options. Psychosocial, emotional, personal historical, cultural and family contextual factors play an important role in an individual's capacity to utilize genetic information optimally, and in the emotional reactions precipitated by the knowledge of a genetic risk, frequently impacting negatively on quality of life. Adverse psychological and behavioural reactions can be minimized when genetic testing is provided within an integrated psychological framework that identifies and addresses emotional distress and when programmes offer psychological support throughout the genetic testing process.

Box 17.3 Common cancer genetic disorders with psychological issues

Breast Cancer (BRCA1 gene mutation)

Several population-based studies and meta-analyses indicate that the average risk by age 70 years for breast cancer was 57–65% and for ovarian cancer was 39–40%.[1] One population-based study indicated that the risk for BRCA1 gene mutation carriers to age 80 years was 90% for breast cancer and 24% for ovarian cancer.[2]

1 Antoniou A., Pharoah P.D.P., Narod S. *et al.* (2003) Average risks of breast and ovarian cancer associated with BRCA1 or BRCA2 mutations detected in case series unselected for family history: a combined analysis of 222 studies. *Am J Hum Genet*, 72, 1117–1130.

2 Risch H.A., McLaughlin J.R., Cole D.E. *et al.* (2006) Population BRCA1 and BRCA2 mutation frequencies and cancer penetrances: a kin-cohort study in Ontario, Canada. *J Natl Cancer Inst*, 98, 1694–1706.

Breast Cancer (BRCA2 gene mutation)

Several population-based studies and meta-analyses indicate that the average risk by age 70 years for breast cancer was 45% and for ovarian cancer was 11%.[1] One population-based study indicated that the risk for BRCA2 gene mutation carriers to age 80 years was 41% for breast cancer and 8.4% for ovarian cancer.[2]

1 Antoniou A., Pharoah P.D.P., Narod S. *et al.* (2003) Average risks of breast and ovarian cancer associated with BRCA1 or BRCA2 mutations detected in case series unselected for family history: a combined analysis of 222 studies. *Am J Hum Genet*, 72, 1117–1130.

2 Risch H.A., McLaughlin J.R., Cole D.E. *et al.* (2006) Population BRCA1 and BRCA2 mutation frequencies and cancer penetrances: a kin-cohort study in Ontario, Canada. *J Natl Cancer Inst*, 98, 1694–1706.

Familial Adenomatous Polyposis (FAP)

(APC gene) and AFAP (Attenuated FAP) and have 100% penetrance. Genetic testing is offered from puberty for FAP and mid-teens for AFAP.[1,2]

1 Gryfe R. (2009) Inherited colorectal cancer syndromes. *Clin Colon Rectal Surg*, 22, 198–208.

2 Semotiuk K., Berk T., Gallinger. S. (2008) The clinical approach to a patient with multiple polyps. *Curr Colorectal Cancer Rep*, 4, 19–23.

Lynch Syndrome, known as Hereditary Non-Polyposis Colon Cancer (HNPCC)

Carries a 52–82% risk of colorectal cancer and a 25–60% of uterine cancer for those with a gene mutation.[1,2]

1 Baglietto L., Lindor N.M., Dowty J.G. *et al.* (2010) Risks of Lynch syndrome cancers for MSH6 mutation carriers. *J Natl Cancer Inst*, 102, 193–201.

2 Kempers M.J., Kuiper R.P., Ockeloen C.W. *et al.* (2011) Risk of colorectal and endometrial cancers in EPCAM deletion-positive Lynch syndrome: a cohort study. *Lancet Oncol*, 12, 49–55.

Key points

- Genetic counselling and testing services should have an integrated psychosocial component, with resources available for further consultation if necessary.
- A 'stepped care' model of intervention is ideal, wherein low levels of distress are managed by information, education and peer support that is embedded in the clinical genetic counselling process, and higher levels of distress are evaluated by a mental health professional for targeted psychotherapeutic intervention.
- Be aware that any genetic counselling and testing affects not just an individual, but the entire family.
- Cognitive processing of genetic risk information is often influenced by emotional and psychological factors, such as the degree of loss in the patient's family. Sensitivity to these issues can positively impact on the accuracy of the information understood by the patient.
- Although genetic risk information and testing results remain a lifelong issue for a patient and their family, most individuals have low levels of distress and positive coping behaviours.

Suggestions for further reading

Sharpe, N.F., Carter R.F. (eds) (2006) *Genetic Testing: Care, Consent, and Liability*, John Wiley & Sons, Inc., Hoboken, NJ, 594 pp.

Patenaude A.F. (2005) *Genetic Testing for Cancer: Psychological Approaches for Helping Patients and Families*, American Psychological Association, Washington, DC.

Eveline M., Bleiker A., Hahn D.E.E., Aaronson, N.K. (2003) Psychosocial issues in cancer genetics – current status and future directions. Division of Psychosocial Research and Epidemiology, The Netherlands Cancer Institute, Amsterdam. *Acta Oncologica*, 42, 276–286.

Thewes B., Meiser B., Tucker K., Schnieden V. (2003) Screening for psychological distress and vulnerability factors in women at increased risk for breast cancer: A review of the literature. *Psychology, Health & Medicine*, 8, 289–304.

Vadaparampil S.T., Wey J.P., Kinney A.Y. (2004) Psychosocial aspects of genetic counseling and testing. *Seminars in Oncology Nursing*, 20, 186–195.

References

1. Schlich-Bakker K.J., ten Kroode H.F., Ausems M.G. (2006) A literature review of the psychological impact of genetic testing on breast cancer patients. *Patient Education and Counseling*, 62, 13–20.
2. Bowen D., McTiernan A., Burke W. *et al.* (1999) Participation in breast cancer risk counseling among women with a family history. *Cancer Epidemiology, Biomarkers & Prevention*, 8, 581–585.
3. Codori A.M., Petersen G.M., Miglioretti D.L. *et al.* (1999) Attitudes toward colon cancer gene testing: Factors predicting test uptake. *Cancer Epidemiology, Biomarkers & Prevention*, 8, 345–351.
4. Rees G., Fry A., Cull A. (2001) A family history of breast cancer: Women's experiences from a theoretical perspective. *Social Science & Medicine*, 52, 1433–1440.
5. Leventhal H., Kelly K., Leventhal E. (1995) Population risk, actual risk, perceived risk, and cancer control: A discussion. *Journal of the National Cancer Institute Monographs*, 25, 81–85.
6. Kash K.M., Lerman C. (1998) Psychological, social, and ethical issues in gene testing, in *Psycho-Oncology*, 2nd edn (ed. J.C. Holland), Oxford University Press, New York, NY, pp. 196–207.
7. Stiefel F., Lehmann A., Guex P. (1997) Genetic detection: The need for psychosocial support in modern cancer prevention. *Supportive Care in Cancer*, 5, 461–465.
8. Black W.C., Nease R.F., Jr, Tosteson A.N. (1995) Perceptions of breast cancer risk and screening effectiveness in women younger than 50 years of age. *Journal of the National Cancer Institute*, 87, 720–731.
9. Esplen M.J., Toner B., Hunter J. *et al.* (2000) A supportive-expressive group intervention for women with a family history of breast cancer: Results of a phase II study. *Psycho-Oncology*, 9, 243–252.

10. Kash K.M., Holland J.C., Halper M.S. *et al.* (1992) Psychological distress and surveillance behaviors of women with a family history of breast cancer. *Journal of the National Cancer Institute*, 84, 24–30.
11. Lerman C., Lustbader E., Rimer B. *et al.* (1995) Effects of individualized breast cancer risk counseling: A randomized trial. *Journal of the National Cancer Institute*, 87, 286–292.
12. Wellisch D.K., Gritz E.R., Schain W. *et al.* (1991) Psychological functioning of daughters of breast cancer patients. Part I: Daughters and comparison subjects. *Psychosomatics*, 32, 324–336.
13. van Oostrom I., Meijers-Heijboer H., Lodder L.N. *et al.* (2003) Long-term psychological impact of carrying a BRCA1/2 mutation and prophylactic surgery: A 5-year follow-up study. *Journal of Clinical Oncology*, 21, 3867–3874.
14. Esplen M.J., Urquhart C., Butler K. *et al.* (2003) The experience of loss and anticipation of distress in colorectal cancer patients undergoing genetic testing. *Journal of Psychosomatic Research*, 55, 427–435.
15. Lerman C., Peshkin B.N., Hughes C. *et al.* (1998) Family disclosure in genetic testing for cancer susceptibility: Determinants and consequences. *Journal of Health Care Law & Policy*, 1, 352–371.
16. Esplen M.J., Hunter J., Leszcz M. *et al.* (2004) A multicenter study of supportive-expressive group therapy for women with BRCA1/BRCA2 mutations. *Cancer*, 101, 2327–2340.
17. Vernon S.W., Gritz E.R., Peterson S.K. *et al.* (1997) Correlates of psychologic distress in colorectal cancer patients undergoing genetic testing for hereditary colon cancer. *Health Psychology*, 16, 73–86.
18. Metcalfe K.A., Esplen M.J., Goel V. *et al.* (2004) Psychosocial functioning in women who have undergone bilateral prophylactic mastectomy. *Psycho-Oncology*, 13, 14–25.
19. Esplen M.J., Stuckless N., Hunter J. *et al.* (2009) The BRCA Self-Concept Scale: A new instrument to measure self-concept in BRCA1/2 mutation carriers. *Psycho-Oncology*, 18, 1216–1229.
20. Lerman C., Hughes C., Croyle R.T. *et al.* (2000) Prophylactic surgery decisions and surveillance practices one year following BRCA1/2 testing. *Preventive Medicine*, 31, 75–80.
21. Watson M., Foster C., Eeles R. *et al.* (2004) Psychosocial impact of breast/ovarian (BRCA1/2) cancer-predictive genetic testing in a UK multi-centre clinical cohort. *British Journal of Cancer*, 91, 1787–1794.
22. Coyne J.C., Benazon N.R., Gaba C.G. *et al.* (2000) Distress and psychiatric morbidity among women from high-risk breast and ovarian cancer families. *Journal of Consulting and Clinical Psychology*, 68, 864–874.
23. Wellisch D.K., Lindberg N.M. (2001) A psychological profile of depressed and nondepressed women at high risk for breast cancer. *Psychosomatics*, 42, 330–336.
24. Smith K.R., West J.A., Croyle R.T. *et al.* (1999) Familial context of genetic testing for cancer susceptibility: Moderating effect of siblings' test results on psychological distress one to two weeks after BRCA1 mutation testing. *Cancer Epidemiology, Biomarkers & Prevention*, 8, 385–392.
25. Schwartz M.D., Peshkin B.N., Hughes C. *et al.* (2002) Impact of BRCA1/BRCA2 mutation testing on psychologic distress in a clinic-based sample. *Journal of Clinical Oncology*, 20, 514–520.
26. Butow P.N., Lobb E.A., Meiser B. *et al.* (2003) Psychological outcomes and risk perception after genetic testing and counselling in breast cancer: A systematic review. *The Medical Journal of Australia*, 178, 77–81.
27. Meiser B. (2005) Psychological impact of genetic testing for cancer susceptibility: An update of the literature. *Psycho-Oncology*, 14, 1060–1074.
28. Cappelli M., Surh L., Humphreys L. *et al.* (1999) Psychological and social determinants of women's decisions to undergo genetic counseling and testing for breast cancer. *Clinical Genetics*, 55, 419–430.
29. Marteau T.M., Croyle R.T. (1998) Psychological responses to genetic testing. *British Medical Journal*, 316, 693–696.
30. Maheu C., Thorne S. (2008) Receiving inconclusive genetic test results: An interpretive description of the BRCA1/2 experience. *Research in Nursing & Health*, 31, 553–562.
31. Ardern-Jones A., Kenen R., Lynch E. *et al.* (2010) Is no news good news? Inconclusive genetic test results in BRCA1 and BRCA2 from patients and professionals' perspectives. *Hereditary Cancer in Clinical Practice*, 8, 1.
32. Foster C., Watson M., Moynihan C. *et al.* (2004) Juggling roles and expectations: Dilemmas faced by women talking to relatives about cancer and genetic testing. *Psychology & Health*, 19, 439–455.
33. Williams J.K., Schutte D.L., Holkup P.A. *et al.* (2000) Psychosocial impact of predictive testing for Huntington disease on support persons. *American Journal of Medical Genetics*, 96, 353–359.
34. Tercyak K.P., Peshkin B.N., Streisand R. *et al.* (2001) Psychological issues among children of hereditary breast cancer gene (BRCA1/2) testing participants. *Psycho-Oncology*, 10, 336–346.

35. Kash K.M. (1995) Psychosocial and ethical implications of defining genetic risk for cancers. *Annals of the New York Academy of Sciences*, 768, 41–52.
36. Meiser B., Eisenbruch M., Barlow-Stewart K. *et al.* (2001) Cultural aspects of cancer genetics: Setting a research agenda. *Journal of Medical Genetics*, 38, 425–429.
37. Forman A.D., Hall M.J. (2009) Influence of race/ethnicity on genetic counseling and testing for hereditary breast and ovarian cancer. *Breast Journal*, 15(suppl 1), S56–62.
38. Hughes C., Gomez-Caminero A., Benkendorf J. *et al.* (1997) Ethnic differences in knowledge and attitudes about BRCA1 testing in women at increased risk. *Patient Education and Counseling*, 32, 51–62.
39. Armstrong K., Micco E., Carney A. *et al.* (2005) Racial differences in the use of BRCA1/2 testing among women with a family history of breast or ovarian cancer. *Journal of the American Medical Association*, 293, 1729–1736.
40. Satia J.A., McRitchie S., Kupper L.L. *et al.* (2006) Genetic testing for colon cancer among African Americans in North Carolina. *Preventive Medicine*, 42, 51–59.
41. Chin T.M., Tan S.H., Lim S.E. *et al.* (2005) Acceptance, motivators, and barriers in attending breast cancer genetic counseling in Asians. *Cancer Detection and Prevention*, 29, 412–428.
42. Benkendorf J.L., Reutenauer J.E., Hughes C.A. *et al.* (1997) Patients' attitudes about autonomy and confidentiality in genetic testing for breast-ovarian cancer susceptibility. *American Journal of Medical Genetics*, 73, 296–303.
43. Decruyenaere M., Evers-Kiebooms G., Denayer L. *et al.* (2000) Predictive testing for hereditary breast and ovarian cancer: A psychological framework for pre-test counselling. *European Journal of Human Genetics*, 8, 130–136.
44. Kasparian N.A., Wakefield C.E., Meiser B. (2007) Assessment of psychosocial outcomes in genetic counseling research: An overview of available measurement scales. *Journal of Genetic Counseling*, 16, 693–712.
45. Esplen M.J., Cappelli M., Wong J. *et al.* (eds) (2011) Development of a Psychosocial Risk Screening Tool for Genetic Testing. 12th International Meeting on Psychosocial Aspects of Hereditary Cancer (IMPAHC), Amsterdam, the Netherlands.
46. Tercyak K.P., Demarco T.A., Mars B.D. *et al.* (2004) Women's satisfaction with genetic counseling for hereditary breast-ovarian cancer: Psychological aspects. *American Journal of Medical Genetics Part A*, 131, 36–41.
47. van Oostrom I., Meijers-Heijboer H., Duivenvoorden H.J. *et al.* (2007) Comparison of individuals opting for BRCA1/2 or HNPCC genetic susceptibility testing with regard to coping, illness perceptions, illness experiences, family system characteristics and hereditary cancer distress. *Patient Education and Counseling*, 65, 58–68.
48. van Oostrom I., Meijers-Heijboer H., Duivenvoorden H.J. *et al.* (2007) Prognostic factors for hereditary cancer distress six months after BRCA1/2 or HNPCC genetic susceptibility testing. *European Journal of Cancer*, 43, 71–77.
49. Thewes B., Meiser B., Tucker K. *et al.* (2003) Screening for psychological distress and vulnerability factors in women at increased risk for breast cancer: A review of the literature. *Psychology, Health & Medicine*, 8, 289–303.
50. Graves K.D., Wenzel L., Schwartz M.D. *et al.* (2010) Randomized controlled trial of a psychosocial telephone counseling intervention in BRCA1 and BRCA2 mutation carriers. *Cancer Epidemiology, Biomarkers & Prevention*, 19, 648–654.
51. McInerney-Leo A., Biesecker B.B., Hadley D.W. *et al.* (2004) BRCA1/2 testing in hereditary breast and ovarian cancer families: Effectiveness of problem-solving training as a counseling intervention. *American Journal of Medical Genetics Part A*, 130A, 221–227.
52. Miller S.M., Roussi P., Daly M.B. *et al.* (2005) Enhanced counseling for women undergoing BRCA1/2 testing: Impact on subsequent decision making about risk reduction behaviors. *Health Education & Behavior*, 32, 654–667.
53. Appleton S., Watson M., Rush R. *et al.* (2004) A randomised controlled trial of a psychoeducational intervention for women at increased risk of breast cancer. *British Journal of Cancer*, 90, 41–47.
54. Wakefield C.E., Meiser B., Homewood J. *et al.* (2007) Development and pilot testing of two decision aids for individuals considering genetic testing for cancer risk. *Journal of Genetic Counseling*, 16, 325–339.
55. Stacey D., O'Connor A.M., DeGrasse C. *et al.* (2003) Development and evaluation of a breast cancer prevention decision aid for higher-risk women. *Health Expectations*, 6, 3–18.
56. van Roosmalen MS, Stalmeier PF, Verhoef LC, *et al.* (2004) Randomized trial of a shared decision-making intervention consisting of trade-offs and individualized treatment information for BRCA1/2 mutation carriers. *Journal of Clinical Oncology*, 22, 3293–3301.

57. van Roosmalen M.S., Stalmeier P.F., Verhoef L.C. *et al.* (2004) Randomised trial of a decision aid and its timing for women being tested for a BRCA1/2 mutation. *British Journal of Cancer*, 90, 333–342.
58. Wellisch D.K., Hoffman A,. Goldman S. *et al.* (1999) Depression and anxiety symptoms in women at high risk for breast cancer: Pilot study of a group intervention. *American Journal of Psychiatry*, 156, 1644–1645.
59. Phelps C., Bennett P., Iredale R. *et al.* (2006) The development of a distraction-based coping intervention for women waiting for genetic risk information: A phase 1 qualitative study. *Psycho-Oncology*, 15, 169–173.
60. Carlson L.E., Speca M., Patel K.D. *et al.* (2003) Mindfulness-based stress reduction in relation to quality of life, mood, symptoms of stress, and immune parameters in breast and prostate cancer outpatients. *Psychosomatic Medicine*, 65, 571–581.
61. Beck A T. (1976) *Cognitive Therapy and the Emotional Disorders*, International Universities Press, New York.
62. Hunter J.J., Maunder R.G., Gupta M. (2007) Teaching consultation-liaison psychotherapy: Assessment of adaptation to medical and surgical illness. *Academic Psychiatry*, 31, 367–374.
63. Maunder R.G., Hunter J.J. (2008) Attachment relationships as determinants of physical health. *Journal of the American Academy of Psychoanalysis and Dynamic Psychiatry*, 36, 11–32.
64. Esplen M.J., Hunter J. (2011) Therapy in the setting of genetic predisposition to cancer, in *Handbook of Psychotherapy in Cancer Care* (eds M. Watson, D. Kissane) John Wiley & Sons, Ltd, Chichester, pp. 201–212.
65. Spiegel D., Spira J. (1991) *Supportive-expressive Group Therapy: A Treatment Manual of Psychosocial Intervention for Women with Recurrent Breast Cancer*, Psychosocial Treatment Laboratory, Stanford University School of Medicine, Stanford, CA.
66. Spiegel D., Bloom J.R., Kraemer H.C. *et al.* (1989) Effect of psychosocial treatment on survival of patients with metastatic breast cancer. *Lancet*, 2, 888–891.
67. Esplen M.J., Toner B., Hunter J. *et al.* (1998) A group therapy approach to facilitate integration of risk information for women at risk for breast cancer. *Canadian Journal of Psychiatry*, 43, 375–380.

CHAPTER 18

Psychosocial and Physical Health in Post-treatment and Extended Cancer Survivorship

Patricia A. Ganz[1,2] *and Annette L. Stanton*[1,3,4]
[1]Division of Cancer Prevention and Control Research, Jonsson Comprehensive Cancer Center, Los Angeles (UCLA), CA, USA
[2]Schools of Medicine and Public Health, UCLA, Los Angeles, CA, USA
[3]Department of Psychology, UCLA, Los Angeles, CA, USA
[4]Department of Psychiatry and Biobehavioral Sciences, UCLA, Los Angeles, CA, USA

Introduction and background

The concept of cancer survivorship was introduced more than 25 years ago by Fitzhugh Mullan in a special article published in the *New England Journal of Medicine* describing the 'seasons of survival' after a cancer diagnosis.[1] Subsequently, with the founding of a grass-roots advocacy organization in the United States in 1986, the National Coalition for Cancer Survivorship (NCCS) defined a survivor as anyone with a diagnosis of cancer from the moment of diagnosis and for the remainder of life, whether that life was lived in increments of weeks, months, years, or decades.[2] This definition, while very broad and inclusive of a substantial number of individuals with a relatively short survival time after diagnosis, raises the awareness of the need to consider issues of long-term survival from the very start of cancer treatment. For example, fertility preservation is something that can only be realistically addressed prior to the administration of chemotherapy or radiation that may cause sterility. Once treatment commences, this option may be completely lost. Other potential long-term and late effects, such as serious organ toxicities, must also be anticipated as part of treatment planning.

Nevertheless, there has not been universal acceptance of this concept or the use of the word 'survivor', to which many individuals who have been diagnosed with cancer object. Recently, since the release of the Institute of Medicine report on adult cancer survivors in 2006,[3] and with an expanding published literature on health care practice and research related to cancer survivors,[4] there has been greater emphasis on the post-treatment phase of the cancer care trajectory or what some have called 're-entry'. Although this term was probably first used to describe the return of childhood cancer survivors back to the school environment after curative therapy,[5] the term is also relevant for adults with cancer who emerge from an extended period of multimodal therapy, including prolonged adjuvant chemotherapy. Until recently, limited research has focused on this period of time in the cancer experience, even though there has been accumulating descriptive information on long-term cancer survivors, especially among children.

Clinical Psycho-Oncology: An International Perspective, First Edition. Edited by Luigi Grassi and Michelle Riba.

In this chapter, we focus on the post-treatment psychosocial and physical health issues facing adult cancer patients who have completed their initial curative cancer treatments, and who must now move on with their lives integrating a life-altering experience, which often includes serious physical and emotional compromise. Although individuals often demonstrate extraordinary resilience, many suffer substantially and are never the same thereafter. We highlight what is known, acknowledging that much of the research is in its infancy and has been conducted largely in breast cancer survivors and primarily in North America. Where appropriate, we identify gaps in the literature where additional research is required.

Trajectory of recovery after treatment ends: Major issues and analysis of the evidence

Psychosocial distress and recovery

Along with many other studies, prospective research on large samples of individuals in the years prior to and following a cancer diagnosis[6,7] documents the considerable psychosocial and physical impact of the earliest phase of cancer survivorship: cancer diagnosis and treatment. Many fewer studies characterize the cancer experience during the months immediately following completion of primary medical treatments (i.e. re-entry) and the longer term. For the purpose of this chapter, the re-entry phase will be defined as the point from treatment completion through 12–18 months, and extended survivorship as proceeding beyond that point (some researchers define long-term survivorship as starting at least five years after diagnosis).

As illustrated by three studies, research demonstrates that individuals diagnosed with cancer follow distinct psychological trajectories after cancer diagnosis. In a sample of women (n = 171) diagnosed with breast cancer in the Netherlands who reported their general psychological distress at five points beginning prior to surgery through six months after completion of treatment, four patterns of distress emerged: 36% of women reported no or minimal distress across all assessments, 33% reported elevated distress from diagnosis through medical treatment whereupon distress declined, 15% evidenced heightened distress starting at treatment completion and continuing through six months following treatment (i.e. re-entry phase), and 15% reported high distress throughout the study period.[8] In 298 breast cancer patients in the United States, 39% reported low depressive symptoms from just prior to surgery through six months, 45% had depressive symptoms just above the clinically suggestive cut-off prior to surgery which increased slightly over six months, 11% had elevated depressive symptoms prior to surgery which declined and then increased again in the fifth and sixth month, and 4.5% began with depressive symptoms slightly below the cut-off which increased to peak at the third month after surgery and then declined to pre-surgical levels.[9] In a study of Chinese colorectal cancer patients (n = 234) assessed within three months of cancer diagnosis and three and 12 months later, 67% scored below a cut-off suggestive of clinically significant anxiety/depressive symptoms across all assessments, 14% began with significant distress and then recovered, 12% reported significant distress at the second assessment which increased through the 12-month assessment, and 7% had clinically significant distress across all assessments.[10]

Findings from these studies covering the first 6–12 months after cancer diagnosis or treatment suggest that most individuals diagnosed with cancer evidence either stable, positive psychological status or clear psychological recovery over time. These groups likely possess sufficient personal, social and medical resources to recover well in their natural environments. Other individuals demonstrate compromised psychological status during the treatment and/or re-entry phase or evidence chronic psychological problems; whether this chronic distress trajectory begins prior to cancer diagnosis or after diagnosis is not known.

In light of the finding that the re-entry phase prompts a peak in psychological distress for some individuals with cancer, it is important to characterize the specific challenges of that phase. Completing primary medical treatments can bring a sense of relief, but the individual often is left with many concerns and questions, such as: Does having this new twinge of pain or feeling so tired mean that the cancer is back? Everyone is celebrating my ending treatment – why do I feel so down? I put all my energy into getting through treatment – what can I do now to feel better and to be healthy? My medical team and my friends were so supportive during treatment – how do I get support now? My family expects me to go back to my old roles – when am I going to recover? Major problems during the re-entry phase include fear of cancer recurrence and continuing treatment side-effects, such as fatigue/sleep disturbance, sexual problems, urinary/bowel problems, and cognitive difficulties (e.g.[11–16]). Some cancer survivors find that the psychological impact of having cancer strikes them only once medical treatments are complete.

Health care professionals often provide minimal preparation to patients for the re-entry phase, contributing to continuing needs for information and psychosocial care. Proactive attempts are necessary to help patients know what to expect, when to contact the medical team, and how to manage enduring psychosocial and physical problems. Continued monitoring of and attention to survivors' concerns as they emerge during the re-entry phase also are needed.

With regard to longer-term psychological quality of life, a study of women with breast cancer beginning at four months after diagnosis and extending through four years demonstrated that the largest proportion of women (43%) evidenced positive psychological quality of life, which changed little over the four years.[17] Other groups reported lower quality of life with little change (18%) or rapid improvement (27%) over time, and the smallest proportion (12%) had compromised mental quality of life that declined further over the four years and improved modestly at the end of the study. In a prospective cohort of more than 45 000 women, 759 were diagnosed with breast cancer during a four-year study period.[6] After statistical control for multiple covariates, women diagnosed with cancer experienced a decline in several domains of quality of life compared to women who did not receive a cancer diagnosis. Women affected by cancer reported that emotional problems interfered with their functioning up to four years after diagnosis, although general mental health was comparable for affected and unaffected women.

As with shorter-term studies, these investigations suggest that psychological status is favourable over the long term for a substantial proportion of cancer survivors, but that some individuals struggle with persistent problems (e.g. depressive symptoms). Even when quality of life is generally positive, specific psychosocial problems can persist, including fear of cancer recurrence, fatigue and sexual problems.[6,18] It also is important to note that survivors of various cancers (e.g. breast, lung, prostate, colon) often find benefit and meaning in their experience. Survivors cite interpersonal benefits such as enhanced intimacy, a greater sense of compassion for others, and a heightened awareness of being valued by friends and loved ones. Survivors also report that experiencing a cancer diagnosis contributes to their appreciating life and the present moment, re-evaluating or re-affirming life priorities and goals, acknowledging personal strengths (e.g. If I can get through cancer, I can get through anything), deepening spirituality, and improving healthy behaviours. Although cancer survivors can perceive others' well-intentioned recommendations to 'look on the bright side' as minimizing their experience, survivors themselves being able to come to their own sense of benefit and meaning or being prompted by a professional's sensitive questions about the meaning of the experience in their lives can be useful.

The experience of cancer carries psychological impact not only for the affected individual, but also for the interpersonal network including intimate partners, other family members and loved ones, friends and co-workers. In the small literature addressing the post-treatment phase, caregivers' concerns include fear of recurrence and sexual problems, among others.[19] Psychosocial interventions that include the patient's primary caregiver can improve several aspects of caregivers' adjustment (e.g. caregiver burden, self-efficacy).[20] Whether the interventions have enduring effects and are best delivered during or following medical treatments require study.

Contributors to psychosocial outcomes

What factors predict risk for compromised psychosocial health during re-entry and beyond (e.g.[6,11,21,22])? We address the importance of cultural and developmental contexts in a subsequent section. With regard to medical factors, undergoing systemic treatments for cancer (e.g. chemotherapy, endocrine therapies) or having comorbid physical diseases are related to compromised quality of life for survivors. Personal attributes and resources also are important. For example, having high optimism (i.e. a general expectancy for positive outcomes) predicts more positive psychological adjustment in survivors. Using active strategies for coping with cancer, such as problem-solving and expressing emotions, can be useful, whereas consistently trying to avoid thoughts and feelings about the cancer often predicts poorer adjustment over time. Social isolation and a lack of emotional support magnify psychological problems during survivorship.

Physical symptoms and recovery

Curative cancer treatments are often complex, multimodal, toxic and often prolonged over many months. With the advent of organ-sparing approaches (e.g. breast conservation, bladder conservation, limb sparing in sarcomas), as well as other combined modality treatments with chemotherapy and radiation (e.g. cervical cancer, head and neck cancers), local therapy for cancer has become more complicated, often including at least two modalities and sometimes three. While cosmetic and functional outcomes may be preserved with these strategies, and survival outcomes may be improved, the duration and toxicity of local therapy is increased. Longer and more toxic therapies in turn may lead to side-effects such as prolonged fatigue, local pain, and sometimes lymphoedema. When chemotherapy is given for an extended time, as in neoadjuvant or adjuvant therapy, many constitutional symptoms (e.g. fatigue, insomnia, pain, cognitive complaints) will persist for many months after treatment ends, often slowly resolving over the course of 12–18 months, and persisting in a subset of patients. The more intensive the treatment regimens, including combined modality therapies and transplant, the more likely these symptoms will persist. Chemotherapy agents such as the taxanes or platinum analogues can contribute to neuropathy and musculoskeletal complaints which may diminish over the short term but linger for years after treatment completion. Although patients are warned of the acute effects of chemotherapy agents, including nausea, vomiting, hair loss and fatigue, which are nearly universal during treatment, they are often unprepared for their persistence and slow resolution after treatment ends.

In addition to these problems, women treated for a particular cancer can encounter specific side-effects and late effects. Many women who are pre-menopausal will endure either transient or permanent amenorrhoea as a result of some chemotherapy drugs, especially aklylating agents. For young women with breast cancer, lymphoma, and leukaemia, the commonly used treatment regimens will increase the risk for infertility and premature menopause. The frequency with which this occurs relates to the age of the woman receiving treatment,[23,24] as well as the intensity and duration of treatment. Women receiving high dose chemotherapy with stem cell transplant (e.g. lymphoma and leukaemia patients) will be at much greater risk for premature menopause. Whole body radiation may also contribute to premature onset of menopause. In addition, women requiring extensive pelvic surgery for gynaecological cancers as well as pelvic radiation will also experience premature menopause. Premature menopause is often accompanied by menopausal symptoms (e.g. hot flushes, sweats, vaginal dryness), which are usually more severe than those experienced with natural menopause.[25,26] In some women, short-term oestrogen therapy may be available to help manage these symptoms. Weight gain is a frequent concomitant of premature menopause,[27] which may be disturbing to women physically and emotionally, and may lead to discomfort with body image.

In men treated for prostate cancer, local therapies such as radiation or radical prostatectomy may lead to a variety of complaints and symptoms including urinary incontinence and erectile dysfunction.[28–31] Androgen deprivation therapy, commonly used with locally advanced prostate cancer or in patients who have a rising prostate specific antigen (PSA) level, may further reduce libido and lead to increased fatigue, weight gain and loss of muscle mass. In addition, osteoporosis and cardiovascular disease may be more serious consequences of this therapy. Although less numerous, testicular cancer survivors represent another group for whom multiple advances in therapy have improved survival and long-term health outcomes. Depending on whether or not radiation is used as part of treatment (as in seminoma), or only chemotherapy, most men function at a high level after curative treatment. More serious late effects are seen in patients with combined therapy, especially second malignancies and cardiovascular disease.[32] Those treated with chemotherapy alone may be at risk for hypertension and cardiovascular disease.[33]

Colorectal cancer survivors make up another large segment of the survivor population. Many of these men and women will have only limited impairments, especially if only surgery is involved. Adjuvant chemotherapy regimens used today often include oxaliplatin, which may cause persistent neuropathy. Given that the average age of colorectal cancer diagnosis is age 71, these individuals must also contend with the concomitant effects of comorbid conditions that may be exacerbated by cancer treatments. Alterations in bowel function (diarrhoea and faecal incontinence) can be troubling, often severely constricting social activities. Patients treated for rectal cancer with neoadjuvant chemotherapy and radiation may suffer from the local effects of these therapies, including sexual difficulties (erectile dysfunction in men) as well as changes in bladder function and capacity. When a stoma is required for curative resection, body image changes and management of the stoma can also affect physical and emotional recovery.

Sociocultural and developmental factors influencing psychosocial and physical recovery

The cancer experience in sociocultural context

Much of the knowledge base on how sociocultural contexts shape psychosocial and physical adjustment during cancer survivorship has been generated in the United States, and even there, it is limited. Although cancer appears universally associated with deep fear, cultural groups diverge sharply on beliefs about causes and prognosis of cancer, extent of stigma associated with cancer in general and with specific cancers, expected roles for the health care provider, patient and family in information-giving and decision-making, and norms for psychological responses to cancer and the acceptability of seeking psychosocial care. Certainly, these cultural beliefs and norms can affect psychosocial adjustment in cancer survivors. For example, high perceived stigma and self-blame associated with cancer are related to poorer psychological adjustment. Cultural factors also condition the meaning of quality of life itself, with differential valuing of effective individual functioning, spiritual well-being, and family harmony, for example.

Although the relevant literature is small, some evidence suggests that quality of life is compromised in ethnic minorities diagnosed with cancer relative to their majority group counterparts (e.g.[34,35]). Research demonstrates that lower socioeconomic status explains some of this disparity. However, the finding persists even when socioeconomic status is controlled statistically in a number of studies. Many other factors, which are receiving empirical attention, might help explain disparities in quality of life after cancer. For example, evidence is accruing for lack of access to survivorship information and resources, specific culturally grounded beliefs, and barriers to effective patient–physician communication as contributors to this disparity.

Although physicians worldwide now inform the majority of cancer patients of their diagnosis and treatment options, in countries lacking adequate resources, the focus often is on establishing the necessary conditions for effective cancer detection and treatment. Under these circumstances, survivorship and accompanying psychosocial care remain foreign concepts. Even in countries where established programmes for psychosocial care exist (e.g. Australia, Canada, United Kingdom, United States), post-treatment care is less well developed than care during the early phases of diagnosis and treatment. As programmes for follow-up care develop and evolve, culturally competent survivorship care can be integrated into training (see [36,37]).

The cancer experience in developmental context

The experience of cancer and its sequelae can be strongly influenced by the time in life in which the cancer occurs. The most consistent demographic predictor of compromised quality of life in adult survivors is relatively young age. Depending on the specific cancer treatment regimen and the environmental context, particularly prominent challenges for younger adult cancer survivors include managing sexual and fertility concerns, depressive symptoms, persistent side-effects (e.g. premature menopause), intimate relationships and career goals. For older men and women who have accomplished most of their life goals (e.g. child-rearing, work achievements, other personal goals), the cancer experience is usually less disruptive, and is something they are likely to be familiar with – close friends, family and associates have likely been diagnosed and treated for cancer. In contrast, the 30-year-old woman who is not partnered and is working in an unsatisfying job may find her post-treatment survivorship challenged by difficult questions regarding career and life goals, as well as a sense of isolation, in that so few people her age have encountered a life-threatening event. These experiences, coupled with the fear of recurrence and toxicity from her treatments, may make it difficult for her to move forward achieving life goals that she might desire at this time, such as marriage, childbearing, or advanced education. Further, fighting the cancer may take several years of time and attention, focused primarily on the health care setting, which may cause cancer patients to disengage from social activities fitting to their developmental phase. It may be challenging to resume these activities after cancer treatment ends due to both physical and emotional changes that have occurred as part of the cancer experience. Clearly, cancer survivorship outcomes must be examined within the framework of how the disease and its treatments disrupt normative developmental processes.

Organizing the survivorship care team

Strategies for delivery of post-treatment survivorship care are in development. Since the 2005 Institute of Medicine report calling for greater attention to the post-treatment phase of cancer care,[3] various organizations and clinical care settings have been working to develop and evaluate models of care for delivery of services to cancer survivors.[38] There are substantial barriers to organizing this care, as many oncologists currently believe that they are providing adequate survivorship care,[39] although much of what they may be providing is surveillance for cancer recurrence only. There is an acute need for incorporation of health promotion and chronic disease prevention, as well as psychosocial services for the post-treatment population.[40,41] Cancer survivors, however, are often reluctant to discontinue care with their treating oncology provider, and do not necessarily trust that their primary care provider will be knowledgeable about the late effects of cancer treatment. Indeed, a recent national survey among providers of oncology care and primary care noted that oncologists did not think that primary care providers were skilled in caring for cancer survivors, and primary care providers were not completely confident that they had sufficient knowledge and preparation.[42]

Currently, various modes of delivery are being considered, including a consultative model provided outside the oncology practice by nurses or physicians, often in a multidisciplinary setting with mental health, nutrition and rehabilitation support. Another model, common in busy tertiary centres, is use of either a nurse practitioner or physician assistant who works within the oncology practice, but sees patients for a transition visit when they complete their primary treatment, and then may continue to follow them thereafter with subsequent referral back to the primary care physician. In other settings, primary care physicians are being integrated into the oncology health care delivery team to provide general medical services to survivors. Finally, some oncology practices are stratifying cancer patients into low- and high-risk groups, with return of low-risk patients to primary care within a short time after primary treatment (e.g. patients with DCIS or early stage colon cancer).

In European settings, there is growing interest in adapting rehabilitation programmes to the post-treatment needs of cancer survivors. This may be a fortuitous strategy in that rehabilitation medicine focuses on needs assessment and tailored interventions, including the physical, emotional and vocational concerns of the patient. In that there are many chronic physical needs after cancer treatment, including pain and mobility problems, physical and occupational therapy may be very helpful. In addition, these programmes usually include attention to the psychological needs of patients. Formal rehabilitation programmes were used early on in the development of cancer services in the United States 40 years ago, with the establishment of the National Cancer Act; however, diminished financial reimbursement for such programmes have limited their use in recent years, and this may be an important strategy to encourage in order to muster more broad-based community support for survivorship services.

The evidence base is growing with regard to specific psychological and behavioural interventions for cancer survivors during the re-entry phase and into extended survivorship. Although findings are not completely consistent, randomized, controlled trials document the efficacy of interventions using cognitive-behavioural, stress management, or psychoeducational approaches with cancer survivors in the re-entry phase on such outcomes as depressive symptoms, fatigue, fear of cancer recurrence, sexual health, and general quality of life (e.g.[43–48]). Although most studies have focused on women with breast cancer, behavioural and cognitive interventions also can be effective into extended cancer survivorship for such persistent problems as insomnia, fatigue, distress, fear of cancer recurrence, post-traumatic stress symptoms, menopausal symptoms and pain (e.g.[49–53]). Approaches to promote physical activity and other positive health behaviours after cancer treatment completion also have demonstrated benefit on aerobic fitness, quality of life, fatigue and treatment-related symptoms.[54,55] More work is necessary to disseminate evidence-based approaches to the larger community of cancer survivors, as well as to develop more efficient and accessible psychological and behavioural interventions. As access to Internet-based resources grows, programmes specifically targeted to post-treatment survivors, such as the National Cancer Institute's Facing Forward series (http://www.cancer.gov/cancertopics/coping/life-after-treatment) and the National Coalition for Cancer Survivorship and collaborators' Journey Forward (www.journeyforward.org) have the capacity to reach large populations.

Conclusions

With more than 25 million cancer survivors worldwide, there is a growing need for research and clinical programmes to address the unique concerns of this population. Even though survivors may be eager to get on with life after cancer treatment and most recover well, almost all harbour some fear of recurrence, whether it surfaces only at the time of a medical test or new symptom or it becomes so intrusive that it interferes with enjoyment of life. In addition, other physical and psychological morbidities associated with cancer treatments should not be minimized. Increasingly, we have become aware of the late effects of cancer treatments in adults, which include second malignancies and accelerated appearance of age-related health problems (e.g. congestive heart failure). As more adults are cured of their cancer, mental health practitioners must become familiar with the after-effects of cancer treatment and incorporate strategies to help survivors maximize their well-being. Depression, symptoms of post-traumatic stress, and cognitive difficulties are likely to occur with some frequency and can warrant a mental health referral. Many survivors may only have contact with the general health care system, and those health care providers need to be aware of the lasting physical and mental health consequences of cancer treatment so that survivors' psychosocial needs can be addressed in the aftermath of treatment and beyond.[40]

Clinical case illustration

Maria is a 35-year-old, married woman with one three-year-old child. She was diagnosed with stage II triple negative breast cancer that was found while she was nursing her eight-month-old son. She recently completed breast-conserving surgical treatment, six cycles of chemotherapy, and radiotherapy to the breast. Although she was tested to see if she was a breast cancer gene mutation carrier (i.e. for *BRCA1/2*) and was found to not harbour a mutation, she still has concerns that she may be at high risk for another breast cancer and should have opted for bilateral mastectomies. At her first scheduled follow-up appointment with Dr Lopez, her treating medical oncologist, Maria is told that she will be seen by the nurse and social worker during this appointment, to receive a cancer treatment summary and a survivorship care plan to describe what she can expect during her recovery from treatment in the months ahead. In response to the oncologist's query about 'any current concerns', she reported, 'I don't know what's wrong with me. Since my last radiation treatment, I can't seem to shake this feeling that something terrible is going to happen. I'm worn out, I'm not thinking very well at work, and I don't think I'm taking very good care of my son who is a very busy toddler...I'm also having this pain in my arm and am wondering if I am going to recover the ability to comb and wash my hair with my right side where the surgery was done.' Dr Lopez evaluated Maria's range of motion with her right arm and noted limitation in elevation above 90 degrees and was worried about the development of a frozen shoulder. He discussed the need for a physical therapy referral and some pain medicine, and reassured Maria that these measures would substantially improve her function. He then assured Maria that many women have similar concerns after they complete treatment and suggested that she first have her transition visit with the nurse and social worker, which would provide her with important information about the usual trajectory of physical and emotional recovery after breast cancer treatment, and in addition offered a referral to the psychologist connected to the practice.

After her meeting with the nurse and social worker, Maria felt better, but continued to mention concerns related to sleep, anxiety and fear of recurrence. The social worker reinforced the potential benefit of meeting with a psychologist with special expertise in working with people diagnosed with cancer. She also informed her about a local cancer support group, but Maria stated that she did not want to take evening time away from her family to attend. In an initial session, Maria discussed her concerns with Dr Hanover, the psychologist, and Dr Hanover conducted an assessment that suggested no clinically significant depression, anxiety, or suicidality. Over eight sessions, Dr Hanover worked with Maria to normalize her concerns, develop reasonable expectancies about the pace of her recovery, become willing to ask her husband and others for help in daily tasks so that she could devote more time to her son, and develop strategies to compensate for problems with attention and concentration. They also discussed Maria's fears about what life would bring and identified one close friend who was a calming presence for her. With Dr Hanover's help, Maria also implemented an evidence-based protocol for sleep problems and gradually resumed her pre-treatment exercise routine. At the end of the eight sessions, Maria reported being 'scared but not petrified' about her upcoming mammogram, feeling as if she had 60% of her energy back, and being 'much less hard' on herself about the pace of her recovery and about 'having bad days sometimes'. She was cherishing her time with her family and friends and looking forward to a planned weekend away with her husband.

Clinical comment

Some of Maria's concerns were addressed proactively in a psychoeducational session at treatment completion and provision of support resources and materials to help her know what to expect during the re-entry phase, as well as acknowledgement by her oncologist that her feelings and concerns were normal. The nurse and social worker provided her with verbal and written information about the follow-up surveillance plan as well as the usual course of physical and emotional recovery. The interaction with the social worker was supportive and the recommendation for further psychological counselling was well received as a result. Had Maria been more seriously depressed or anxious, a psychiatric consultation also may have been recommended, with a treatment protocol that would have included additional evidence-based approaches (e.g. cognitive-behavioural therapy, antidepressant medication). Additional problems could be addressed by other members of a multidisciplinary team. In cases where resources are less available, toll-free cancer support phone lines and print or Internet-delivered materials could be offered.

Key points

- When cancer treatment ends, patients are often left with substantial physical and emotional symptoms and concerns. It may take some time for these to resolve; information and reassurance are critical, including symptom management interventions.
- Ideally, all patients completing curative intent therapy should receive a written summary of the treatment they received, including likely short- and long-term effects from the treatments, and their likely temporal resolution. This should be accompanied by a care plan that indicates recommended psychosocial care and health promotion and disease-prevention activities (e.g. physical activity, weight loss, bone health) and indicates what cancer surveillance studies would be appropriate, if any.
- Inclusion of mental health services at this time in the survivorship trajectory is extremely important because of the significant anxiety and depression that can occur at this time point. When everyone thinks the treatment has ended, the patient often experiences increased distress and may feel uncomfortable looking for social support. Professionally facilitated support groups and individual counselling can be particularly helpful at this juncture as a result. It is important to have some linkage to these services so that when one screens for distress it is possible to refer to professionals who have experience of working with cancer patients.

Key references

Hewitt M., Greenfield S., Stovall E. (2006) *From Cancer Patient to Cancer Survivor: Lost in Transition,* National Academies Press, Washington, DC.

Adler N.E., Page A.E.K. (2007) *Cancer Care for the Whole Patient: Meeting Psychosocial Health Needs,* Institute of Medicine, National Academies Press, Washington, DC.

Feuerstein, M., Ganz, P.A. (eds) (2011) *Health Services for Cancer Survivors,* Springer, New York.

References

1. Mullan F. (1985) Seasons of survival: Reflections of a physician with cancer. *New England Journal of Medicine,* 313, 270–273.
2. Stovall E. (2005) Remarks of Ellen Stovall, NCI/ACS Survivorship Symposium, June 2002. *Cancer,* 104, 2643–2645.
3. Hewitt M., Greenfield S., Stovall E. (2006) *From Cancer Patient to Cancer Survivor: Lost in Transition,* National Academies Press, Washington, DC.
4. Feuerstein M. (2007) Defining cancer survivorship. *Journal of Cancer Survivorship,* 1, 5–7.
5. McCarthy A.M., Williams J., Plumer C. (1998) Evaluation of a school re-entry nursing intervention for children with cancer. *Journal of Pediatric Oncology Nursing,* 15, 143–152.
6. Michael Y.L., Kawachi I., Berkman L.F. *et al.* (2000) The persistent impact of breast carcinoma on functional health status: Prospective evidence from the Nurses' Health Study. *Cancer,* 89, 2176–2186.
7. Polsky D., Doshi J.A., Marcus S. *et al.* (2005) Long-term risk for depressive symptoms after a medical diagnosis. *Archives of Internal Medicine,* 165, 1260–1266.
8. Henselmans I., Helgeson V.S., Seltman H. *et al.* (2010) Identification and prediction of distress trajectories in the first year after a breast cancer diagnosis. *Health Psychology,* 29, 160–168.
9. Dunn L.B., Cooper B.A., Neuhaus J. *et al.* (2011) Identification of distinct depressive symptom trajectories in women following surgery for breast cancer. *Health Psychology* 30, 683–692.
10. Hou W.K., Law C.C., Yin J. *et al.* (2010) Resource loss, resource gain, and psychological resilience and dysfunction following cancer diagnosis: A growth mixture modeling approach. *Health Psychology,* 29, 484–495.
11. Ganz P.A., Kwan L., Stanton A.L. *et al.* (2004) Quality of life at the end of primary treatment of breast cancer: First results from the moving beyond cancer randomized trial. *Journal of the National Cancer Institute,* 96, 376–387.
12. Costanzo E.S., Lutgendorf S.K., Mattes M.L. *et al.* (2007) Adjusting to life after treatment: Distress and quality of life following treatment for breast cancer. *British Journal of Cancer,* 97, 1625–1631.
13. Armes J., Crowe M., Colbourne L. *et al.* (2009) Patients' supportive care needs beyond the end of cancer treatment: A prospective, longitudinal survey. *Journal of Clinical Oncology,* 27, 6172–6179.
14. Stanton A.L., Ganz P.A., Rowland J.H. *et al.* (2005) Promoting adjustment after treatment for cancer. *Cancer,* 104, 2608–2613.
15. Bower J.E. (2008) Behavioral symptoms in patients with breast cancer and survivors. *Journal of Clinical Oncology,* 26, 768–777.

16. Talcott J.A., Manola J., Clark J.A. *et al.* (2003) Time course and predictors of symptoms after primary prostate cancer therapy. *Journal of Clinical Oncology*, 21, 3979–3986.
17. Helgeson V.S., Snyder P., Seltman H. (2004) Psychological and physical adjustment to breast cancer over 4 years: Identifying distinct trajectories of change. *Health Psychology*, 23, 3–15.
18. Mols F., Vingerhoets A.J.J.M., Coebergh J.W. *et al.* (2005) Quality of life among long-term breast cancer survivors: A systematic review. *European Journal of Cancer*, 41, 2613–2619.
19. Kim Y., Given B.A. (2008) Quality of life of family caregivers of cancer survivors. *Cancer*, 112, 2556–2568.
20. Northouse L.L., Katapodi M.C., Song L. *et al.* (2010) Interventions with family caregivers of cancer patients: Meta-analysis of randomized trials. *CA: A Cancer Journal for Clinicians*, 60, 317–339.
21. Lynch B.M., Steginga S.K., Hawkes A.L. *et al.* (2008) Describing and predicting psychological distress after colorectal cancer. *Cancer*, 112, 1363–1370.
22. Roesch S.C., Adams L., Hines A. *et al.* (2005) Coping with prostate cancer: A meta-analytic review. *Journal of Behavioral Medicine*, 28, 281–293.
23. Goodwin P.J., Ennis M., Pritchard K.I. *et al.* (1999) Risk of menopause during the first year after breast cancer diagnosis. *Journal of Clinical Oncology*, 17, 2365–2370.
24. Ganz P.A., Land S.R., Geyer C.E. *et al.* (2011) Menstrual history and quality-of-life outcomes in women with node-positive breast cancer treated with adjuvant therapy on the NSABP B-30 Trial. *Journal of Clinical Oncology*, 29, 1110–1116.
25. Ganz P.A., Kwan L., Stanton A.L. *et al.* (2011) Physical and psychosocial recovery in the year after primary treatment of breast cancer. *Journal of Clinical Oncology*, 29, 1101–1109.
26. Crandall C., Petersen L., Ganz P.A. *et al.* (2004). Association of breast cancer and its therapy with menopause-related symptoms. *Menopause* 11, 519–530.
27. Goodwin P.J., Ennis M., Pritchard K.I. *et al.* (1999) Adjuvant treatment and onset of menopause predict weight gain after breast cancer diagnosis. *Journal of Clinical Oncology*, 17, 120–129.
28. Litwin M.S., Flanders S.C., Pasta D.J. *et al.* (1999) Sexual function and bother after radical prostatectomy or radiation for prostate cancer: Multivariate quality-of-life analysis from CaPSURE (Cancer of the Prostate Strategic Urologic Research Endeavor). *Urology*, 54, 503–508.
29. Litwin M.S., Melmed G.Y., Nakazon T. (2001) Life after radical prostatectomy: A longitudinal study. *Journal of Urology*, 166, 587–592.
30. Talcott J.A., Rieker P., Clark J.A. *et al.* (1998) Patient-reported symptoms after primary therapy for early prostate cancer: Results of a prospective cohort study. *Journal of Clinical Oncology*, 16, 275–283.
31. Chen R.C., Clark J.A., Talcott J.A. (2009) Individualizing quality-of-life outcomes reporting: How localized prostate cancer treatments affect patients with different levels of baseline urinary, bowel, and sexual function. *Journal of Clinical Oncology*, 27, 3916–3922.
32. van den Belt-Dusebout A., de Wit R., Gietema J.A. *et al.* (2007) Treatment-specific risks of second malignancies and cardiovascular disease in 5-year survivors of testicular cancer. *Journal of Clinical Oncology*, 25, 4370–4378.
33. Haugnes H.S., Wethal T., Aass N. *et al.* (2010) Cardiovascular risk factors and morbidity in long-term survivors of testicular cancer: A 20-year follow-up study. *Journal of Clinical Oncology*, 28, 4649–4657.
34. Janz N.K., Mujahid M.S., Hawley S.T. *et al.* (2008) Racial/ethnic differences in adequacy of information and support for women with breast cancer. *Cancer*, 113, 1058–1067.
35. Yanez B., Thompson E.H., Stanton A.L. (2011) Quality of life among Latina breast cancer patients: A systematic review of the literature. *Journal of Cancer Survivorship*, 5, 191–207.
36. Moore R.J., Spiegel D. (2004) *Cancer, Culture, and Communication*, Kluwer Academic/Plenum, New York.
37. Findley P.A. (2007) Global considerations, in *Handbook of Cancer Survivorship*, (ed. M. Feuerstein), Springer, New York, pp. 449–480.
38. Hahn E.E., Ganz P.A. (2011). Survivorship programs and care plans in practice: Variations on a theme. *Journal of Oncology Practice*, 7, 70–75.
39. Ganz P.A., Kwan L., Somerfield M.R. *et al.* (2006) The role of prevention in oncology practice: Results from a 2004 survey of American Society of Clinical Oncology Members. *Journal of Clinical Oncology*, 24, 2948–2957.
40. Adler N.E., Page A.E.K. (2007) *Cancer Care for the Whole Patient: Meeting Psychosocial Health Needs*, Institute of Medicine, National Academies Press, Washington, DC.
41. Ganz P.A. (2011) The 'three Ps' of cancer survivorship care. *BMC Medicine*, 9, 14.

42. Potosky A., Han P., Rowland J. *et al.* (2011) Differences between primary care physicians' and oncologists' knowledge, attitudes and practices regarding the care of cancer survivors. *Journal of General Internal Medicine*, http://dx.doi.org/10.1007/s11606-011-1808-4.
43. Penedo F.L., Traeger L., Dahn J. *et al.* (2007) Cognitive behavioral stress management intervention improves quality of life in Spanish monolingual Hispanic men treated for localized prostate cancer: Results of a randomized controlled trial. *International Journal of Behavioral Medicine*, 14, 164–172.
44. Lengacher C.A., Johnson-Mallard V., Post-White J. *et al.* (2009) Randomized controlled trial of mindfulness-based stress reduction (MBSR) for survivors of breast cancer. *Psycho-Oncology*, 18, 1261–1272.
45. Scheier M.F., Helgeson V.S., Schulz R. *et al.* (2007) Moderators of interventions designed to enhance physical and psychological functioning among younger women with early-stage breast cancer. *Journal of Clinical Oncology*, 25, 5710–5714.
46. Marcus A.C., Garrett K.M., Cella D. *et al.* (2010) Can telephone counseling post-treatment improve psychosocial outcomes among early stage breast cancer survivors? *Psycho-Oncology*, 19, 923–932.
47. Dolbeault S., Cayrou S., Bredart A. *et al.* (2009) The effectiveness of a psycho-educational group after early-stage breast cancer treatment: Results of a randomized French study. *Psycho-Oncology*, 18, 647–656.
48. Stanton A.L., Ganz P.A., Kwan L. *et al.* (2005) Outcomes from the moving beyond cancer psychoeducational, randomized, controlled trial with breast cancer patients. *Journal of Clinical Oncology*, 23, 6009–6018.
49. Espie C.A., Fleming L., Cassidy J. *et al.* (2008) Randomized controlled clinical effectiveness trial of cognitive behavior therapy compared with treatment as usual for persistent insomnia in patients with cancer. *Journal of Clinical Oncology*, 26, 4651–4658.
50. Gielissen M.F.M., Verhagen S., Witjes F. *et al.* (2006) Effects of cognitive behavior therapy in severely fatigued disease-free cancer patients compared with patients waiting for cognitive behavior therapy: A randomized controlled trial. *Journal of Clinical Oncology*, 24, 4882–4887.
51. Gil K., Mishel M., Belyea M. *et al.* (2006) Benefits of the uncertainty management intervention for African American and white older breast cancer survivors: 20-month outcomes. *International Journal of Behavioral Medicine*, 13, 286–294.
52. DuHamel K.N., Mosher C.E., Winkel G. *et al.* (2010) Randomized clinical trial of telephone-administered cognitive-behavioral therapy to reduce post-traumatic stress disorder and distress symptoms after hematopoietic stem-cell transplantation. *Journal of Clinical Oncology*, 28, 3754–3761.
53. Ganz P.A., Greendale G.A., Petersen L. *et al.* (2000) Managing menopausal symptoms in breast cancer survivors: Results of a randomized controlled trial. *Journal of the National Cancer Institute*, 92, 1054–1064.
54. Demark-Wahnefried W., Pinto B.M., Gritz E.R. (2006) Promoting health and physical function among cancer survivors: Potential for prevention and questions that remain. *Journal of Clinical Oncology*, 24, 5125–5131.
55. Speck R.M., Courneya K.S., Mâsse L.C. *et al.* (2010) An update of controlled physical activity trials in cancer survivors: A systematic review and meta-analysis. *Journal of Cancer Survivorship*, 4, 87–100.

CHAPTER 19
End-of-life Care

William Breitbart[1], Harvey Max Chochinov[2] and Yesne Alici[3]
[1]Department of Psychiatry and Behavioral Sciences, and Pain and Palliative Care Service, Department of Medicine, Memorial Sloan-Kettering Cancer Center; Department of Psychiatry, Weill Medical College of Cornell University, New York, NY, USA
[2]Manitoba Palliative Care Research Unit, Cancer Care Manitoba; Departments of Psychiatry and Family Medicine, University of Manitoba, Winnipeg, Manitoba, Canada
[3]Geriatric Psychiatry Treatment Unit, Central Regional Hospital, Butner, NC, USA

Introduction

One of the most challenging roles for clinicians caring for the terminally ill is to help guide patients physically, psychologically and spiritually through the dying process. Psycho-oncologists who care for the terminally ill are often faced with patients who are experiencing psychological distress. While emotional distress is natural and expected in individuals confronting the end of their lives, the differentiation between a normal and appropriate reaction to dying versus a more serious psychiatric disorder can be a major clinical challenge. Patients with advanced cancer have an enormous burden of both physical as well as psychological symptoms.[1] In fact, surveys suggest that psychological symptoms such as depression, anxiety and hopelessness are as frequent, if not more so, than pain and other physical symptoms.[1] The psycho-oncologist, as a consultant to or member of a palliative care team, has a unique role and opportunity to offer competent and compassionate care to those with terminal illnesses. The role of the psycho-oncologist, in the care of the dying, extends beyond the management of psychiatric symptoms and syndromes (e.g. depression, suicide, anxiety, delirium, fatigue and pain) into existential issues, family and caregiver support, bereavement, doctor–patient communication, and education and training. Psycho-oncologists can play an important role in the management of social, psychological, ethical, legal and spiritual issues that complicate the care of dying patients.

The purpose of this chapter is to review the most salient aspects of care of terminally ill cancer patients for psycho-oncologists across the globe. In this chapter, we review basic concepts and definitions of palliative care and the experience of dying; assessment and management of common psychiatric disorders in the terminally ill, including suicide, desire for hastened death, and physician assisted-suicide. A brief description of psychotherapeutic modalities used in palliative care settings, and concepts of dignity-conserving care are also included. Bereavement and spirituality aspects of end-of-life care are reviewed in Chapters 20 and 21 respectively.

Palliative care

Historical perspectives

Modern palliative care is an outgrowth of the hospice movement that began in the 1840s with Calvaires in Lyon, France, and progressed through 1900 and the establishment of the St Joseph's Hospice in London, finally culminating with the progenitor of all modern hospices, St Christopher's Hospice, established in 1967 by Cicely Saunders. The first hospice in the United States was

Clinical Psycho-Oncology: An International Perspective, First Edition. Edited by Luigi Grassi and Michelle Riba.

established in 1974 in Connecticut. By 1975, a large number of independent hospices had been developed in Australia, Canada and the United Kingdom. Modern palliative care evolved from that hospice movement into a mixture of academic and non-academic clinical care delivery systems that have components of home care and hospital-based services.[1]

Defining palliative care

The term *palliation* is derived from the Latin root word *palliare,* which means 'to cloak' or 'to conceal'. *Pallium* also refers to the cloth that covers or cloaks burial caskets. These root words suggest that the dying patient, although not amenable to cure, can be 'cloaked' or 'embraced' in the comforting arms of the caregiver.[1]

In 1990, the World Health Organization (WHO) defined *palliative care* as the active total care of patients whose disease is not responsive to curative treatment. According to the WHO definition the goal of palliative care is achievement of the best quality of life for patients and their families, and that many aspects of palliative care are also applicable earlier in the course of the illness in conjunction with anti-cancer treatment. This definition was the first to suggest applicability even at stages of disease that precede the end of life.[2]

The World Health Organization definition of palliative care has been revised and expanded through the years.[3] The most recent and comprehensive definition of palliative care as outlined by the World Health Organization[3] provides a framework for palliative care in all settings. According to the WHO (2009), palliative care:

- provides relief from pain and other distressing symptoms.
- affirms life and regards dying as a normal process.
- intends neither to hasten nor to postpone death.
- integrates psychological and spiritual aspects of patients care.
- offers a support system to help patients live as actively as possible until death.
- offers a support system to help families cope during the patient's illness and in their own bereavement.
- is interdisciplinary and uses a team approach including physicians, nurses, mental health professionals, clergy and volunteers to address the needs of patients and their families.
- will enhance quality of life and may also positively influence the course of illness.
- is applicable early in the course of illness, in conjunction with other therapies that are intended to prolong life, and includes those investigations needed to better understand and manage distressing complications.

Palliative care programmes/ models of care delivery

Fully developed, model palliative care programmes ideally include all of the following components: (1) a home care programme (e.g. hospice programme); (2) a hospital-based palliative care consultation service; (3) a day care programme or ambulatory care clinic; (4) a palliative care inpatient unit (or dedicated palliative care beds in hospital); (5) a bereavement programme; (6) training and research programmes; and (7) Internet-based services.

Palliative care is not restricted to those who are dying or those who are enrolled in hospice programmes, but rather can be applied cost-effectively to the control of symptoms and provision of support to those living with life-threatening illnesses. Palliative care programmes can reduce hospital and intensive care unit expenditures by clarifying the goals of care and assisting patients and families to select treatments that are consistent with these goals.[4] Palliative care has been successfully instituted for patients with cancer as national policy in countries that are neither wealthy nor industrialized.

Definition of a 'good' death

A meaningful dying process is one throughout which the patient is physically, psychologically, spiritually and emotionally supported by his or her family, friends and caregivers. In 1972 Weisman described four criteria for what he called an 'appropriate death': (1) internal conflicts, such as fears about loss of control, should be reduced as much as possible; (2) the individual's personal sense of identity should be sustained; (3) critical relationships should be enhanced or at least maintained, and conflicts should be resolved, if possible; and (4) the person should be encouraged to set and attempt to reach meaningful goals, even though limited, such as attending a graduation, a wedding, or the birth of a child, as a way to provide a sense of continuity into the future.[1]

Steinhauser and colleagues examined components of a good death from the perspective of patients, families and health care providers where participants identified six major elements of a good death:

- Effective pain and symptom management
- Clear decision-making
- Preparation for death
- Completion (e.g. life review, saying goodbye, resolving conflicts, spending time with family and friends)
- Contributing to others (e.g. giving gifts, time or imparting knowledge)
- Affirmation of the whole person.

The WHO[3] outlined guidelines characterizing a 'good' death as one that is (1) free from avoidable distress and suffering for patient, family and caregivers, (2) in general accord with the patient's and family's wishes, and (3) reasonably consistent with clinical, cultural and ethical standards. These guidelines and the aforementioned considerations for achieving a good death can serve as general principles for clinicians in caring for the dying.

Assessment and management of commonly encountered psychiatric disorders in the palliative care setting

Anxiety disorders

The terminally ill patient presents with a complex mixture of physical and psychological symptoms in the context of a frightening reality, making the identification of anxiety symptoms requiring treatment challenging. Patients with anxiety complain of tension or restlessness, or they exhibit jitteriness, autonomic hyperactivity, vigilance, insomnia, distractibility, shortness of breath, numbness, apprehension, worry, or rumination. Often the physical manifestations of anxiety are the symptoms that the patient most often presents with and they overshadow the psychological or cognitive ones.[1] The consultant must use these symptoms as a cue to inquire about the patient's psychological state, which is commonly one of fear, worry, or apprehension.

The assumption that a high level of anxiety is inevitably encountered during the terminal phase of illness is neither helpful nor accurate. In deciding whether to treat anxiety during the terminal phase of illness, the clinician should assess the patient's level of distress, problematic patient behaviour such as non-compliance due to anxiety, family and staff reactions to the patient's distress, and balance the risks and benefits of treatment.[1]

Prevalence

Prevalence of anxiety disorders among terminally ill cancer ranges from 15–28%.[1] Prevalence studies report a higher prevalence of mixed anxiety and depressive symptoms rather than anxiety alone. In the Canadian National Palliative Care Survey, younger patients, those with a lower performance status, smaller social networks, and less participation in organized religious services were more likely to have an anxiety disorder.[5] It was also noted that palliative care patients with a DSM-IV anxiety and/or depressive disorder reported more severe distress from several physical symptoms, social concerns and existential issues.[5]

Assessment

Anxiety can occur in terminally ill patients as an adjustment disorder, a disease- or treatment-related condition, or an exacerbation of a pre-existing anxiety disorder.[1] Adjustment disorder with anxiety is related to adjusting to the existential crisis and the uncertainty of the prognosis and the future.[1] When faced with terminal illness, patients with pre-existing anxiety disorders are at risk for reactivation of symptoms. Generalized anxiety disorder or panic disorders are apt to recur, especially in the presence of dyspnoea or pain. Persons with phobias can experience a difficult time if the disease or treatment confronts them with their fears (e.g. claustrophobia, fear of needles, fear of isolation). Post-traumatic stress disorder (PTSD) may be activated in dying patients as they relate their situation to some prior frightening experience. Patients with PTSD may present with high levels of anxiety, insomnia, frequent panic attacks, comorbid depressive symptoms, and avoidance of medical settings that trigger traumatic memories.[6]

Symptoms of anxiety in the terminally ill patient may arise from a medical complication of the illness or treatment. Hypoxia, sepsis, poorly controlled pain, medication side-effects such as akathisia, and withdrawal states often present as anxiety.[6] In the dying patient, anxiety can represent impending cardiac or respiratory arrest, pulmonary embolism, sepsis, electrolyte imbalance, or dehydration. Delirium can present with anxiety and restlessness in palliative care settings. Disturbance in level of consciousness, attentional disturbances, and fluctuation of symptoms are important diagnostic indicators of delirium as opposed to a diagnosis of anxiety disorder.[1]

Despite the fact that anxiety in terminal illness commonly results from medical complications, it is important to consider psychological factors that may play a role. As disease progresses, patients' anxiety may include fears about the disease process, the clinical course, financial consequences, possible treatment outcomes, and death. Patients frequently fear the isolation and separation of death. Claustrophobic patients may fear the idea of being confined and buried in a coffin. These issues can be disconcerting to consultants, who may find themselves at a loss for words that are consoling to the patient. Often all that is required in these situations are the clinician's basic listening and reflective skills.[1]

Treatment

The most effective management of anxiety involves a combination of psychotherapy and pharmacological management.

Pharmacological treatment

For patients who feel persistently anxious, the first-line anti-anxiety drugs are the benzodiazepines. For patients with severely compromised hepatic function, the use of shorter-acting benzodiazepines such as lorazepam, oxazepam or temazepam are preferred, since these drugs have no active metabolites.[7] Dying patients can be administered diazepam rectally when no other route is available, with dosages equivalent to those used in oral regimens. It is important to note that a Cochrane review of pharmacotherapy for anxiety in palliative care settings concluded that there was lack of high level evidence on the role of anti-anxiety medications in terminally ill patients. The excessive use of benzodiazepines may result in mental status changes. In anxious patients with severely compromised pulmonary function, the use of benzodiazepines that suppress central respiratory mechanisms may be unsafe. Although low doses of an antipsychotic or an antihistamine can be useful, the anticholinergic effects of antihistamines make them problematic in the debilitated patient prone to develop delirium, and none of the antipsychotics have been systematically studied in the treatment of anxiety among patients receiving palliative care.[7] Sedating antidepressants such as trazodone or mirtazapine may help patients with persistent anxiety, insomnia and anorexia. The utility of antidepressants and buspirone for anxiety disorders is often limited in the dying patient because they require weeks to achieve therapeutic effect. Opioid drugs are primarily indicated for the control of pain but are also effective in the relief of dyspnoea and associated anxiety.[1] Continuous intravenous infusions of morphine or other opioid analgesics allow for careful titration and control of respiratory distress, anxiety, pain and agitation (APPI). However, when respiratory distress is not a major problem, it is preferable to use the opioid drugs solely for analgesia and to add more specific anxiolytics to control concomitant anxiety.

Non-pharmacological treatment

Non-pharmacological interventions for anxiety and distress include supportive psychotherapy, behavioural interventions, and cognitive behavioural therapy that are used alone or in combination. Brief supportive psychotherapy is often useful in dealing with both crises and existential issues confronted by the terminally ill.[1] Supportive-expressive group therapy has been shown to reduce distress and subsyndromal symptoms of PTSD in women with advanced breast cancer.[1] Inclusion of the family in psychotherapeutic interventions should be considered, particularly as the patient with advanced illness becomes increasingly debilitated and less able to interact. Relaxation, guided imagery and hypnosis may help reduce anxiety and thereby increase the patient's sense of control.

The goals of psychotherapy with the patient are to establish a bond that decreases the sense of isolation experienced with terminal illness; to help the patient face death with a sense of self-worth; to correct misconceptions about the past and present; to integrate the present illness into a continuum of life experiences; and to explore issues of separation and loss as well as the unknown that lies ahead. The therapist should emphasize past strengths and support previously successful ways of coping. In doing so the person is better equipped to mobilize inner resources, modify plans for the future and perhaps even accept the inevitability of their own death.[7]

Depression

Epidemiology

Depression is common in palliative care settings, yet it is underdiagnosed and undertreated. Most studies on the prevalence of major depression in advanced cancer patients suggest that the prevalence of depression in patients with advanced disease ranges from 9–26%.[5] The wide variability is explained by the lack of agreement as to appropriate diagnostic criteria, differences in patient populations, and variation in assessment methods.

Family history of depression and history of previous depressive episodes increase the terminally ill patient's risk of developing a depressive episode.[6] Loss of meaning, and low scores on measures of spiritual well-being have been associated with higher levels of depressive symptoms.[1] Inability to come to terms with a terminal diagnosis has also been found to correlate closely with feelings of hopelessness, a sense of suffering, and depression.[8] Depression is associated with poor treatment compliance, reduced quality of life, poor survival, and desire for hastened death among terminally ill patients.[9] Many studies have also found a correlation between depression, pain, and functional status.[5] Younger age and poor social support have also been identified as risk factors for depression in the terminally ill. Certain factors associated with the patient's illness or its treatment may be associated with depression. Tumours arising within or metastasizing to the central nervous system can cause depression. Metabolic complications such as hypocalcaemia, often associated with breast and lung cancers, can also be associated with depression. Glucocorticosteroids, chemotherapeutic agents (vincristine, vinblastine, asparaginase, intrathecal methotrexate, interferon, interleukin), amphotericin, whole brain radiation to central nervous system (CNS), and paraneoplastic syndromes can all cause depressive symptoms.[1]

Assessment

Depressed mood and sadness can be appropriate responses as the terminally ill patient faces death. On the other hand, minimization of depressive symptoms as 'normal reactions' and the difficulties of accurately diagnosing depression in the terminally ill lead to underdiagnosis of depression. Among the many barriers to the recognition of depression in terminally ill patients is the clinician's own sense of hopelessness that can lead to therapeutic nihilism when caring for dying patients.[1]

Preferences for life-sustaining medical therapy are frequently influenced by depressive symptoms. Consequently, treatment of depression can impact these preferences. It is important to encourage those patients who are severely depressed to hold off decisions about life-sustaining therapy until after their depressive symptoms are treated.

The diagnosis of a major depressive syndrome in a terminally ill patient often relies more on the psychological or cognitive symptoms of major depression than the neurovegetative symptoms. Feelings of hopelessness, worthlessness, or suicidal ideation must be explored in detail. Although many dying patients lose hope for a cure, they are able to maintain hope for better symptom control. For many patients hope is contingent on the ability to find continued meaning in their day-to-day existence. Hopelessness that is pervasive and accompanied by a sense of despair is more likely to represent a symptom of a depressive disorder. Even mild and passive forms of suicidal ideation are very often indicative of significant degrees of depression in terminally ill patients.[1]

Several screening instruments have been studied for detection of depression in palliative care settings, a detailed description of these instruments can be found elsewhere. Chochinov and colleagues studied brief screening instruments to measure depression in the terminally ill, including a single-item interview assessing depressed mood ('Have you been depressed most of the time for the past 2 weeks?'), a two-item interview assessing depressed mood and loss of interest in activities, a visual analogue scale for depressed mood, and the Beck Depression Inventory. Most noteworthy, the single-item question correctly identified the diagnosis of every patient, substantially outperforming the questionnaire and visual analogue measures. The single-item depression question has been incorporated into routine clinical assessments in a variety of clinical settings to identify depression among medically ill patients. Although the sensitivity and specificity of the single-item question as a screen for depression has been shown by others in diverse cohorts, conflicting results have been observed in palliative care populations in the United Kingdom and in Japan. This is not surprising as while some patients may readily verbalize that they are depressed, patients from different cultural backgrounds, no matter how despairing, may never acknowledge it, or may label it something else (e.g. nervousness).[1] Guidelines for distress management from the National Comprehensive Cancer Network suggest the use of a visual assessment scale (VAS) as well as patient self-report of depression, sadness and loss of interest in usual activities (yes or no) as a screen for depression. Both methods are reasonable as screening tools.[1]

Treatment

Depression is frequently undertreated at the end of life. Undertreatment is due in part to the concern that severely medically ill patients will not be able to tolerate the side-effects of antidepressants.[1] However, recent evidence from the increasing prevalence of antidepressant utilization among cancer patients suggests that clinicians have become more vigilant in recognition and treatment of depression in the medically ill.[1]

A combination of pharmacotherapy, supportive psychotherapy, cognitive-behavioural therapy and psychoeducation is the mainstay of treatment for depression in palliative care settings. It is also important to treat the distressing physical symptoms (such as pain, dyspnoea, nausea) concurrently while managing depression in patients with advanced disease.

Pharmacological treatment

Antidepressant medications are the mainstay of pharmacological management for gravely ill patients meeting diagnostic criteria for major depression and have established efficacy. A Cochrane review supported the use of antidepressants in this patient population, but emphasized the methodological weaknesses in reviewed studies.[10] Factors such as prognosis and the time frame for treatment may play an important role in determining the type of pharmacotherapy for depression in the terminally ill. A depressed patient with several months of life expectancy can afford to wait the 2–4 weeks it may take to respond to a standard antidepressant. The depressed dying patient with less than 3 weeks to live may do best with a rapid-acting psychostimulant.[1] A review of the 19 controlled trials of methylphenidate in medically ill older adults and patients in palliative care settings has concluded that the use of low-dose methylphenidate is appropriate in the treatment of depression, fatigue, or apathy in this patient population with monitoring for response and adverse effects.[11] Patients who are within hours to days of death and in distress are likely to benefit most from the use of sedatives or narcotic analgesic infusions.[1]

Non-pharmacological treatment

Psychotherapeutic interventions, in the form of either individual or group counselling, have been shown to effectively reduce psychological distress and depressive symptoms in advanced-stage cancer patients. Both supportive psychotherapy and cognitive-behavioural interventions have been shown to decrease depressive symptoms in patients with mild to moderate levels of depression. An extensive review of psychotherapeutic interventions for depression in the terminally ill can be found elsewhere.[12] Several novel psychotherapies (e.g. meaning-centred psychotherapy) have been developed for the treatment of depression, hopelessness, loss of meaning and demoralization at the end of life. Pastoral counselling may additionally be helpful, and chaplaincy service should be offered to the patient and family members if it is available.

Suicide, assisted suicide, and desire for hastened death

Suicide, suicidal ideation, and desire for hastened death are important and serious consequences of unrecognized and/or inadequately treated clinical depression. Although clinical depression has been demonstrated to be a critically important factor in desire for hastened death[13] (through suicide or other means), understanding more fully why some patients with a terminal illness wish or seek to hasten their death remains an important element in the practice of palliative care. The issues of managing suicidality and DHD raise clinical, legal, ethical and moral issues for health care professionals. In addition, there are a multitude of complex risk factors that may contribute to the manifestation of DHD or suicidality. Guidelines for the assessment and management of DHD and suicidality for health care providers and the ability to deliver empirically supported psychosocial and pharmacological interventions assist health care providers to meet these challenges and result in better outcomes for patients.

In cancer patients, less severe forms of suicidal ideation, such as a fleeting wish to die, are relatively common and not necessarily a cause for concern. Suicidal ideation becomes problematic when it becomes persistent or involves actual suicidal intent, plan, or behaviour. Other terms closely related to suicidality are physician-assisted suicide, which involves a physician providing the means for the patient to end his or her life, such as by prescribing a lethal dose of medication. Despite the continued legal prohibitions against assisted suicide in most of the world, a substantial number of patients think about and discuss those alternatives with their physicians, family and friends. Euthanasia is the term used when a physician administers a fatal overdose of medication with or without the patient's consent.[13]

Suicide

Psycho-oncologists should be competent in the identification and assessment of patients who are at risk for suicide, as cancer patients are more likely to express suicidal ideation and commit suicide than both the general population and other medically ill populations most frequently in the advanced stages of disease[13] (see Tables 19.1 and 19.2).

Several patient-related factors have been associated with suicidality. Older age is significantly associated with suicide risk. While men with cancer may have over twice the risk of suicide compared to the general population, the relative risk of suicide in women with cancer is less clear. The highest suicide risk is attributed to males with respiratory cancers which may also be related to the presence of other risk factors (i.e. alcohol and tobacco use) or pre-existing psychological problems. Lack of social support has also been associated with higher rates of suicide in cancer patients. Several studies have found a significant correlation between lower levels of social support and a higher DHD and suicide in advanced cancer patients.[13]

Depressive symptoms play a significant role in suicidality among terminally ill patients. Individuals with major depressive disorder are 25 times more likely to commit suicide than the general population, and half of all suicides involve depressive symptoms. Hopelessness is a key variable linking depression and suicide in the terminally ill, possibly

Table 19.1 Guidelines for assessment of suicide in palliative care settings.[13]

Be vigilant to recognize your own responses	• Be aware of how your responses influence discussions • Monitor your attitude, behaviour and responses • Demonstrate positive regard for the patient • Seek supervision
Be open to hearing concerns	• Gently ask about and encourage expression of emotional concerns • Be alert to recognize verbal and non-verbal distress cues • Attentively listen without interrupting • Discuss desire for death using patient's words • Permit sadness, silence and tears • Express empathy verbally and non-verbally • Acknowledge differences in responses to illness
Assess contributing factors	• Prior psychiatric history • Family psychiatric history • Prior suicide attempts • History of alcohol or substance abuse • Lack of social support • History of poor impulse control • Feelings of burden • Family conflict • Depression and anxiety • Existential concerns, loss of meaning and dignity • Cognitive impairment • Physical symptoms, especially severe pain
Respond to specific issues	• Acknowledge patient or family fears and concerns • Address and manage modifiable contributing factors (such as pain) • Develop a plan to manage more complicated issues
Conclude discussion	• Summarize and review important points • Clarify patient perceptions • Provide opportunity for questions • Assist in facilitating discussion with others • Provide appropriate referrals
After discussion	• Document discussion in medical records • Communicate with members of the treatment team

Adapted from Breitbart *et al.* (2010).[12]

a stronger predictor of suicidal ideation than severity of depression among patients with terminal cancer. In Scandinavia, the highest incidence of suicide was found in cancer patients who were offered no further treatment and no further contact with the health care system.[1] Being left to face illness alone creates a sense of isolation and abandonment that is critical to the development of hopelessness. Loss of control and a sense of helplessness in the face of terminal illness are important factors in suicide vulnerability. Personality factors such as concerns about loss of autonomy, dependency, and a strong need to control the circumstances of one's death are important predictors of suicide.[13] Anxiety is one of the most common reasons for psychiatric consultation in terminally ill cancer patients, but has received less attention as a predictor of suicide. A recent study of anxiety in 200 terminally ill

Table 19.2 Questions to ask patients and family when assessing suicidal risk.[14]

Acknowledge that these are common thoughts that can be discussed	• Most patients with cancer have passing thoughts about suicide, such as 'I might do something if it gets bad enough'. Have you ever had thoughts like that? • Have you had any thoughts of not wanting to live? • Have you had those thoughts in the past few days?
Assess level of risk	• Do you have thoughts about wanting to end your life? How? • Do you have a plan? • Do you have any strong social supports? • Do you have pills stockpiled at home? • Do you own or have access to a weapon
Obtain prior history	• Have you ever had a psychiatric disorder, suffered from depression, or made a suicide attempt? • Is there a family history of suicide?
Identify substance abuse	• Have you had a problem with alcohol or drugs?
Identify bereavement	• Have you lost anyone close to you recently?
Identify contributing factors (e.g. depression, pain, cognitive impairment)	• Do you have pain that is not being relieved? • How has the disease affected your life? • How is your memory and concentration? • Do you feel hopeless? • What do you plan for the future?

Adapted from *Quick Reference for Oncology Clinicians: The Psychiatric and Psychological Dimensions of Cancer Symptom Management* (2006).[13]

cancer patients revealed that high levels of anxiety was significantly associated with increased rates of suicide.[13]

Cognitive disorders, especially delirium, can increase risk of suicide in terminally ill cancer patients. Delirium or any cognitive impairment often impairs one's ability to reason and increases risk of impulsive behaviour.[1]

Uncontrolled pain plays an important role in vulnerability to suicide in cancer patients. Most cancer suicides were preceded by inadequately managed or poorly tolerated pain. In advanced cancer patients, the presence of pain increases the likelihood of the co-occurrence of several risk factors for suicide including depression, delirium, loss of control, hopelessness and desire for hastened death. It was also reported that persistent or uncontrolled pain fuels the majority of requests for physician-assisted suicide.[13] Aggressive pain management should be the first line of treatment in cases of cancer patients with suicidal ideation. In addition to pain, other physical symptoms such as fatigue also have a relationship with suicide, as they can induce psychological distress and escalate to suicidal thoughts or behaviours.

Frequency of suicidal ideation

It is widely believed that most terminally ill patients experience occasional thoughts of suicide as a means of escaping the threat of being overwhelmed by their illness ('If it gets too bad, I always have a way out') and will reveal this to a sensitive interviewer. In a study of 200 terminally patients in a palliative care setting, Chochinov and colleagues found that 44.5% patients reported at least a fleeting desire to die, but that these thoughts did not reflect a persistent or committed desire to die. A more explicit and sustained desire for death was reported, however, by 8.5% of patients. Of the patients reporting this persistent desire for death, 58.8% received a diagnosis of depression, whereas only 7.7% of patients who did not report a strong desire to die were clinically depressed.[13]

Assessment and management of the suicidal terminally ill patient

Assessment of suicide risk and appropriate intervention are critical. Early involvement of the psycho-oncology team with high-risk individuals can often avert suicide in the cancer setting. Patients often reconsider and reject the idea of suicide after they have an opportunity to express underlying issues to an attentive physician, particularly fears of loss of control over aspects of their death. Suicidal ideation is often driven by unbearable symptoms that may not have been recognized and should become the focus of palliative care.

A careful evaluation includes a search for the meaning of suicidal thoughts, as well as an exploration of the seriousness of the risk. The clinician's ability to establish rapport and elicit a patient's thoughts is essential as he or she assesses history, degree of intent, and quality of internal and external controls. One must listen sympathetically, not appearing critical or stating that such thoughts are inappropriate. Allowing the patient to discuss suicidal thoughts often decreases the risk of suicide. The myth that asking about suicidal thoughts 'puts the idea in their head', is one that should be dispelled, especially in cancer. Patients often reconsider and reject the idea of suicide when the physician acknowledges the legitimacy of their option and the need to retain a sense of control over aspects of their death. Practitioners should use assessment as a therapeutic opportunity to ask patients about their concerns about the future, provide accurate information in order to allay unwarranted fears, convey willingness to discuss these feelings, and allow patients to express feelings that may be difficult to discuss with others.[13] Prior to any assessment, patients should be made aware of limits of confidentiality and be advised that members of a patient's treatment team may share patient information in an effort to provide optimal care.

Specific recommendations and guidelines for managing suicide and DHD have been developed to assist practitioners with challenging discussions about this sensitive topic.[15] A therapeutic response to suicide and DHD includes empathy, active listening, management of realistic expectations, permission to discuss psychological distress, and providing a referral to other professionals when appropriate. Systematic reviews of randomized, controlled trials have shown that this approach ameliorates distress and promotes psychological well-being.

Comprehensive evaluations of the severity and intensity of suicidal ideation will then help to inform appropriate intervention and treatment planning. Initial interventions should focus on determining imminent risk and making necessary plans and arrangements for patient safety. Appropriate interventions may include psychiatric hospitalization for severely suicidal patients, the use of suicide prevention resources, contracting with the patient for safety, limiting access to potential means such as pills or guns, and involvement of family or friends in monitoring the patient.[13] However, it should be noted that psychiatric hospitalization may not be ideal or realistic for severely medically ill patients. Thus, the medical hospital or home is the setting in which management most often takes place. Crisis intervention and the mobilization of support systems may act as external controls and strongly reduce the risk of suicide.[13]

The second level of interventions should utilize specific risk factors to inform targeted intervention strategies that may reduce suicidality, such as the aggressive management of depression, pain, physical symptoms, delirium and cognitive impairment. A variety of psychotherapeutic modalities have been found to be helpful in managing and reducing suicidal ideation in cancer patients. Cognitive behavioural techniques can be tailored to manage cancer patients' physical symptoms and challenge cognitive distortions driving suicidal ideation and hopelessness.[13] Both individual and group supportive psychotherapy for cancer patients can provide additional support by assuaging feelings of isolation, bolstering coping skills, and addressing existential concerns. Conversations about advanced care directives have the potential to facilitate discussion of end-of-life issues and concerns among patients and their families. Additionally, if patients are feeling burdensome to caregivers, facilitating communication about their relationships may be helpful. Interventions focusing on enhancing patients' sense of meaning, and dignity, as well as spiritual and existential concerns are utilized as described in detail below. An intervention based in mindfulness theory, teaching patients to focus on the moment may help to alleviate distress and fears about the future.

Ultimately, palliative care clinicians are not able to prevent all suicides in terminally ill patients for whom they provide care. Intervention should emphasize an aggressive attempt to prevent suicide that is driven by the desperation of physical and psychological symptoms, such as uncontrolled pain and unrecognized or untreated delirium or depression. Prolonged suffering caused by poorly controlled symptoms can lead to such desperation, and it is the appropriate role of the psycho-oncologist to provide effective management of physical and psychological symptoms as an alternative to desire for death, suicide, or request for physician-assisted suicide.

Desire for hastened death (DHD)

Desire for hastened death may be thought of as a unifying construct underlying requests for assisted suicide or euthanasia, as well as suicidal thoughts in general. Rather than involving a wish to harm oneself, DHD represents a person's wish to die sooner than might occur by natural disease progression, often in the context of advanced or terminal illness. DHD may be characterized by: (1) a passive wish (fleeting or persistent) for death without active plans, (2) a request for assistance in hastening death, or (3) an active desire and plan to commit suicide.[13]

A systematic review of the literature surrounding suicide and DHD in cancer patients identified the following most common risk factors associated with DHD: feeling like a burden to others, loss of autonomy, a wish to control one's death, physical symptoms (e.g. severe pain), depression and hopelessness, existential concerns, and fear of the future.[15]

Several studies have demonstrated that depression plays a significant role in the terminally ill patient's desire for hastened death.[1] Breitbart and colleagues studied the relationships among depression, hopelessness and desire for death in terminally ill cancer patients. Patients with major depression were four times more likely to have a high desire for hastened death. Both depression and hopelessness acted synergistically increasing patients' desire for hastened death. Several additional studies identified hopelessness as a strong predictor of DHD in advanced cancer and physician-assisted suicide.[1] Hopelessness and depression both appear to be independent and significant predictors of DHD, and the presence of both is likely the strongest clinical marker for DHD.

Desire for hastened death also appears to be a function of psychological distress and social factors such as social support, spiritual well-being, quality of life, and perception of oneself as a burden to others. Concerns about burdening others are significantly associated with DHD in terminally ill cancer patients. A study of Oregonian patients who died by assisted suicide found that 63% of patients felt that they had become a significant burden to family, friends, or other caregivers.[16] Similar perceptions of being a burden to others were significantly associated with a wish to hastened death among cancer patients receiving hospice care.

Existential distress (e.g. loss of meaning, purpose, or dignity; awareness of incomplete life tasks; regret; and anxiety surrounding the existence of a higher power) is particularly relevant for cancer patients with advanced disease and may contribute to DHD. DHD has been found to be higher in terminally ill cancer patients reporting low spiritual well-being and, in particular, those who endorsed a loss of sense of meaning and dignity. Kissane and colleagues have described a syndrome of 'demoralization' in the terminally ill which is proposed to be distinct from depression, and consists of a triad of hopelessness, loss of meaning, and a desire for death. These data prompted clinicians to develop interventions in the terminally ill that address depression, hopelessness, loss of meaning, or what many palliative care practitioners refer to as 'spiritual suffering'.[13]

It is also important to consider the role of the practitioner in the intensity of a patient's desire for hastened death. Clinicians' perceptions of lower optimism and greater emotional suffering among patients and their willingness to assist with hastened death have been found to be associated with a stronger wish for hastened death among patients.

The response of a clinician to despair at the end of life as manifest by a patient's expression of desire for death or request for assisted suicide has important and obvious implications for all aspects of care and affects patients, family and staff. These issues must be addressed both rapidly and thoughtfully, offering the patient a non-judgmental willingness to discuss the factors contributing to the kind of suffering and despondency that leads to such a desire for death.[1]

Aggressive management of physical and psychological distress (such as depression) plays an important role in management of desire for hastened death and physician-assisted suicide among terminally ill patients as demonstrated by a recent study by Breitbart and colleagues.[17]

Several psychosocial interventions using cognitive techniques to restructure beliefs underlying hopelessness or demoralization, others focusing on enhancing patients' sense of meaning, and dignity have also been proposed, and studied in terminally ill patients with desire for hastened death as described later in this chapter.[13]

Legal and ethical issues in physician-assisted suicide

Physician-assisted suicide remains among the most controversial topics in palliative care, and thus several important legal and ethical issues should be considered. First, this area continues to change and evolve both within the field of palliative care and the judicial system. Second, there is potential for emotionally charged ethical dilemmas, as demonstrated by high-profile media coverage of assisted suicide cases (e.g. the Dr Jack Kevorkian and Terry Shiavo cases). Finally, the controversial nature of assisted suicide is likely to play a role in providers' assessment of and responses to patients' wishes to die, impacting subsequent treatment decisions.[13]

The debate around the issue of legalizing euthanasia and/or physician-assisted suicide (PAS) for terminally ill patients has encouraged research into the frequency and correlates of requests for hastened death. Studies have looked at (a) physicians who have engaged in these practices in jurisdictions where they are either legal or illegal, (b) family members of deceased individuals, and (c) the clinical records of patients who have requested euthanasia.[18] More recently there have also been studies focusing on the attitudes of patients who actually have life-threatening illnesses. In a Canadian study by Wilson and colleagues, researchers assessed cancer patients' attitudes toward the legalization of euthanasia and physician-assisted suicide. Among 379 patients receiving palliative care, the majority (62.8%) believed that euthanasia and/or PAS should be legalized, while only 26% firmly opposed legalization. Primary reasons for supporting legalization included the desire to have autonomy and control at the end of life, to avoid suffering, loss of resilience, and concerns about the futility of coping with a terminal illness, isolation and communication difficulties, as well as symptoms of depression and hopelessness. The psychological concern that occurred in over 50% of these participants was the sense of self-perceived burden to others. About 40% of respondents reported that they could envision future circumstances in which they might personally request a hastened death. Researchers concluded that even patients who were currently comfortable could have a fear of symptoms that might arise later in the progression of their illness, and for them, simply knowing that euthanasia or PAS was available could be a source of relief or control. In reality, however, most would never choose to exercise that option. In Canada, both voluntary euthanasia and PAS remain violations of the criminal code. Wilson and colleagues also found that had euthanasia or PAS been legally available, 5.8% of the participants believed that they would have taken direct action to end their lives; a much higher figure than in Oregon, where fewer than 0.1% of dying patients choose PAS, but closer to the 7.4% incidence of hastened deaths in the Netherlands among patients with advanced cancer.[18]

The legalization of assisted suicide remains under the jurisdiction of each state in the United States. As a result of the 1997 Death with Dignity Act, Oregon is the only state in the United States that has legalized physician-assisted suicide, permitting physicians to write prescriptions for lethal doses of medication for terminally ill residents who make this request. The US Supreme Court upheld legalization with the *Gonzales v. Oregon* decision in 2006 (*Gonzales v. Oregon*, 546 U.S. 243 (2006)). In spite of the heated debate, the practice of assisted suicide by providers is still relatively rare. Since assisted suicide was legalized in Oregon, 292 patients (87% of whom had cancer) have died by this method.[19] Assisted suicide and euthanasia are also legal in the Netherlands, comprising about 1–5% of all deaths and 7.4% of deaths among cancer patients, and these rates have remained stable over the past decade.[20] Those opposing legalization have expressed concerns that requests for assisted suicide are often due to the potentially treatable clinical correlates of DHD. On the other hand, it has been shown that aspects of the quality of end-of-life care, including an increase in referrals to palliative care, have improved since assisted suicide was legalized in the state of Oregon.

Regardless of position on the issue of assisted suicide, comprehensive and detailed assessment of palliative care patients is critical to determine if conditions related to DHD can be modified to enhance patients' quality of life, ameliorate unnecessary suffering, and ensure that patients are not requesting assisted suicide impulsively or without a clear understanding of possible alternative solutions.[13]

Delirium

In the palliative care literature, delirium occurring in the last days of life is often referred to as 'terminal delirium', 'terminal restlessness' or 'terminal agitation'. Despite being the most common neuropsychiatric complication of advanced illness, delirium is often underdiagnosed, and untreated in palliative care settings. Delirium is a harbinger of impending death among terminally ill patients, also a significant source of distress for patients, families and staff. Delirium presenting with hypoactive subtype, irreversible aetiologies, and greater cognitive impairment is often associated with death within a period of days to weeks.[21] Delirium can interfere dramatically with the recognition and control of other physical and psychological symptoms such as pain in later stages of illness. Palliative care clinicians should thus be familiar with the assessment and management of delirium, as well as the controversies regarding the goals of management in the terminally ill.[21]

Prevalence

Prevalence rates range from 25–85%, most studies suggesting a rate as high as 52–88% among terminally ill cancer patients.[21]

The experience of delirium for patients, families and staff

Delirium causes significant distress in patients, families and staff.[21,22] In a study of terminally ill cancer patients, Breitbart and colleagues[22] found that 54% of patients recalled their delirium experience after recovery from delirium. The most significant factor predicting distress for patients was the presence of delusions. Patients with hypoactive delirium were just as distressed as patients with hyperactive delirium. Spouse distress was predicted by the patients' performance status, and nurse distress was predicted by delirium severity and perceptual disturbances.

Assessment and reversibility of delirium in the terminally ill

Clinically, the diagnostic 'gold standard' is the clinician's assessment utilizing the DSM-IV-TR criteria for delirium. Of the several instruments available for diagnosing and monitoring severity of delirium, the Memorial Delirium Assessment Scale (MDAS) and the Confusion Assessment Method have been validated in palliative care settings.[1]

In the palliative care setting, hypoactive subtype of delirium is most common, the subtype that is characterized by psychomotor retardation, lethargy, sedation and reduced awareness of surroundings.

Delirium can have multiple potential aetiologies. In patients with advanced cancer, for instance, delirium can be due to the direct effects of cancer on the CNS, indirect CNS effects of the disease or treatments (medications, electrolyte imbalance, failure of a vital organ, infection, vascular complications), and/or pre-existing CNS disease (e.g. dementia).[21] Given the large numbers of drugs terminally ill patients require and the fragile state of their physiological functioning, even routinely ordered hypnotic agents may be enough to tip patients over into delirium.

The standard approach to managing delirium remains relevant in the terminally ill, including a search for underlying causes, correction of those factors, and management of the symptoms of delirium. The ideal and often achievable outcome is a patient who is awake, alert, calm, cognitively intact, not psychotic, and communicating coherently with family and staff. In the terminally ill patient who develops delirium in the last days of life, the management differs, presenting a number of dilemmas, and the desired clinical outcome may be significantly altered by the dying process.[21]

In confronting delirium in the terminally ill or dying patient, a differential diagnosis should be formulated as to the likely aetiology. However, there is an ongoing debate as to the appropriate extent of diagnostic evaluation that should be pursued in a dying patient with a terminal delirium.[21] Reversibility of delirium is often possible even in the patient with advanced illness, but it may not be reversible in the last 24–48 hours of life, with the outcome probably attributable to irreversible processes such as multiple organ failure occurring in the final hours of life. Most palliative care clinicians would undertake diagnostic studies only when a clinically suspected aetiology can be identified easily, with minimal use of invasive procedures, and treated effectively with simple interventions that carry minimal burden or risk of causing further distress. Diagnostic workup in pursuit of an aetiology for delirium may be limited by either practical constraints such as the setting (home, hospice) or the focus on patient comfort, so that unpleasant or painful diagnostics may be avoided. Most often, however, the aetiology of terminal delirium is multifactorial or may not be determined. A prospective study of delirium in patients on a palliative care unit found that 68% of delirious cancer patients could be improved, despite a 30-day mortality of 31%.[21] The aetiology of delirium was multifactorial in the great majority of cases in that study. Although delirium occurred in 88% of dying patients in the last week of life, delirium was reversible in approximately 50% of episodes. Causes of delirium that were most associated with reversibility included dehydration and psychoactive or opioid medications. Hypoxic and metabolic encephalopathies were less likely to be reversible in terminal delirium.[21] Even in terminal delirium a diagnostic workup should include basic assessment of potentially reversible causes of delirium while minimizing any investigation that would be burdensome for the patient. A full physical examination should be conducted to assess for evidence of sepsis, faecal impaction, dehydration, or major organ failure. Medications that could contribute to delirium should be reviewed. Oximetry can rule out hypoxia, one set of blood draws can screen for metabolic disturbances and haematological abnormalities. Imaging studies of the brain and assessment of the cerebrospinal fluid may be appropriate in some instances if they have the potential to identify lesions amenable to palliative treatment.

Interventions

Pharmacological

A detailed review of the use of psychotropic medications in the treatment of delirium in patients with advanced disease is available elsewhere.[21] While no medications have been approved by the US Food and Drug Administration (FDA) for treatment of delirium, treatment with antipsychotics or sedatives is often required to control the symptoms of delirium in palliative care settings. Low doses of neuroleptic medication are usually sufficient in treating delirium in the terminally ill, but high doses have sometimes been required. Haloperidol remains the drug of first choice and may be given orally or parenterally. A Cochrane review on drug therapy for delirium in the terminally ill concluded that haloperidol is the most suitable medication for the treatment of patients with delirium near the end of life, with chlorpromazine as an acceptable alternative.[21] Many palliative care clinicians use low dose atypical antipsychotics in the management of delirium in terminally ill patients. A Cochrane review comparing the efficacy and the adverse effects of haloperidol and atypical antipsychotics concluded that haloperidol, risperidone and olanzapine were all effective in managing delirium, and that extrapyramidal adverse effects did not differ significantly between atypical antipsychotics and haloperidol.[21] Psychostimulants have also been suggested in the treatment of hypoactive subtype of delirium, alone or in combination of antipsychotics.

Although neuroleptic drugs are generally very beneficial in reducing agitation, anxiety and confusion in delirium, this is not always possible in terminal delirium. A significant group (at least 10–20%)

of terminally ill patients experience delirium that can only be controlled by sedation to the point of a significantly decreased level of consciousness. The goal of treatment in those cases is quiet sedation only with midazolam, propofol, or other sedating agents.[21]

Non-pharmacological

In addition to seeking out and potentially correcting underlying causes for delirium, environmental and supportive interventions are important in patients with terminal delirium. In fact, in the dying patient these may be the only steps taken. The presence of family, frequent reorientation, correction of hearing and visual impairment, reversal of dehydration, and a quiet well-lit room with familiar objects all are helpful in reducing the severity and impact of delirium in seriously ill patients.

Psychotherapy interventions in palliative care

The potential benefits of psychotherapy for seriously medically ill patients are frequently underestimated by clinicians. This bias against psychotherapeutic interventions tends to be even more pronounced in patients who are terminally ill. However, psychotherapeutic interventions have been demonstrated to be useful and effective for patients struggling with advanced life-threatening medical illness.[23] In the following section we briefly describe different psychotherapeutic interventions and their relative applicability and efficacy for patients near the end of life.

Individual psychotherapies

Traditional insight-oriented psychotherapy has had limited application among dying patients. Insight-oriented psychotherapy is based on the development of a trusting relationship between the psychotherapist and the patient and an exploration of various unconscious conflicts and issues. This approach may be too demanding for most patients nearing death, but elements of psychodynamic therapy have an important role in all palliative psychotherapies.

Cognitive-behavioural and interpersonal therapies have been widely studied in the medically ill.[23] In full extended form they too may not be practical in imminently dying patients, but there are important cognitive and interpersonal elements in the psychotherapy modalities devised for patients in palliative care settings.

Existential therapies

Existential therapies explore ways in which suffering can be experienced from a more positive and meaningful perspective. *Logotherapy* is one approach with the primary tenet that one always has control over one's attitude or outlook, no matter the enormity of the adversity. The goal is to decrease patients' suffering and encourage them to live life to its fullest by engaging in activities that bring the greatest amount of meaning and purpose to their lives.[1] The focus is on goals to achieve, tasks to fulfil, and responsibilities toward others. Rather than covering up patients' distress, logotherapy acknowledges and fully explores patients' suffering. Although it was not designed for patients who were imminently dying it has been reported to help terminally ill patients have a greater sense of freedom to change their attitudes and to see themselves and their lives as meaningful and worthwhile.[1]

Another form of existential therapy useful with dying patients is the *life narrative*. This treatment explores the meaning of the physical illness in the context of the patient's life trajectory. It is designed to create a new perspective of dealing with the illness, emphasize past strengths, increase self-esteem, and support effective past coping strategies. The therapist emphatically summarizes the patient's life history and response to the illness to convey a sense that the therapist understands the patient over time. Life narrative can bolster patients' psychological and physical well-being. Life narrative has traditionally been used for treating depressed patients whose depression is a response to physical illness. However, the written form of this approach can be too demanding for patients at the end stage of their illness.[1]

A similar method of intervention is the *life review*, which provides patients with the opportunity to identify and re-examine past experiences and achievements to find meaning, resolve old conflicts and make amends, or resolve unfinished business. The process of life review can be achieved through written or taped autobiographies, by reminiscing, through storytelling about past experiences or discussion of the patient's career or life work, and by creating family trees. Life review has traditionally been used in the elderly as a means of conflict resolution and to facilitate a dignified acceptance of death (APPI). For dying patients, their stories have a special meaning. In negotiating one's way through serious illness and its treatment, the telling of one's own story takes on a renewed urgency. This approach has not, however, been widely utilized in palliative care settings.[1]

Group psychotherapy

Group interventions may offer benefits less available in individual therapies, such as a sense of universality, sharing a common experience and identity, a feeling of helping oneself by helping others, hopefulness fostered by seeing how others have coped successfully, and a sense of belonging to a larger group (self-transcendence, meaning, common purpose). However, patients in advanced stages of terminal illness are often too sick to participate in group therapy.[1]

Emerging psychotherapeutic interventions in the terminally ill

Treatment of spiritual suffering

Palliative care practitioners have recognized the importance of spiritual suffering in their patients and have begun to design interventions to address it. Rousseau[24] has developed an approach for the treatment of spiritual suffering that centres on facilitating religious expression while also controlling physical symptoms; providing a supportive presence; encouraging life review to assist in recognizing purpose, value and meaning; exploring guilt, forgiveness and reconciliation; reframing goals; and encouraging meditative practices. Although this approach blends basic principles common to many psychotherapies, it should be noted that this intervention contains a heavy emphasis on facilitating religious expression and confession and thus, although very useful to many patients, is not applicable to all and is not an intervention that all clinicians feel comfortable providing.

Meaning-centred psychotherapy

Like many clinical interventions in the field of psycho-oncology, meaning-centred psychotherapy (MCP) arose from a need to deal with a challenging clinical problem, that of despair, hopelessness and desire for hastened death in advanced cancer patients who were, in fact, not suffering from a clinical depression, but rather confronting an existential crisis of loss of meaning, value and purpose in the face of a terminal prognosis.[25] Breitbart and colleagues have applied Viktor Frankl's concepts of meaning-based psychotherapy (logotherapy) to address spiritual suffering in dying patients.[25] This 'meaning-centred group psychotherapy' is an eight-session group psychotherapy that utilizes a mixture of didactics, discussion and experiential exercises focusing on particular themes related to meaning and advanced cancer. It is designed to help patients with advanced cancer sustain or enhance a sense of meaning, peace and purpose in their lives even as they approach the end of life. A high degree of meaning corresponds with higher satisfaction with quality of life, better tolerance of severe physical symptoms, lower rates of depression, hopelessness and desire for hastened death.[25] In a recent randomized-controlled trial, comparing meaning-centred group psychotherapy (MCGP) and supportive group psychotherapy among advanced cancer patients, Breitbart and colleagues have shown that the MCGP resulted in significant improvements in spiritual well-being, sense of meaning, anxiety and desire for hastened death. A detailed review of MCGP can be found elsewhere.[25]

Demoralization

Kissane and colleagues[26] described a syndrome of 'demoralization' in the terminally ill that is distinct from depression and consists of a triad of hopelessness, loss of meaning and existential distress expressed as a desire for death. It is associated with life-threatening medical illness, disability, bodily disfigurement, fear, loss of dignity, social isolation and feelings of being a burden.[23] Because of the sense of impotence and hopelessness, those with the syndrome predictably progress to a desire to die or commit suicide. Kissane and colleagues[26] formulated a treatment approach for demoralization syndrome that emphasizes a multidisciplinary, multimodal approach consisting of (1) ensuring continuity of care and active symptom management; (2) ensuring dignity in the dying process; (3) using various types of psychotherapy to help sustain a sense of meaning, limit cognitive distortions, and maintain family relationships (i.e. meaning-based, cognitive-behavioural, interpersonal and family psychotherapy interventions); (4) using life review and narrative and attention to spiritual issues; and (5) administering pharmacotherapy for comorbid anxiety, depression and delirium.[1]

Dignity-conserving care

Ensuring dignity in the dying process is a critical goal of palliative care. Despite use of the term *dignity* in arguments for and against a patient's self-governance in matters pertaining to death, there is little empirical research on how this term has been used by patients who are nearing death. Chochinov and colleagues examined how dying patients understand and define *dignity* in order to develop a model of dignity in the terminally ill. A semi-structured interview was designed to explore how patients cope with their illness and their perceptions of dignity. Three major categories emerged, which included illness-related concerns (concerns related to the illness itself that threaten or impinge on the patient's sense of dignity), dignity-conserving repertoire (internally held qualities or personal approaches that patients use to maintain their sense of dignity), and social dignity inventory (social concerns or relationship dynamics that enhance or detract from a patient's sense of dignity). These broad categories and their carefully defined themes and subthemes form the foundation for an emerging model of dignity among the dying.[1] The concept of dignity and the notion of dignity-conserving care offer a way of understanding how patients face advancing terminal illness and present an approach that clinicians can use to explicitly target the maintenance of dignity as a therapeutic objective. Patient dignity inventory, a 25-item scale, has been designed and validated by Chochinov and colleagues[27] to provide a measure of dignity-related distress and serve as a screening tool to assess a broad range of issues that have been reported to influence sense of dignity. This inventory could assist clinicians in identifying sources of distress and in delivering dignity-conserving end-of-life care.[27] A detailed description of dignity-conserving care is beyond the scope of this chapter, and can be found elsewhere.[28]

Model of dignity for the terminally ill[28]

Accordingly, Chochinov has developed a short-term dignity-conserving care intervention for palliative care patients coined dignity therapy, which incorporates various facets from this model most likely to bolster the dying patients' will to live, lessen their desire for death or overall level of distress, and improve their quality of life. The dignity model establishes the importance of generativity as a significant dignity theme. As such, the sessions are taped, transcribed and edited, and the transcription is returned to the patient within 1–2 days. The creation of a tangible product that will live beyond the patient acknowledges the importance of generativity as a salient dignity issue. The immediacy of the returned transcript is intended to bolster the patient's sense of purpose, meaning and worth while giving them the tangible experience that their thoughts and words continue to be valued. In most instances, these transcripts will be left for family or loved ones and form part of a personal legacy that the patient will have actively participated in creating and shaping.[1]

End-of-life care among older adults

Older adults dying from cancer are at risk of suffering due to the inherent physical, psychological, social and spiritual changes that occur as we age. It is essential for psycho-oncologists to understand the impact of various changes and life transitions that occur in older age to deliver quality care at the end of life. In a comprehensive review of the literature, Thompson and Chochinov[29] examined potential sources of distress in an elder's physical, psychological, social and spiritual well-being to shed light on the unique challenges and needs facing this age group. Thompson and Chochinov concluded that drawing on the inner strengths, and resources, previous life experience, and life-acquired wisdom would help older adults feel valued, help them to cope with the inherent changes of ageing and facing life's end, promote dignity-conserving care,[29] and greatly reduce the potential for suffering at the end of life.

Cross-cultural issues in care of the dying

Ethnicity and culture strongly influence attitudes toward death and dying. Although fears of cancer and other debilitating diseases are universal, it appears that individuals from mainstream Western cultures generally use different coping strategies than those used in non-Western cultures.[1] Wide differences also exist within countries.

In a study of ethnic attitudes in the United States toward patient autonomy regarding disclosure of the diagnosis and prognosis of a terminal illness and toward end-of-life decision-making, researchers have found that different cultures have distinct opinions about how much information physicians should provide concerning diagnoses and prognoses. For instance it was shown that African Americans (88%) and European Americans (87%) are significantly more likely than Mexican Americans (65%) or Korean Americans (47%) to believe that a patient should always be informed of a diagnosis of metastatic cancer. They also found that African Americans (63%) and European Americans (69%) are more likely than Korean Americans (35%) and Mexican Americans (48%) to believe a patient should be informed of a terminal prognosis and be actively involved in decisions concerning use of life-sustaining technology.[1] Therefore it is recommended that physicians should ask their patients whether they wish to be informed of their diagnoses and prognoses and to be involved in treatment decisions or prefer to let family members or caregivers handle such matters.[1]

Important differences between cultures include those that exist in the roles of religion, family, alternative healing traditions and folk healers, attitudes toward pain and suffering, beliefs about afterlife, and customs regarding the deceased's body and burial preparations.[1] At the same time, one should beware of cultural stereotypes and not assume that every member of a particular ethnic or cultural group holds identical shared values.

Conclusion

As the possibility of cure becomes increasingly remote in the care of the person with terminal illness, the focus of treatment shifts to symptom control and enhancement of quality of life. Psycho-oncologists can play an important role in the care of terminally ill patients. The role of the psycho-oncologist in the care of terminally ill or dying persons is critical to both adequate symptom control and integration of the physical, psychological and spiritual dimensions of human experience in the last weeks of life. The psycho-oncologist working in the palliative care setting must be knowledgeable in the assessment and management of major psychiatric complications such as anxiety, depression and delirium, and also must be adept in dealing with issues of existential despair and spiritual suffering. Cultural issues, communication issues, ethical issues, and issues of bereavement are all areas requiring attention and awareness. As part of an interdisciplinary team, the psycho-oncologist plays an essential role in the provision of comprehensive palliative care including not only control of pain and other physical symptoms but also assessment and management of psychiatric and psychosocial complications.

Key points

- The role of the psycho-oncologist, in the care of the dying, extends beyond the management of psychiatric symptoms and syndromes (e.g. depression, suicide, anxiety, delirium, fatigue and pain) into family and caregiver support, bereavement, doctor–patient communication, education and training, social, psychological, ethical, legal, existential and spiritual issues that complicate the care of dying patients.

- Palliative care is not restricted to those who are dying or those who are enrolled in hospice programmes, but rather can be applied cost-effectively to the control of symptoms and provision of support to those living with life-threatening illnesses. Palliative care programmes can reduce hospital and intensive care unit expenditures by clarifying the goals of care and assisting patients and families to select treatments that are consistent with these goals. Palliative care has been successfully instituted for patients with cancer as national policy in countries that are neither wealthy nor industrialized.
- Depressed mood and sadness can be appropriate responses as the terminally ill patient faces death. On the other hand, minimization of depressive symptoms as 'normal reactions' and the difficulties of accurately diagnosing depression in the terminally ill lead to underdiagnosis of depression.
- Psycho-oncologists should be competent in the identification and assessment of patients who are at risk for suicide, as cancer patients are more likely to express suicidal ideation and commit suicide than both the general population and other medically ill populations most frequently in the advanced stages of disease.
- Regardless of position on the issue of assisted suicide, comprehensive and detailed assessment of palliative care patients is critical to determine if conditions related to DHD can be modified to enhance patients' quality of life, ameliorate unnecessary suffering, and ensure that patients are not requesting assisted suicide impulsively or without a clear understanding of possible alternative solutions.

Clinical case

Mr A is a 63-year-old lawyer from Bern, Switzerland, who was referred to the psychiatry consult team for suicidal ideation. Mr A was admitted to the hospital six weeks ago, following a seizure while on a family vacation in Boston. His brain imaging revealed a temporal lobe lesion. The biopsy was consistent with glioblastoma multiforme. After discussing his prognosis with the oncology team Mr A told his family that he would not pursue any further treatment, and that he would inquire about physician-assisted suicide 'to end my misery sooner than later'. 'After all, if I only have months to live, I see no meaning, value, or purpose in living beyond today.' Mr A became furious when he was informed that physician-assisted suicide was illegal in the state of Massachusetts. Mr A insisted that as a Swiss citizen he had the right to request physician aid in dying regardless of what part of the world he was. The oncology team requested a psychiatry consult for assessment of suicidal ideation and desire for hastened death.

During interview with the psychiatry consult team Mr A revealed to the psychiatrist that he had been experiencing severe headaches, and had been reluctant to take any pain medications due to his fear of 'feeling like zombie'. He had not been able to sleep due to pain for several weeks. Mr A also reported that he did not want to be a 'burden' to his family anymore, and that his 'hastened death' would 'end the misery' for all of them. When asked about any thoughts of taking his own life, Mr A admitted to having a stash of sleeping pills 'in case the doctors did not' carry out his wishes for an assisted suicide. Further evaluation suggested that Mr A was moderately cognitively impaired, with mild arousal disturbance, disinhibition and mood lability. He was hopeless, worthless, guilty, and demoralized, feeling his life had no meaning as he faced the inevitability of disability and death. 'I don't want to lose my dignity.'

The psychiatrist recommended aggressive symptom control including treatment of pain, mood disturbance and cognitive impairment (mild delirium). Mr A's desire for hastened death was primarily attributed to his mood disturbance, delirium, uncontrolled pain, loss of meaning and 'feeling like a burden' to others. It was also communicated to the oncology team that even in countries where assisted suicide was legally authorized the physician's primary task would be to rule out and treat underlying treatable risk factors for desire for hastened death. The psychiatrist's role was to advocate for better pain control, initiate treatment for cognitive impairment with mild delirium and mood disorder-depression. Finally, when the patient was more cognitively stable, bedside narrative meaning-making and legacy enhancing techniques, adapted from such structured psychotherapies as meaning-centred psychotherapy, and dignity conserving therapy, were utilized to help diminish the patient's desire for hastened death, demoralization, and hopelessness.

References

1. Breitbart W., Chochinov H., Alici Y. (2010) Palliative care, in *APPI Textbook of Psychosomatic Medicine*, 2nd edn (ed. J. Levenson), American Psychiatric Publishing, Arlington, VA.
2. World Health Organization (WHO) (1990) Cancer Pain Relief and Palliative Care: Report of a WHO

Expert Committee (Technical Bulletin 804), WHO, Geneva.

3. World Health Organization (WHO) (2011) Definition of palliative care. Available at: http://www.who.int/cancer/palliative/definition/en/ (accessed 4 September 2011).
4. Chochinov H.M. (2011) Death, time and the theory of relativity. *Journal of Pain Symptom Management*, 42, 460–463.
5. Wilson K.G., Chochinov H.M., Skirko M.G. *et al.* (2007) Depression and anxiety disorders in palliative cancer care. *Journal of Pain Symptom Management*, 133, 118–129.
6. Miovic M., Block S. (2007) Psychiatric disorders in advanced cancer. *Cancer*, 110, 1665–1676.
7. Levin T.T., Alici Y. (2010) Anxiety disorders, in *Psycho-Oncology*, 2nd edn (ed. J.C. Holland), Oxford University Press, New York, pp. 324–330.
8. Thompson G.N., Chochinov H.M., Wilson K.G. *et al.* (2009) Prognostic acceptance and the well-being of patients receiving palliative care for cancer. *Journal of Clinical Oncology*, 27, 5757–5762.
9. Breitbart W., Rosenfeld B., Pessin H. *et al.* (2000) Depression, hopelessness, and desire for death in terminally ill patients with cancer. *Journal of the American Medical Association*, 284, 2907–2911.
10. Gill D., Hatcher S. (2000) Antidepressants for depression in medical illness. *Cochrane Database Systematic Review*, 4, CD001312.2000.
11. Hardy S.E. (2009) Methylphenidate for the treatment of depressive symptoms, including fatigue and apathy, in medically ill older adults and terminally ill adults. *American Journal of Geriatric Pharmacotherapy*, 7, 34–59.
12. Breitbart W., Pessin H., Kolva E. (2010) Suicide and desire for hastened death in people with cancer, in *Depression and Cancer* (eds D. Kissane, M. Maj, N. Sartorius), John Wiley & Sons, Inc., Hoboken, NJ, pp. 125–150.
13. Breitbart W. (2006) *Quick Reference for Oncology Clinicians: The Psychiatric and Psychological Dimensions of Cancer Symptom Management*, IPOS Press, Charlottesville, VA.
14. Hudson P.L., Kristjanson L.J., Ashby M. *et al.* (2006) Desire for hastened death in patients with advanced disease and the evidence base of clinical guidelines: A systematic review. *Palliative Medicine*, 20, 693–701.
15. Sullivan A.D., Hedberg K., Hopkins D. (2001) Legalized physician-assisted suicide in Oregon, 1998–2000. *New England Journal of Medicine*, 344, 605–607.
16. Chochinov H.M., Tataryn D., Clinch J.J. *et al.* (1999) Will to live in the terminally ill. *Lancet*, 354, 816–819.
17. Breitbart W., Rosenfeld B., Gibson C. *et al.* (2010) Impact of treatment for depression on desire for hastened death in patients with advanced AIDS. *Psychosomatics*, 51, 98–105.
18. Wilson K.G., Chochinov H.M., McPherson C.J. *et al.* (2007) Desire for euthanasia or physician-assisted suicide in palliative cancer care. *Health Psychology*, 26, 314–323.
19. Oregon Department of Health Services (2007) *Death with Dignity Act Annual Report 2006 – Year 9 Summary.*
20. Onwuteaka-Philipsen B.D., van der Heide A., Koper D. *et al.* (2003) Euthanasia and other end-of-life decisions in the Netherlands in 1990, 1995, and 2001. *Lancet*, 362[9381], 395–399.
21. Breitbart W., Alici Y. (2008) Agitation and delirium at the end of life: "We couldn't manage him." *Journal of the American Medical Association*, 300, 2898–2910.
22. Breitbart W., Gibson C., Tremblay A. (2002) The delirium experience: Delirium recall and delirium-related distress in hospitalized patients with cancer, their spouses/caregivers, and their nurses. *Psychosomatics*, 43, 183–194.
23. Kissane D., Treece C., Breitbart W., Chochinov H.M. (2009) Dignity, meaning, and demoralization, in *Handbook of Psychiatry in Palliative Medicine*, 2nd edn (eds H.M. Chochinov, W. Breitbart), Oxford University Press, New York, pp. 324–340.
24. Rousseau P. (2000) Spirituality and the dying patient. *Journal of Clinical Oncology*, 18, 2000–2002.
25. Breitbart W., Applebaum A. (2011) Meaning-centered group psychotherapy, in *Handbook of Psychotherapy in Cancer Care* (eds M. Watson, D. Kissane), Wiley-Blackwell, Chichester, pp. 137–148.
26. Kissane D., Clarke D.M., Street A.F. (2001) Demoralization syndrome: A relevant psychiatric diagnosis for palliative care. *Journal of Palliative Care*, 17, 12–21.
27. Chochinov H.M., Hassard T., McClement S. *et al.* (2008) The patient dignity inventory: A novel way of measuring dignity-related distress in palliative care. *Journal of Pain Symptom Management*, 36, 559–571.
28. Chochinov H.M. (2002) Dignity-conserving care – a new model for palliative care: Helping the patient feel valued. *Journal of the American Medical Association*, 287, 2253–2260.
29. Thompson G.N., Chochinov H.M. (2010) Reducing the potential for suffering in older adults with advanced cancer. *Palliative and Supportive Care*, 8, 83–93.

Suggested websites (accessed January 2012)

American Academy of Hospice and Palliative Medicine (AAHPM) and the American Board of Hospice and Palliative Medicine (ABHPM) http://www.aahpm.org

Center to Advance Palliative Care (CAPC) http://www.capc.org

End-of-Life / Palliative Educational Resource Center (EPERC) http://www.eperc.mcw.edu

National Consensus Project for Quality Palliative Care (NCP) http://www.nationalconsensusproject.org

National Hospice and Palliative Care Organization http://www.nhpco.org/templates/1/homepage.cfm

CHAPTER 20

Grief and Bereavement

Sue Morris[1] *and Susan Block*[2]

[1]Dana-Farber/Brigham and Women's Cancer Center; Department of Psychosocial Oncology and Palliative Care, Dana-Farber Cancer Institute, Boston, MA, USA

[2]Department of Psychosocial Oncology and Palliative Care, Harvard Medical School Center for Palliative Care; Dana-Farber Cancer Institute and Brigham and Women's Hospital, Boston, MA, USA

Introduction

Bereavement is a complex, multidimensional process that involves the physical, psychological, spiritual, and sociological domains of the human experience.[1] Working with the bereaved can be both an extremely rewarding and challenging experience for clinicians because it forces us to confront our own mortality and the strongly held 'fix it' mentality of the medical profession. Individual differences, both within and between cultures, increase the complexity of bereavement and the need for a patient-centred approach in which support can be tailored to meet the individual needs of the bereaved. Offering bereavement follow-up to families, including at a minimum, an expression of condolence, should be incorporated by health professionals into their routine practice.

Background

The death of a significant loved one is believed to be the most powerful stressor in everyday life and has the potential to cause marked distress in all those closely connected to the deceased.[2] It is well documented that bereaved people are more at risk of serious mental health problems such as depression, sleep disturbance, increased alcohol, tranquillizer and tobacco consumption, and are at increased risk of suicide.[3,4] While it is estimated that approximately 80–90% of bereaved people cope with their losses without requiring professional intervention,[5] a significant number of individuals experience suffering from prolonged or complicated grief.

Defining normal and complicated grief responses has been the focus of recent attention. Healthy grieving has been thought to be a process involving multiple stages in which the bereaved gradually withdraws emotional energy from the deceased. Pathological grief, on the other hand, has been conceptualized as a failure to 'let go' of the deceased.[6] Recent research has shown that the hypothesized stages of grief actually are a good reflection of the theoretical models originally proposed by Freud, Bowlby, Kübler Ross and Parkes.[7,8] The focus of clinical intervention, however, has shifted to helping the bereaved adapt to their life without their loved one while at the same time maintaining a bond or connection with the deceased.[6]

When dealing with a recent death, one of the hardest things for bereaved individuals is 'not knowing' what to expect especially if the death was their first significant loss. Often, the bereaved question whether their experience is 'normal' and wonder whether they are going crazy. Psychosocial professionals, therefore, are in a unique position not only to assess bereavement risk of family members prior to the death of the patient and provide early bereavement support, but to help educate families about what they might experience

Clinical Psycho-Oncology: An International Perspective, First Edition. Edited by Luigi Grassi and Michelle Riba.

in the first few months post-loss in an attempt to increase their sense of control, understanding, and adaptation.

Major issues

Definitions of normal and abnormal grief are culturally specific and the following conceptualizations stem from research and clinical experience from Western countries.

Understanding grief

Bereavement is considered a normal human experience and studies have shown that the majority of individuals adapt to their loss over the course of time. Nonetheless, grief remains an intensely painful period for the bereaved where adjustments can take months or even years and varies considerably among individuals and across cultures.[4]

From a psychological perspective, loss, change and control are three of the major components of grief that are relevant when working with the bereaved.[9] With the death of a loved one, the bereaved individual not only loses the person themselves but also all the other things that person represented. These other losses can range from practical roles to their hopes and dreams for the future. Further, change is an inevitable result of loss; how much a person's life changes following the death of a loved one tends to reflect how much their lives overlapped, both physically and emotionally. Finally, the concept of control is significant because not only do the bereaved have little or no control over the circumstances surrounding the death of their loved one, but they may feel overwhelmed by their grief at times to the point that it seems as though their grief has total control over them. Part of supporting someone as they grieve is to help them regain a sense of control in their life and restore balance.

An individual's view of the world, including views about life and death, also greatly affects the bereavement experience.[9] Most people expect that children will outlive their parents and that adults will live well into old age. When someone dies prematurely or suddenly, many basic assumptions about the world are challenged, often resulting in a discrepancy for the bereaved between what they expected to happen in their life and what actually happened. The greater the discrepancy, the more difficult it can be to adapt to the death of a loved one. This is one reason why the death of a child is considered to be one of the most difficult losses because it challenges our beliefs about life and death and the way we think the world 'should' be.

Often bereaved individuals and society at large internalize a view that grief should be something they can 'get over quickly' and return to 'normal', in the same way that one would recover from a common cold. This view of grief is obviously incorrect: grief is not an illness with a prescribed cure. For any bereaved person, life is changed forever following the death of a loved one. The process of grieving involves adaptation and the role of the clinician therefore is to help facilitate this adjustment so that the bereaved individual can continue to live a fulfilling life, even though it may not be the life originally planned or expected.

What is normal grief?

In the days and weeks following the death of a loved one, many people describe their emotions as paralysing. Not only is grief characterized by a deep sadness but also by an intense yearning or pining to be with the loved person again. The bereaved often experience feelings of numbness, shock and disbelief regardless of whether the death was expected or sudden. They typically describe themselves as being on 'automatic pilot' where they are just 'going through the motions', taking care of funeral and financial matters as well as visiting with family and friends. Concentration difficulties and appetite and sleep disturbance are common during this initial period.

Approximately four to six weeks after the death, many bereaved people state that they feel as though they are getting worse. This feeling often coincides with the gradual withdrawal of support from family and friends as their lives return to normal routines. The additional expectation that the bereaved should be getting over the death and moving on amplifies distress. Intense feelings of sadness, yearning for the deceased, anxiety about

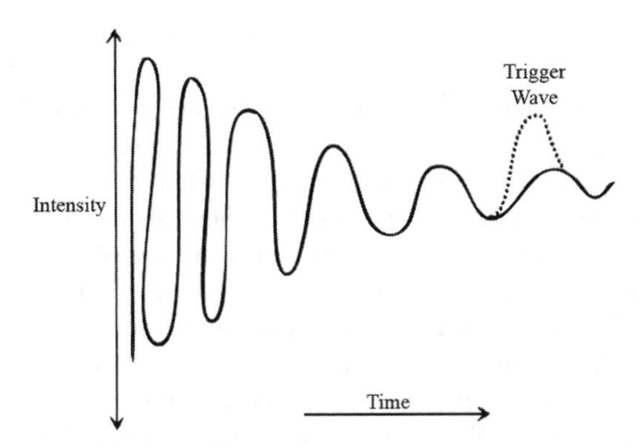

Figure 20.1 The wave-like pattern of grief.
© Sue Morris. Reprinted by permission of Constable & Robinson Ltd.

the future, disorganization and feelings of emptiness are common as the full reality of the loss is comprehended. Often the events of their loved one's last days are replayed over and over in an attempt to make sense of what has happened. For the bereaved, this can be a particularly difficult and isolating period.

The wave-like pattern of grief

Grief is often described as coming in waves which provides a useful framework to help the bereaved understand their experience, and in turn, increase their sense of control.[9]

Most people report that the intensity and frequency of the waves decrease over time even though there will be triggers for grief that result in an intensification of emotion (see Figure 20.1). Such triggers can range from hearing a favourite song on the radio to the change in seasons or the passing of a significant date such as a birthday or anniversary. Conceptualizing grief as a series of waves helps to illustrate the differences between people's grief and explain why some people seem to struggle more than others following the death of a loved one. Thinking ahead about potential triggers and making a plan to deal with them also helps the bereaved take control.

Dual Process Model

The Dual Process Model of coping with bereavement views normal grief as an oscillation between confronting the loss (loss orientation), and compartmentalizing it so the bereaved individual can deal with the changes in their life subsequent to the death (restoration orientation).[8] The authors postulate that the key theoretical mechanism in healthy grieving is the confrontation-avoidance mechanism in which a balance between the two poles needs to be achieved after a major bereavement. Examples of loss orientation stressors include yearning for the deceased and separation distress whereas examples of restoration orientation stressors include mastering new skills and reconciling one's self to a changed identity.

Resolution

Normal bereavement can manifest as intense symptoms that subside slowly but usually cause little impairment to functioning by six months post-death.[7] A study of 233 bereaved individuals living in Connecticut, found that yearning was the dominant negative grief indicator, and acceptance was the most frequently endorsed item. The sequence of stages – disbelief, yearning, anger, depression, and acceptance peaked in the hypothesized order, usually within approximately six months post-loss. The authors concluded that individuals who score high on these grief indicators beyond six months might benefit from further evaluation.

Risk factors for poor bereavement outcomes

Identifying those at risk for a poor bereavement outcome is an essential task of the psychosocial clinician. Screening significant family members and implementing psychosocial services prior to the death of the patient, is believed to mitigate a difficult bereavement that may develop into prolonged grief disorder.

A number of risk factors have been identified in the literature and include:[4,10,11]

- History of psychiatric disorders
- History of childhood separation anxiety
- Perceived lack of or poor social supports
- History of abuse or neglect in childhood
- Concurrent stresses
- Previous losses
- High initial distress
- Unexpected diagnosis and unanticipated death
- Lack of preparation for death

- Highly dependent relationship with the deceased
- Conflict with the deceased/unresolved issues
- Death of a child
- Witnessing difficult deaths.

Prolonged grief

For the minority of people who do suffer intense and debilitating grief following the death of a loved one, some presentations may meet the criteria for a distinct mental disorder. At present, complicated or prolonged grief is not recognized as a mental disorder in the DSM-IV or ICD-10 although criteria to identify bereaved persons at heightened risk have been proposed for DSM-V and ICD-11.[12] Agreement on standardized criteria for complicated grief would allow clinicians and researchers better ways to identify those at risk and develop both preventive measures and treatment programs for prolonged grief.

Prolonged grief disorder criteria

The proposed prolonged grief disorder (PGD) criteria specify that a bereaved individual must experience yearning or pining for the deceased and at least five out of nine additional cognitive, emotional or behavioural symptoms on a daily basis or to a disabling degree. These symptoms include:

- confusion about one's role in life
- difficulty accepting the loss
- avoidance of reminders of the reality of the loss
- an inability to trust others since the loss
- bitterness or anger related to the loss
- difficulty moving on
- numbness
- a feeling that life is unfulfilling or meaningless since the loss
- feeling stunned, dazed or shocked by the loss.

The diagnosis should not be made until at least six months have elapsed since the death and the symptoms must cause clinical impairment in social, occupational or other important areas of functioning.[12]

Bereavement versus depression

Only a small minority of bereaved persons develop significant depression, but when a full depressive syndrome occurs early in the grieving process, it is likely to result in prolonged and substantial morbidity.[13]

The diagnosis of major depression in a grieving person represents a clinical challenge. Helpful clinical clues to the diagnosis of major depression in this context include generalized feelings of hopelessness, helplessness, worthlessness, guilt, lack of enjoyment and pleasure, and active suicidal thoughts, as well as persistence of the initial and severe symptoms of early grief. Treatment with antidepressants and psychotherapy represents a reasonable diagnostic and therapeutic approach in equivocal cases.

Caring for the bereaved

Psychosocial clinicians can play an active role in assessing and managing the bereaved before and after the death of the patient. The following guidelines are recommended, adapting them as necessary to the cultural context of the bereaved.

Before death

1 Help family members prepare for their loved one's death. Provide clear and accurate information about the dying process to help decision-making especially in complex situations.

2 Assess the coping skills and vulnerabilities of the family members.

3 Make a referral to an appropriate community clinician prior to the death for individuals who present with risk factors for complicated grief.

The quality of the dying process also impacts the caregiver's bereavement. Preparation for death, including an opportunity to say goodbye, helps bereavement adjustment as does the opportunity for family members to participate in providing care at the end of life. Involvement of palliative care clinicians, to assure good symptom control and emotional support for patient and family is often helpful. Hospice use has been shown to reduce major depressive disorder and mortality among patients' spouses.[14,15] A recent study found that the bereaved caregivers of patients with advanced cancer who die in a hospital or ICU were at an increased risk for developing prolonged grief disorder and post-traumatic stress disorder than caregivers of patients who die at home with hospice.[11]

After death

1 Family members not present at the death of the patient should be contacted as soon as possible by the physician to inform them of the death, express condolences, answer questions, and offer them the opportunity to view the body.

2 Sending a letter of condolence is an essential component of quality end-of-life care that should be incorporated into routine practice for clinicians. Condolence letters can be sent from both individual clinicians and teams that have been involved in the care of the patient. Ideally these letters should be sent within the first few weeks following the death. Not only do these letters benefit the family but they can also help staff process their grief. Table 20.1 lists guidelines for writing condolence letters or sympathy cards.

Table 20.1 Guidelines for writing condolence letters or sympathy cards.

1	Use simple language.
2	Refer to the deceased (and bereaved) by name and title as you knew them.
3	Avoid euphemisms, for example *passed away; passed on,* unless indicated by the culture of the bereaved.
4	Articulate how you have been affected, for example *saddened to hear; sorry to learn.*
5	If you knew the deceased well, write something that reflects their personality or the history you shared. If possible add a personal memory.
6	Remember that for many bereaved, learning more about their loved one and the way they touched people's lives, helps them as they grieve.
7	If appropriate, mention what you will miss about them.
8	If possible, emphasize the good job the family member did in supporting the patient.
9	Be mindful that you do not know how the bereaved is feeling even if you have had a similar experience.
10	Do not promise anything to the bereaved that you cannot honour.
11	It is always better to send a late card or letter than not one at all. If some time has elapsed since the death of the patient, acknowledge the delay, for example *I am sorry that this card arrives late, but I wanted to get in touch to express my deepest sympathy*, or *I only recently learnt of X's death – please accept my condolences.*

3 Bereavement telephone calls also provide an opportunity for the clinician to check in with the bereaved, to say goodbye to the family and to make follow-up recommendations for support if needed, especially as the bereaved often find it difficult to initiate contact.[3]

Psychological strategies to help the bereaved

Research findings about the effectiveness of psychological interventions for normal and complicated grief are mixed with the general consensus that intervention is more effective for those with more complicated forms of grief.[16] Results vary according to the study design, including subject inclusion criteria and the type of intervention targeted. Effective treatments for complicated grief, such as complicated grief therapy (CGT), based on cognitive-behavioural models, are beginning to emerge. A randomized trial in 95 people with complicated grief found a higher response with CGT than with interpersonal psychotherapy.[17] Interventions that normalize the bereavement experience, provide an opportunity for the bereaved to tell their story, receive support and target adjustment to the loss, have been shown to be effective. Support groups are a valuable resource for many bereaved individuals and can help facilitate grief resolution.[18] Other studies have shown reductions in grief symptoms with crisis intervention and brief dynamic psychotherapy.[3]

When working with the bereaved, whether in a group or in individual therapy, the overall aims are: (1) to help the bereaved adjust to life without the deceased, and (2) to help them maintain a connection with the deceased by changing the focus of their relationship from one of physical connection to that of memory. It's essential to gain a clear understanding of their current level of functioning and the circumstances of their bereavement. If you are meeting the bereaved for the first time post-death, the following routine issues need to be addressed:

1 the bereaved's story

2 what they have lost with the death of the deceased

3 their cultural, religious and social background

4 social support

5 past psychiatric history, including current and past use of alcohol and drugs
6 concurrent stressors
7 coping skills
8 anything left unsaid or unresolved with the deceased
9 their goals for seeking support.

Strategies to help the bereaved based on self-help principles and cognitive behaviour therapy[9] can be grouped into five categories:

1 Education about the nature of grief and what to expect
2 Self-care activities
3 Opportunities to express their loss and acknowledge the death
4 Facing new or difficult situations and tackling barriers
5 Maintaining a connection with the deceased.

Education about the nature of grief and what to expect

It is important that the bereaved have accurate information about the nature of grief and the course it might take including:

- Grief is unique
- Grief follows a wave-like pattern
- There is no one way to grieve
- Grief is not an illness with a prescribed cure
- It is normal to feel sad when a significant loved one dies
- Grieving is healthy as it gives you the time to adjust to life without the deceased
- Children benefit from being included and learning that grief is a normal response to loss.

Self-care activities

Encourage the bereaved to pay attention to their physical and mental health soon after the death of a loved one including:

- Establishing a simple daily routine
- Trying to eat at regular times even if they have little appetite
- Limiting alcohol intake
- Making an appointment to see their family doctor for a check-up
- Daily physical activity or exercise
- Writing a daily 'to-do' list of what needs to be done and prioritizing
- Creating folders for any paperwork that needs to be completed.

Opportunities to express their loss and acknowledge the death

Not everyone who is grieving will have the support of loved ones who are able to listen repeatedly to the bereaved's story and bear their level of distress. The clinician often fills an important role in being able to do so or by recommending other possibilities for support which include:

- Attending a support group
- Individual therapy
- Journal-writing – including writing about the events surrounding the death
- Writing to their loved one
- Arranging a visit with the health professionals who cared for their loved one as a way to say 'goodbye' and have any questions answered
- Making a memory book that tells their loved one's story.

Facing new or difficult situations and tackling barriers

Strategies adapted from the cognitive behaviour therapy model can help bereaved individuals gradually face new and difficult situations that may be preventing them from moving forward.[9,19] These strategies can be tailored to the individual's specific circumstances and target unhelpful thoughts or behaviours, including:

- Help with making difficult decisions;
- Gradual exposure to situations that are difficult or avoided;
- Planning for the 'firsts';
- Challenging of unhelpful thoughts especially those leading to feelings of guilt and anger based on cognitive behaviour therapy.[9] For example, *What would your loved one tell you to do if they were here now? What are the alternatives to what you thought? Where is the evidence for what you thought?*;
- Encouraging the bereaved to increase their social connections.

Maintaining a connection with the deceased

Helping the bereaved develop a new relationship with the deceased while at the same time continuing to live a fulfilling life is an important goal of bereavement support or counselling. Often the bereaved fear that they will forget their loved one and question whether they will ever be happy again. Suggestions to help them maintain a connection with their loved one include answering the following questions:

- What was their loved one's story?
- How would they like to be remembered?
- Who were they to you?
- What did you learn from them?
- What history do you share?
- What would they say to you now as you go on with your life?

Other suggestions that help people remain connected to the deceased include supporting a significant cause in their memory, making a DVD of favourite photos, celebrating their birthday, planting a tree in their memory, and developing new traditions around the holidays.

When a parent of a young child dies, other adults should be encouraged to assume the responsibility of creating and maintaining a connection between the deceased parent and child. Encouraging patients who are terminally ill to record messages or video clips for children can be a wonderful gift for the child at a later date.

Pharmacological interventions

Treatment of sleep disruption

Sleep disruption is a common symptom of grief. Short-term prescription of a sleep agent may be effective in promoting sleep. For individuals who are overwhelmed by anxiety, a short-term prescription of an anxiolytic can be useful as a crisis measure. However, these medications generally should not be prescribed at high doses or for long periods.

Treatment of complicated/prolonged grief

Because complicated grief can lead to prolonged dysfunction, and its symptoms often overlap with those of major depression, patients with complicated grief should be referred to a psychiatrist for evaluation. Medications have not generally been found to be helpful in treatment of complicated grief; however, one open-label trial of paroxetine demonstrated a 53% reduction in symptoms of complicated grief.[20]

Treatment of bereavement-related depression

Bereaved patients who have symptoms of depression for at least two weeks, six to eight weeks after a major loss, should be considered candidates for a therapeutic trial of antidepressants. Open-label trials of desipramine, nortriptyline and bupropion SR have demonstrated positive outcomes; however, depressive symptoms tend to respond better than bereavement symptoms. Treatment with antidepressants is associated with improvement in symptoms of depression, but appears to be less effective in ameliorating the symptoms of grief.[21,22]

Case study

Mrs Tanner is a 53-year-old widow who contacted the bereavement program for support following the death of her husband two weeks prior. Her husband had been diagnosed with lung cancer several months ago and had died sooner than she expected. During the initial interview she described a reasonably happy marriage though stated that the last few years had been rocky. She and her husband have three children, two of whom are away at college and the third is in his final year of high school. She was tearful throughout the interview as she told of the events surrounding her husband's last days and her concerns for the future. In particular she said that she couldn't get the image out of her mind of her husband lying in the hospital bed in their bedroom on the day he died. She was concerned that he choked to death because of the noises he made before he died. She also expressed concerns about how she would continue to pay her mortgage and her children's college expenses especially as she only worked part-time. She feared that she would have to sell their home. Toward the end of the interview, she said that she felt angry toward her husband for 'leaving me in this mess' and for them not having the opportunity to get their marriage back on track.

Based on Mrs Tanner's initial presentation, what bereavement risk factors are present? What hypotheses might you entertain? What options might you consider for her care?

Table 20.2 lists Mrs Tanner's bereavement risk factors taken from her initial presentation. Evaluation

Table 20.2 Mrs Tanner's bereavement risk assessment.

Risk Factor	Yes	No	Unsure
History of psychiatric disorders			X
History of childhood separation anxiety			X
Lack of or poor social supports			X
History of abuse or neglect in childhood			X
Concurrent stresses	X		
Previous losses			X
High initial distress	X		
Unexpected diagnosis and unanticipated death	X		
Lack of preparation for death	X		
Highly dependent relationship with deceased			X
Conflict with the deceased/unresolved issues	X		
Death of a child		X	
Witnessing difficult deaths	X		

of risk factors provides the clinician with an understanding of potential difficulties, and suggests treatment approaches and follow up that is likely to be helpful. Because bereavement follow-up is often haphazard, the clinician may only have one visit with the bereaved to make suggestions about his/her care.

Tentative hypothesis

Mrs Tanner may be at risk of complicated grief given the fact that she has at least six risk factors.

Possible options for care

It is too soon to tell whether or not Mrs Tanner will develop a prolonged grief reaction but the clinician can make recommendations to help reduce its likelihood. Such recommendations include: a referral for individual counselling, a meeting with her husband's physician to gain perspective on his symptoms at the end of his life to reduce the likelihood of post-traumatic stress, and information about support groups, especially with other widows. It would also be recommended that Mrs Tanner check in with her family doctor who can monitor her progress and also refer her to a psychiatrist if she develops symptoms of depression over the next few months.

Cultural guidelines

Bereavement is an experience that is heavily influenced by culture and traditions. As clinicians, our own professional culture, as well as our personal backgrounds, play a role in determining how we understand and respond to the grief of others. Awareness of our own biases is the first step to being able to be helpful to others. Because each loss is unique, and cultural generalizations are limited, a helpful stance for the clinician in working with a bereaved individual from another culture is to assume an attitude of curiosity and openness, learning from the bereaved, as well as from other resources (academic, religious, etc.) about his/her experience and needs. Table 20.3 outlines some general guidelines for working with the bereaved from different cultures.

Table 20.3 Exploring bereavement experiences across cultural differences.

1. What is the cultural background of the bereaved individual?
2. What language is spoken/understood? (Be aware of the subtle differences in the meanings of words if translated)
3. How should the bereaved be addressed?
4. What terms are used to refer to death? Direct terms or euphemisms?
5. How is death and dying viewed in this particular culture?
6. How is grief expressed?
7. Are there specific mourning rituals? What forms do they take? For how long?
8. What is the role of the wider community in the grieving process?
9. What does the bereaved believe happens to the deceased when they die?
10. Are there differences between the way men and women grieve?
11. How are children involved in the grieving process?
12. What is the bereaved's understanding of how and why their loved one died?
13. What help or support do they want from the clinician?

In addition to understanding the person's cultural context, the clinician should also explore the specific nature of the bereaved's grieving experience. While bereavement is highly influenced by culture, there is great individual variability within cultures.

Self-care for clinicians

Grief touches all of us at some stage in our lives, which presents a unique challenge for clinicians who work in the area of death and dying. When working with the bereaved, it is essential that the clinician be aware of his/her own relationship to death, and personal values and beliefs about grieving which are influenced by one's own experiences of loss. It is also important to recognize that clinicians in this field are prone to hold a skewed view of the world given the pain and suffering encountered on a daily basis. Being able to keep this view in perspective requires that the clinician build a repertoire of self-care strategies to maintain a healthy balance between personal and professional lives, and to have settings to reflect on the challenges of caring for the bereaved.

Strategies for self-care

We recommend a number of self-care strategies to help clinicians look after themselves and their colleagues. These strategies include:

- Clearly defined (but flexible) boundaries with patients;
- Continuing education about end-of-life issues and bereavement;
- Set realistic goals and do not promise more than you can deliver;
- Debriefing opportunities at both an informal and institutional level especially for difficult deaths or when conflict exists within the team;
- Team support;
- Creative personal outlets such as exercise, hobbies and other interests;
- Memorial rituals – develop a systematic way to acknowledge deceased patients, write sympathy cards, and identify family members who may be considered at risk of prolonged grief to enable early follow-up.

Conclusion

Bereavement is a normal yet complex human response to the death of a loved one. How grief is expressed varies considerably among individuals and across cultures. While the majority of individuals adapt to their loss without professional intervention, grieving remains an intensely painful and often isolating period for many, often lasting months or even years.

Psychosocial clinicians are in a unique position to help the bereaved not only deal with the death of their loved one and the changes that the loss brings, but also to help families prepare for the death ahead of time. Identifying risk factors and providing early support can help mitigate prolonged or complicated grief.

Key points

- Bereavement is a normal response to the death of a loved one that varies considerably among individuals and across cultures. While the majority of individuals adapt to their loss without professional intervention, grieving remains an intensely painful and isolating period for many, often lasting months or even years.
- Psychosocial clinicians are in a unique position to help the bereaved prepare for the death ahead of time, identify risk factors and provide early support – all of which can help reduce the likelihood of prolonged or complicated grief.

References

1. Sanders C.M. (1999) Risk factors in bereavement outcome, in *Handbook of Bereavement: Theory, Research, and Intervention* (eds M.S. Stroebe, W. Stroebe, R.O. Hansson), Cambridge University Press, Cambridge, pp. 255–267.
2. Holmes T.H., Rahe R.H. (1967) The social readjustment rating scale. *Journal of Psychosomatic Research*, 11, 213–218.
3. Prigerson H.G., Jacobs S.C. (2001) Caring for bereaved patients – all the doctors just suddenly go. *Journal of the American Medical Association*, 286, 1369–1376.
4. Stroebe M., Schut H., Stroebe W. (2007) Health outcomes of bereavement. *Lancet*, 370, 1960–1973.

5. Prigerson H.G. (2004) Complicated grief: When the path of adjustment leads to a dead end. *Bereavement Care*, 23, 38–40.
6. Jordan J.R., Neimeyer R.A. (2007) Historical and contemporary perspectives on assessment and intervention, in *Handbook of Thanatology: The Essential Body of Knowledge for the Study of Death, Dying, and Bereavement* (ed. D. Balk), Association for Death Education and Counseling, The Thanatology Association, pp. 213–225.
7. Maciejewski P.K., Zhang B., Block S.D., Prigerson H.G. (2007) An empirical examination of the stage theory of grief. *Journal of the American Medical Association*, 297, 716–723.
8. Stroebe M., Schut H., Stroebe W. (2005) Attachment in coping with bereavement: A theoretical integration. *Review of General Psychology*, 9, 48–66.
9. Morris S.E. (2008) *Overcoming Grief: A self-help guide using cognitive behavioral techniques*, Constable & Robinson, London.
10. Zhang B., El-Jawahri A., Prigerson H.G. (2006) Update on bereavement research: Evidence-based guidelines for the diagnosis and treatment of complicated bereavement. *Journal of Palliative Medicine*, 9, 1188–1203.
11. Wright A.A., Keating N.L., Balboni T.A. *et al.* (2010) Place of death: Correlations with quality of life of patients with cancer and predictors of bereaved caregivers' mental health. *Journal of Clinical Oncology*, 28, 4457–4464.
12. Prigerson H.G., Horowitz M.J., Jacobs, S.C. *et al.* (2009) Prolonged Grief Disorder: Psychometric validation of criteria proposed for DSM-V and ICD-11. *PLoS Med*, DOI:10.1371/journal.pmed.1000121.
13. Zisook S., Shuchter S.R. (1993) Uncomplicated bereavement. *Journal of Clinical Psychiatry*, 54, 365–372.
14. Bradley E.H., Prigerson H., Carlson M.D.A. *et al.* (2004) Depression among surviving caregivers: Does length of hospice enrollment matter? *American Journal of Psychiatry*, 161, 2257–2262.
15. Christakis N.A., Iwashyna T.J. (2003) The health impact of health care on families: A matched cohort study of hospice use by decedents and mortality outcomes in surviving, widowed spouses. *Social Science & Medicine*, 57, 465–475.
16. Schut H., Stroebe M.S. (2005) Interventions to enhance adaptation to bereavement. *Journal of Palliative Medicine*, 8 (suppl 1), S140–S147.
17. Shear K., Frank E., Houck P.R., Reynolds C.F. (2005) Treatment of complicated grief: A randomized controlled trial. *Journal of the American Medical Association*, 293, 2601–2608.
18. Vachon M.L., Lyall W.A., Rogers J. *et al.* (1980) A controlled study of self-help intervention for widows. *American Journal of Psychiatry*, 137, 1380–1384.
19. Kavanagh D.J. (1990) Towards a cognitive-behavioural intervention for adult grief reactions. *British Journal of Psychiatry*, 157, 373–383.
20. Zygmont M., Prigerson H.G., Houck P.R. *et al.* (1998) A post hoc comparison of paroxetine and nortriptyline for symptoms of traumatic grief. *Journal of Clinical Psychiatry*, 59, 241–245.
21. Zisook S., Shuchter S.R., Pedrelli P. *et al.* (2001) Bupropion sustained release for bereavement: Results of an open trial. *Journal of Clinical Psychiatry*, 62, 227–230.
22. Hensley P.L. (2006) Treatment of bereavement-related depression and traumatic grief. *Journal of Affective Disorders*, 92, 117–124.

CHAPTER 21

Spiritual and Religious Coping with Cancer

David W. Kissane[1], *Carrie E. Lethborg*[2] *and Brian Kelly*[3]

[1]Department of Psychiatry and Behavioral Sciences, Memorial Sloan-Kettering Cancer Center; Department of Psychiatry, Weill Medical College of Cornell University, New York, USA
[2]Department of Oncology, St Vincent's Hospital, University of Melbourne, Victoria, Australia
[3]Department of Psychiatry, University of Newcastle, New South Wales, Australia

Introduction

The diagnosis of cancer commonly precipitates a sense of threat to life, with a variety of related existential challenges.[1] Death anxiety, coping with uncertainty, loss of meaning and purpose, loss of control, enhanced sense of aloneness and fear of what the future holds may all be problematic.[2] For some, this may be accompanied by the development of spiritual doubt, distress or angst as their background beliefs may be called into question. For others, the perceived preciousness of any remaining life may shift priorities, invite consideration of what is important and create a search for deeper meaning. Others still may start to despair, lose their sense of continued purpose and value, and become profoundly demoralized, beginning to desire hastened death.[3] A healthy adaptation to existential distress is a necessary response for all concerned.

Many definitions of spirituality have been offered, with most referring to a connection to something that is larger than the self and which generates some sense of meaning and purpose to life.[4] Unruh and colleagues[5] identified seven themes within multiple definitions of spirituality: (1) a relationship to God or a higher power, a reality greater than self; (2) something not part of the physical body; (3) a connection that transcends ordinary life; (4) not part of the material world; (5) the source of meaning; (6) the integrating life force of the person; and (7) combinations of the above. In contrast, religion is understood as a set of beliefs and practices shared by a community.[6] Many express their spirituality through religion, but in today's secular world with its social movement away from religion, the spiritual self remains important to our humanity.

A seminal revision to coping theory emerged in the last decade of the twentieth century, when Susan Folkman became curious about positive psychological states among the caregivers of men dying from AIDS.[7] In addition to the emotion-based and problem-based approaches to coping described in the original Lazarus and Folkman model,[8] meaning-based coping was recognized as a common adaptive response to adversity.[9] This renewed focus on meaning has presaged recognition of the importance of spirituality in palliative care.

In this chapter, we review the importance of belief, prayer and a spiritual life in cancer care. The role of meaning-based coping in psychotherapy complements the value of religious coping as a meaningful response to the existential challenges of life. Knowledge of the world's major religions

Clinical Psycho-Oncology: An International Perspective, First Edition. Edited by Luigi Grassi and Michelle Riba.

enriches any clinician's approach to end-of-life care through endorsement of the use of rituals that are likely to facilitate adaptive coping. Use of a routine spiritual assessment emerges as an important clinical tool, while therapeutic models that make use of meaning and spirituality become the mainstay of therapy.

Religious coping and the world's major religions

For many across the globe, the world's great religions have provided structured pathways in the existential quest to understand the meaning of life. Each set of beliefs, associated communal traditions and use of language and ritual have evolved as practices that guide people towards some state of inner peace and acceptance of the limitations of human life. The effort to transcend self and connect to something larger brings the person into a reverent stance with their perception of ultimate power.[10]

This framework of spiritual relationship to God serves as a means to ward off death anxiety and any awareness of the limits of human life through what Yalom saw as a coping strategy, operating as a 'belief in the ultimate rescuer', someone greater than self, who helps the individual overcome their finiteness and mortality.[11] This contrasts with the more omnipotent defence achieved through an overvalued idea about the inviolability of self through a sense of specialness, creative accomplishment, heroism, compulsive control or narcissism. We recognize coping mechanisms through such constructs and come to understand the practice of religion as an approach to coping with many deep existential challenges.

The religious construct of the *soul* as a non-embodied aspect of each person is derived from Greek philosophical representations of the immaterial. The Hebrew expressions for the soul (*Nefesh, Neshamah, and Ruach*) are derived from roots meaning 'breath' and 'wind' and reflect a higher order of existence, pure and untainted. Reunion of body and soul in an afterlife was taught by the Pharisees (the Sadducees rejected the notion of an afterlife) as occurring through the resurrection (*Tehiyyath Hamethem*).[12] In Orthodox Judaism, the soul is understood to be immortal and not bounded by time and space. In Catholicism, after death of the body, the soul may be purified in Purgatory before becoming worthy of union with God.[13] Within Protestant tradition, William James saw the 'sick soul' as spoilt by evil deeds, bringing the terror of judgment and punishment of the soul after death.[14] Similarly, within Eastern traditions, Hindu texts (*Upanishads*) represent the immortal soul seeking union with Brahman, while for the Muslim, the 'anguish of the grave' occurs when the soul answers five questions of faith before two angels.[15]

Death anxiety is substantially influenced by these religious beliefs, which impact upon the perceived state of holiness of the soul and dying person, their readiness for communion with God and the saints, and their capacity to gain entry into eternal life or condemnation. While not relevant to the atheist or agnostic person, religious coping can be a profound influence on the emotional well-being of those religiously adherent.

Let us review each of the world's major religions to take stock of their beliefs and consider how these might impact upon the coping of their adherents.

Hinduism

The world's most ancient religion postulates that rebirth occurs with the transmigration of the *jeevatma* or unique personality of an individual into another life, until eventually the *atma* (soul) merges with God.[16] Belief in rebirth counters the fear of death. Pursuit of the teachings of the sacred religious texts (the *shastras*) supports maturation of the soul until it becomes worthy to merge with God.[17]

Buddhism

Beginning in the sixth century BC, Buddhist tradition also believed in repeated rebirth until the calm mind of a diligent and compassionate person allows escape from the continuous cycle of rebirth to attain enlightenment (*nirvana*). Teachings and devotional practices vary between

Theravada, Mahayana and Vajrayana Buddhist traditions.[18]

Confucianism

This philosophy values a person as part of an infinite biological chain of family and society.[19] Social and family-centred rituals teach the right way to relate to others to achieve peace, harmony and happiness.[20] There is a strong tradition of filial duty, with guidance to follow the middle way, always avoiding extremes.[21]

Taoism

The circle of the *yin* and *yang* is the symbol of the supreme reality and the cosmic forces underpinning the state of continuous, natural change.[20] The passive, feminine, soft aspects of life – the yin – are complemented by the active, masculine, strong elements – the yang. Acceptance and tranquillity are achieved through adoption of a dimension of playful amusement at the ceaseless transformations of life.[21]

Judaism

A theistic tradition emerged in the West to contrast with the more animistic traditions of the East. Belief in one God, the sanctity of the human created in the image of God, the immortality of the soul and an afterlife following judgment and purification form the basic orthodox creed.[22] The laws and traditional rituals vary culturally between Central-Eastern Europe (Ashkenazi) and Spanish-African (Sephardic) lands.[23] The Talmud records the fundamental tenets, while the practice of the prescribed rituals varies between Orthodox, Conservative and Reform denominations.[24]

Christianity

Built on Judaic tradition, Jesus Christ was recognized as the Jewish Messiah, whose death achieved a redemptive function and whose resurrection provided evidence of his divinity. Basic tenets are found in the Bible. Belief in the soul, the forgiveness of sin and everlasting life with God in heaven are the essential beliefs sustained by Roman Catholic, Eastern Orthodox and Protestant Reformation traditions.[25]

Islam

Muhammad is accepted as a holy prophet following in the tradition of Moses, Abraham and Jesus, who preached God's judgment on each person based on the quality of their life, culminating in the resurrection of the dead.[26] The religious tenets are contained in the *Qur'an*. Islamic practices spread across Arab nations from Morocco and Egypt through the Middle East to Pakistan and Indonesia.

Secular Humanism

Following the scientific revolution across the past century, atheism has denied the existence of God, placing more emphasis on the moral life as a pathway that is beneficial for the community. Valuing education and respect for our species, yet rejecting the supernatural and religious dogma, humanism emerged as a code of behaviour based on virtue derived from reason.[27] Its adherents remain untroubled by the concerns generated by religion, yet existential reverie about the meaning and purpose of life ensures that spiritual issues remain on the stage of the mind.

As we look back across these philosophical and religious traditions, we can see two broad forms of coping with the existential challenges of our humanity, one taking a broadly spiritual and non-religious approach (Humanism, Confucianism or Taoism), while the other invokes religious coping based on the tenets of the specific religion (Hinduism, Buddhism, Judaism, Christianity or Islam).

Religious prayer, spirituality and meaning

Let us next review the empirical studies of spirituality and meaning-based coping and consider studies of intercessory prayer and other meditative processes.

Studies of prayer

Prayer could be considered one of the oldest supportive interventions and interest in it by cancer patients reflects its societal prevalence.[28] The role of intercessory prayer where others pray for the ill cancer sufferer has had both positive[29] and neutral effects.[30] While Whitford and colleagues suggest that medicine and prayer are not incompatible and people with faith could consider the possibility that God works through physicians, others recommend a prohibition on further trials involving intercessory prayer.[31,32]

The role of personal prayer offers clearer results with a recent meta-analysis finding that private prayer resulted in significant improvements for physical and psychological ailments.[33] Further work on moderator and mediator mechanisms is needed.[34]

Meditation studies

Meditation is another ancient form of self-care and has become increasingly popular through Mindfulness Based Stress Reduction (MBSR) programmes. While some criticism of research methodology exists, MBSR appears potentially beneficial.[35] Indeed, MBSR significantly improves quality of life, symptoms of stress, and sleep quality;[36] increases optimism and positive coping (including acceptance and positive reframing) and decreases negative coping (including denial and behavioural disengagement);[37,38] and lowers depression, anxiety, anger and confusion while increasing vigour.[39] Meditation effects may be mediated through fostering an individual's self-reliance, their inner exploration and greater understanding of life.[40]

Meaning and spirituality

While a sense of meaning and peace is associated with less depression, this is not apparent between religiosity and depression.[41,42] Similarly, meaning correlates with improved quality of life, while faith alone does not.[29,43] Meaning-finding can predict well-being,[44–46] ameliorate distress,[47,48] and assist in making sense of the illness.[49] Finding meaning can involve a period of intense growth, even self-transformation.[50,51] Patients speak of reprioritization of goals, changed lifestyles and values, increased appreciation for nature and others, and spiritual development.[52,53] Strength in the face of adversity coupled with insight into the meaning of life can moderate any sense of loss or helplessness and, in turn, promote adjustment,[54] while providing a buffer against depression and demoralization towards the end of life.[55,56]

Placebo: the power of belief

The use of a 'sugar pill' as a control arm in medication trials demonstrates what benefits the active compound causes above and beyond those obtained from the patient's belief that improvement will occur.[57] Brain imaging studies of placebo interventions have shown activation of information processing and motivational domains.[58,59] The power of the mind in anticipating and beginning to perceive benefit through the meaning that is attributed to an intervention is one component of the placebo response. A placebo pain injection has been as effective as 8 mg of morphine in relieving dental pain following extraction.[60] Up to half of the gain through antidepressants has been attributed to a placebo benefit.[61] Meta-analyses show one third of patients responding positively to placebos,[62] which could be understood as a meaning-based or spiritual response. We recognize that personally held beliefs can be enormously powerful.

Nature of the mystical experience

Tradition has long recognized religious ecstasy as a subjective experience wherein the person describes contact with a transcendent reality, such as an encounter with the divine. Without a sense of personal control, a temporary state of mind occurs which is transformational, in bringing profound change to the individual's world. They recognize the extraordinary and unbelievable nature of the experience (retain insight), display no thought disorder, handle everyday tasks and reach a positive outcome over time.[63] This contrasts with the religious content of delusions in some third of patients with schizophrenia or bipolar disorder.[64]

To exemplify the mystical, the visions of a white lady seen by 14-year-old Bernadette Soubirous in 1858 at a Grotto beside the Gave River at Lourdes, France, have been understood as a mystical vision of Mary, the mother of Jesus.[65] Culturally, these Bigourdanian people lived in the foothills of the Pyrénées, spoke an Occitan dialect and held a number of folk beliefs about traditional nature spirits, the *dames blanches* or *demoiselles*, of the woods. During carnival season, local men dressed in costume as demoiselles, and Bernadette's first vision was thought to be a *demoiselle*. Bernadette recognized the prayer beads carried by the white lady and started to pray with her own rosary. This description as a mystical experience contrasts with a psychotic process by the finite number of the apparitions, absence of disturbed affect, their cultural interpretation as religious phenomena, their non-grandiose impact on the individual's life, and the inability of local physicians to identify epilepsy or brain disease. The spiritual interpretation that followed within the Catholic Church led to acceptance of the visions as non-psychiatric and indeed, supernatural, with the recognition of Lourdes as a place of religious pilgrimage and eventual designation of sainthood upon Bernadette. Nevertheless, differentiation of the mystical from the psychotic can be challenging.

In the next section, we will examine the form that spiritual or religious issues can take amid the existential concerns arising in a person with cancer, while in the following section, we will look at the psycho-oncologist's contribution in responding therapeutically to these issues.

Clinical issues in spiritually-directed patient care

Spiritual well-being is recognized as one of the core domains of quality supportive care of the dying.[66] Spiritual perspectives are important in assuaging distress, can influence treatment choice, adaptation to the illness and how a person cares for him or herself.[67–69] Respect for each person's spirituality is a core ingredient of a helpful therapeutic alliance between patient and clinician in which discussions of diagnosis, prognosis, treatment and needs occur.[70] In addition, a significant proportion of patients seek such discussion with their doctors[71] and patients will often make reference to spiritual or religious concerns that necessitate sensitive clinical exploration. The integration of key spiritual resources into comprehensive clinical care is vital, as is the routine completion of a spiritual assessment as a component of initial history-taking.

Spiritual distress can be located within a broader typology of existential distress as displayed in Table 21.1. Insight into the potential contribution of spiritual concerns is paramount, alongside awareness of the interference that cultural beliefs, folk health practices or religious convictions can make to the completion of appropriate anticancer treatment.

Spiritual assessment by the clinician

Helpful guidelines about how to discuss religious and spiritual issues increase confidence in making this routine.[72] Moving beyond asking only about religious affiliation, a Spiritual Assessment Tool provides an effective structure to assist clinicians.[73] This includes:

1 Enquiring about faith or beliefs (e.g. 'Do you consider yourself spiritual or religious?' 'What is your faith or belief system?');
2 Understanding the strength of these beliefs;
3 Clarifying the nature of any related community and perception of its support; and
4 Appreciating how the patient may wish these issues to be addressed in his/her care?

Complementing each clinician's assessment of spiritual issues, chaplains and spiritual advisors are important members of the overall team to respond to any spiritual concerns. Where services are denominationally based, a person with a secular spirituality may not seek a chaplain's assistance, yet benefit from discussion of existential concerns through other means. Considerable overlap may occur between matters dealt with by chaplains and the core concerns in psychological aspects of care. For example, themes of purpose, meaning and hope, connection with others, and continuity of self may also be addressed in specific psychotherapeutic interventions such as supportive-expressive therapy[74] and dignity therapy[75] among others outlined in the next section.

Spiritual interventions and psycho-oncology treatments can be successfully integrated, rather than viewed as mutually exclusive or contradictory. When distress is more severe, spiritual

Table 21.1 Typology of existential distress, with adaptive and maladaptive pathways.

Nature of existential challenge	Features of successful adaptation	Form of existential distress when problematic	Symptoms experienced	Resulting psychiatric disorders	Suitable therapy approaches
1. Death	Courageous awareness and acceptance of dying; saying goodbye	Death anxiety	Fear of the process of dying or the state of being dead; panic at somatic symptoms; distress at uncertainty	Anxiety disorders, panic disorder, agoraphobia, generalized anxiety disorder, acute stress disorder, adjustment disorder with anxious mood	Psycho-educational, Cognitive-Behavioural Therapy, Existential Psychotherapy, Psychodynamic Therapy
2. Loss	Sadness at reality, yet resigned or accepting	Complicated grief	Intense tearfulness, grief and waves of emotionality, progressing into symptoms of depression	Depressive disorders	Supportive psychotherapy, Grief therapy, Interpersonal psychotherapy
3. Alone-ness	Accompanied and supported by family and friends	Profound loneliness	Isolated, alienated and sense of complete aloneness in life	Dysfunctional family, absence of social support, relationship problems	Interpersonal psychotherapy, Family focused grief therapy, Supportive group therapy, Linking with visiting and community services
4. Freedom	Acceptance of frailty and reduced independence	Loss of control	Angst at loss of control, obsessional behaviours, indecisive, non-adherence to treatments, fear of dependency	Phobic disorders, obsessive-compulsive disorders, substance abuse disorders	Supportive psychotherapy, Interpersonal psychotherapy, Psychodynamic therapy
5. Meaning	Sense of fulfilment	Demoralization	Pointlessness, meaninglessness, futility, loss of role, desire to die	Demoralization syndrome, depressive disorders	Interpersonal psychotherapy, Narrative and dignity conserving therapies, Meaning-centred therapies, Existential psychotherapy
6. Dignity	Sense of worth despite disfigurement or handicap	Worthlessness	Shame, horror, body image concerns, fear of being a burden	Adjustment disorders	Narrative and dignity conserving therapies, Supportive psychotherapy, Grief therapy
7. Mystery	Reverence for what is unknowable, yet sacred	Spiritual doubt and despair	Guilt, loss of faith, loss of connection with the transcendent	Adjustment, anxiety and depressive disorders	Meaning-centred therapy, Life narrative therapies, Religious rituals

Adapted with permission from Kissane DW, Poppito S. (2006) Death and Dying. In: Blumenfeld M & Strain JJ (eds.) Psychosomatic Medicine. Lippincott Williams & Wilkins, Philadelphia, PA, pp. 671–694.

interventions alone should not be seen as a replacement for necessary psychiatric care such as pharmacological treatment of severe depression. Conversely, undertaking psychiatric assessment, diagnosis and treatment does not negate the importance of spiritual concerns and the benefit of spiritual advice. Considerable multidisciplinary collaboration is needed between psychiatrists, psychologists, social workers and cancer clinicians with chaplains and pastoral care practitioners. The psycho-oncologist will commonly be the source of a referral to a chaplaincy service through recognition of spiritually or religiously directed issues amid any existential concerns.

Spiritual distress in the face of death

Fears of death may occur at many points throughout the course of cancer. In the face of advancing disease, such fears and related spiritual and existential distress may become more prominent.

Case example

An 80-year-old woman, staunchly independent despite severe visual impairment, was admitted to hospital with advanced sarcoma after a fall at home, where she had lived alone. She had become withdrawn and angry, refused food and drink, and expressed the conviction that she had been 'abandoned by God'. Her religion had been a source of comfort in coping with her visual impairment until her husband's recent death took away her key care provider. Her grief was prominent in therapy and depressive symptoms intensified, leading to antidepressants. She formed a strong rapport with the hospital chaplain, who helped her re-establish some consolation from her faith. Gradually, her depressive symptoms improved, she became more engaged with her family, and came to accept the decision to move her to inpatient hospice.

The intersection of depression and spirituality is common.[76] Moreover, the stigma of cancer remains prominent, despite progress in understanding its cause, thus adding to the distress.[77] As individuals search for explanations for the onset or progression of cancer, spiritual or religious-based attributions may become interwoven with the sense of shame and stigma that occurs.

Case example

A 65-year-old woman with cervical cancer suffered severe anxiety and unrelieved abdominal pain. Throughout treatment, she described her fear that the cancer was 'God's punishment' for a brief sexual relationship that followed the death of her husband years earlier. She believed her abdominal pain was a reminder of God's wrath. While she rejected the offer of spiritual assistance, discussion of her attributions reduced agitation, she reported 'relief' at unburdening herself, and the ensuing conversation improved understanding of the medical factors influencing her illness.

Demoralization can also arise from spiritual distress when the latter is associated with loss of faith, and the resultant loss of meaning and purpose engenders a sense of futility about continued life.[3] The following example illustrates this:

Case example

A 70-year-old pastor with an advanced cancer expressed distress at the waste that his life had been as a priest. He now doubted that God existed, as a result of which, he considered his years of community service pointless. He saw no meaning to continued life and hoped he would soon die from his cancer. Alongside psychotropic treatment of his depression, a chaplain reviewed with him the nature of spiritual doubt, set reading exercises about saints who had also struggled this way, and prayed regularly with him. Gradually his faith was restored and the meaning of his life was re-established.

Spirituality interfering with appropriate anticancer care

Spiritual beliefs may have a direct bearing on medical decisions through specific religious dictates (e.g. beliefs about blood transfusion for a Jehovah's Witness). Spirituality can also encompass views about health and healing. Pursuit of activities or interventions linked with eastern or indigenous spiritual practices (e.g. meditative practices, herbal or 'natural' remedies) occur alongside conventional treatment. For some, this may accompany a vigorous rejection of standard anticancer treatments. Often these alternative approaches represent a source of hope and control in the face of fear and helplessness invoked by cancer, while for a smaller number they are rooted in deeply held religious and cultural beliefs, practices and explanatory models for illness. A non-judgmental approach is key, exploring respectfully the significance and expectations of such treatments and how these can be combined with the potential benefits of conventional treatments. When resolute denial of illness and rejection of necessary treatment are spiritually or religiously based, this can be extraordinarily challenging for clinicians. This calls for effective teamwork with close involvement of spiritual advisors. Careful attention is needed to family factors that either promote such actions through shared religious convictions or, where family hold views to the contrary, as support in assisting a more adaptive response. This calls for careful negotiation, compromise and collaboration with the patient.

Case example

A 28-year-old, separated Catholic mother of two small children was admitted to hospital with advanced bowel cancer. The nursing staff was increasingly concerned about her and the attendant family. 'They are all in denial!' Her mother had refused discussion of prognosis. The patient was heard to say, 'I am going to survive to see my two wonderful girls grow up – I won't leave them.' Religious icons (e.g. images of saints) had been placed around her room, while they all expressed 'hope for a miracle'. She was initially reluctant to consider anticancer therapy because this would be 'giving up', preferring to 'pray all night' with accompanying anxiety and desperation. She was visited by a priest, who was brought into discussion with the clinical team regarding the significance of her faith. This enabled an approach that respected her hope for 'miracle', but empowered exploration of her fears of chemotherapy toxicity, her distress for her daughters and affirmation of her faith as a source of comfort. Extending these spiritual discussions to her mother was critical to achieving more open discussion.

Need for spiritual resources to assist in cancer care

Religious communities are an important source of social connection, acceptance, and both practical and emotional support. The capacity to maintain religious practices despite illness is fundamental to sustaining these connections, overcoming isolation and promoting a sense of continuity of self despite illness (important to maintaining dignity and morale).[78]

Themes emerging through the process of life review, which can be expressed in spiritual or religious terms, can become a focus for spiritual assistance. Such themes may include forgiveness (of others or self), guilt, responsibility and reconciliation at the impending close of life, which may otherwise contribute to distress if left unaddressed.

Case example

A 63-year-old widow, who had undergone extensive pelvic surgery for advanced bladder cancer, was left depressed, 'not coping with the news' and feeling 'everything was pointless now'. She had had a long period of separation from her strongly religious family (prior to the death of her parents), 'taking a different path' that meant less religious activity. She was subsequently visited by a hospital chaplain, who helped reconcile her with her faith as they talked through her perceived failings and family conflicts. This reconnected her with the family, including a sense of spiritual linkage to her deceased parents. She was surprised at its beneficial emotional impact, obtained a sense of acceptance in 'belonging' within the culture of her faith, and felt supported by others as she faced her own death.

Therapeutic approaches to spiritually directed care

Meaning-centred therapies

These aim to explore and enhance the meaning and purpose in patients' lives and increase their sense of acceptance of the cancer. The focus of these therapies is not on suffering but on the other aspects of their lives that bring meaning – not to ignore their suffering, but to offer a balance to it. The positive outcome of this focus is an increased sense of authenticity, significance, comprehensibility and a consensus between what is meaningful and what is lived.[79]

Greenstein and Breitbart[80] developed a meaning-centred group therapy for patients with advanced cancer, based on principles of logotherapy.[81] With the aim of helping patients increase meaning, peace and purpose, even as they approach life's end, this therapy uses a mix of education, discussion and experiential exercises. A randomized, controlled trial showed significant improvement in spiritual well-being and sense of meaning.[82]

More recently, Meaning and Purpose (MaP) therapy has been developed, again in advanced cancer.[83] This brief (four-session) individual therapy involves therapists making links between meaning (significance) and purpose (intention) with the aim of increasing awareness and encouraging action or direction for future goals.

While meaning-centred therapies begin with a narrative approach,[84,85] they are not only focused on discussing the life story, but in using its meaning to encourage a change in attitude to a person's difficulties, adopt a new perspective on identity, and positively reinterpret the significance of their contribution to life.[86]

Spiritually integrated care

Dignity therapy is an innovative, individualized approach to promoting meaning, purpose and sense of worth among patients at the end of life, through assisting the patient in the creation of a 'generativity document' to be bequeathed to family or others. This approach emphasizes 'personhood' of the patient through life review undertaken with a therapist, and has demonstrated significant benefits in reducing levels of suffering and existential concerns.[87]

Religiously specific approaches/rituals

Religious approaches and rituals assist many people spiritually, based on their specific worldviews. Thus, a Chinese patient may view illness as being caused by an imbalance of yin and yang.[88] To cure the block in their meridians, he/she may prefer Chinese medicine or acupuncture rather than analgesics for pain.[89] They may also view their cancer as resulting from disharmony between them and their environment (time, place, or others).[90,91] They may use various rituals to enhance harmony (e.g. move some furnishings or ask clinicians to perform procedures at a specific time), and they might refuse visitors who do not enhance this harmony.

Native Americans traditionally believe that illness stems from spiritual problems and that cancer is more likely to invade their bodies if they are imbalanced, have negative thinking, or live an unhealthy lifestyle.[92] With this worldview, healing practices are aimed at finding and restoring balance and wholeness to a pure state, believing that the spirit is an inseparable element of healing. Some of the most common aspects of Native American healing include the use of herbal remedies, purifying rituals, shamanism, and symbolic healing rituals to treat illnesses of both the body and spirit.

Prayer is considered to be the most prevalent spiritual therapy used by Western populations.[93] The vast majority (90%) of Americans state that they believe in prayer[94] and 82% say they have prayed for personal health.[95,96] People with cancer have been found to pray more as a response to living with their disease.[97–99]

While we are compelled to consider these beliefs and rituals, so central to specific patient's coping, this does not mean that the clinician is required to use such practices in patient care. Rather, the clinician needs to incorporate questions about religiously specific approaches/rituals in any comprehensive assessment and, where appropriate, affirm the value of these practices.

Integrative Medicine

Given the popularity of complementary therapies, many cancer centres combine Integrative Medicine with traditional medicine. Notable examples include the Memorial Sloan-Kettering Cancer Center (MSKCC) in New York and the Osher Center at the University of California San Francisco (UCSF). The MSKCC Integrative Medicine Service opened in 1999, offering complementary therapies as adjuncts rather than alternatives to traditional treatments. The aims are to help alleviate stress and anxiety, reduce pain, and promote well-being. Services offered include touch therapies such as massage, mind-body therapies such as meditation and self-hypnosis, nutrition consultations, yoga and fitness training, music therapies and acupuncture.

Twelve-step recovery programme

The importance of spiritual aspects of recovery has been embodied in programmes such as the 12-Step Facilitation upon which Alcoholics

Anonymous and other successful substance use recovery programmes have been based, providing an example of 'spiritual recovery' interventions.[100] These encompass the gaining of strength from a transcendent God to combat substance dependence and have developed to be inclusive of more diverse meanings of spirituality, including some models based on indigenous spirituality.[101] While there are potentially deleterious social and personal impacts from more intensely zealous or exclusive spiritual recovery movements, the provision of meaning, renewed sense of purpose, overcoming the erosion of social networks and the establishment of a strong affiliation to a normative culture, with its expectations regarding abstinence, are core elements of the model.

Spiritual approach to the atheist

While patients with a humanist, agnostic or atheistic orientation will not ordinarily seek a spiritual approach, narrative and meaning-centred therapies have much to offer in helping them resolve existential concerns. In the setting of advanced cancer, they may perceive little point to continued life, and not want to go on. Yet the clinician can still ask: Does their life lack meaning? Can they leave a legacy to their families?

Narrative therapies seek to understand the patient's coherent life story, taking stock of accomplishments, recognizing taken-for-granted sources of fulfilment as seen in relational roles, and discerning what is central and most authentic in the life that has been lived.[84] The therapist is both editor and at times scribe in re-organizing this story into a meaningful narrative.[102]

Challenges in delivering spiritually informed clinical care

There are potential pitfalls in clinical approaches to spiritual concerns that will be briefly outlined.

Professional boundaries and the spiritual assessment

Proselytizing is inappropriate; imposing personal beliefs and religious values on a patient breaches ethical standards. Providing premature reassurance such as 'Trust in God and have faith' can leave the person with unexpressed needs, feeling misunderstood and unsupported, and without help to find their own solutions.[72] Clinicians may be asked to declare their own religious affiliation by patients or families requiring a thoughtful approach to managing professional boundaries. While physicians should not feel compelled to reveal their own beliefs, a sensitive strategy is to understand the purpose behind such a query – why is it important to the patient? Responding in a non-defensive manner such as 'I'm interested in why you might ask that. I wonder if you are concerned that I might not understand how important these beliefs are to you?' is one example of a helpful response. Declaring the purpose and rationale for religiously and spiritually oriented questions can deflect awkwardness in taking a spiritual history.

Role confusion

The psycho-oncologist may be well trained in existential philosophy, but not a student of theology; the chaplain may have a refined knowledge of sacred texts, yet not be trained to recognize a clinical depression. Sociologists have described psychiatrists as modern-day priests, hinting at the potential for role confusion in spiritual care provision. Clergy often feel caught with an ethic of confidentiality, where guilt that has been shared in the confessional may also be a dimension of depression. Multidisciplinary Psychosocial Care Teams (PCT) are one means to ensure collaboration between these disciplines, creating a forum to foster mutual understanding of respective roles and ensure that patient care is advantaged through sufficient exchange of clinically relevant concerns.

Intersection of culture and religion

Clinicians need to remain open to each patient's personal experience and the significance of their beliefs, even when the clinician is familiar with that belief system, thus avoiding cultural or religious biases or expectations. Another trap for the unwary lies at the intersection of culture and religion:

the Irish Catholic may well today be agnostic; the Jew a humanist; the Turk could be Muslim or Christian. Thoughtful spiritual assessment will include building a comprehensive understanding of the cultural sources of spirituality alongside any ethnic influences on religious practices. Only by asking can stereotypic assumptions be avoided. Thoughtful clinicians will ask their professional interpreters about any personal experience of religious upbringing and philosophy so as to understand potential influences on their translation.[103]

Key points

- Modern cancer care recognizes the ever-present existential themes that patients confront and seek answers to.
- Person-centred care seeks to respond to these concerns with sensitivity and skill, using a biopsychosocial and spiritual framework to respond to all potential sources of distress.
- Applied psychotherapy makes eclectic use of narrative, meaning-centred, existentially oriented and spiritually informed models to guide its approaches.
- Attention to both spiritual and religious coping is vital to support adaptive processes of adjustment and help achieve optimal quality of life for all concerned.

Suggested further reading

Folkman S. (ed.) (2010) *The Oxford Handbook of Stress, Health and Coping*, Oxford University Press, New York.

Unprecedented coverage of key research issues related to stress and coping: How to mitigate harm and sustain well-being in the face of stress.

Peteet J.R., Lu F.G., Narrow W.E. (eds) (2011) *Religious and Spiritual Issues in Psychiatric Diagnosis. A Research Agenda for DSM-V*, American Psychiatric Association, Arlington, VA.

Experts discuss the impact of religion and spirituality on mental health through consideration of each major category of psychiatric disorder. Two expert commentaries are offered about the philosophical issues represented in each chapter.

Watson M., Kissane D.W. (eds) (2011) *Handbook of Psychotherapy in Cancer Care*, Wiley-Blackwell, Chichester, UK.

Leading psycho-oncology researchers offer expert guidance to applied therapy approaches in cancer care.

References

1. Kissane D.W. (2000) Psychospiritual and existential distress. *Australian Family Physician*, 29, 1022–1025.
2. Kissane D.W., Poppito S. (2006) Death and dying, in *Psychosomatic Medicine* (eds M. Blumenfeld, J.J. Strain), Lippincott Williams & Wilkins, Philadelphia, PA, pp. 671–694.
3. Kissane D.W., Clarke D.M., Street A.F. (2001) Demoralization syndrome – a relevant psychiatric diagnosis for palliative care. *Journal of Palliative Care*, 17, 12–21.
4. Sinclair S., Pereira J., Raffin S. (2006) A thematic review of the spirituality literature within palliative care. *Journal of Palliative Medicine*, 9, 464–478.
5. Unruh A.M., Versnel J., Kerr N. (2002) Spirituality unplugged: A review of commonalities and contentions, and a resolution. *Canadian Journal of Occupational Therapy*, 69, 15–19.
6. Marler P.L., Hadaway C.K. (2002) " Being religious" or "being spiritual" in America: A zero-summed proposition? *Journal for the Scientific Study of Religion*, 41, 289–300.
7. Folkman S. (1997) Positive psychological states and coping with severe stress. *Social Science and Medicine*, 45, 1207–1221.
8. Lazarus R.S., Folkman S. (1984) *Stress, Appraisal and Coping*, Springer, New York.
9. Folkman S. (2001) Revised Coping Theory and the process of bereavement, in *Handbook of Bereavement Research. Consequences, Coping and Care* (eds M.S. Stroebe, R.O. Hansson, W. Stroebe, H. Schut), American Psychological Association, Washington DC, pp. 563–584.
10. Woodruff P. (2001) *Reverence. Renewing a Forgotten Virtue*, Oxford University Press, Oxford.
11. Yalom I.D. (1980) *Existential Psychotherapy*, Basic Books, New York.
12. Grollman E.A. (1993) Death in Jewish thought, in *Death and Spirituality* (ed. K.J. Doka), Baywood, Amityville, NY, pp. 21–32.

13. Miller E.J. (1993) A Roman Catholic view of death, in *Death and Spirituality* (eds K.J. Doka, J.D. Morgan), Baywood, Amityville, NY, pp. 33–49.
14. Klass D. (1993) Spirituality, Protestantism and death, in *Death and Spirituality* (eds K.J. Doka, J.D. Morgan), Baywood, Amityville, NY, pp. 51–73.
15. Jonker G. (1997) The many facets of Islam. Death, dying and disposal between orthodox rule and historical convention, in *Death and Bereavement Across Cultures* (eds C. Parkes, P. Laungani, B. Young), Routledge, London, pp. 147–65.
16. Sharma D. (1990) Hindu attitude toward suffering, dying and death. *Palliative Medicine*, 4, 235–238.
17. Laungani P. (1997) Death in a Hindu family, in *Death and Bereavement Across Cultures* (eds C. Parkes, P. Laungani, B. Young), Routledge, London, pp. 52–72.
18. Truitner K., Truitner N. (1993) Death and dying in Buddhism, in *Ethnic Variations in Dying, Death, and Grief: Diversity in Universality* (eds D. Irish, K. Lundquist, V. Nelsen), Taylor & Francis, Washington, DC, pp. 125–136.
19. Ryan D. (1993) Death: Eastern perspectives, in *Death and Spirituality* (eds K.J. Doka, J.D. Morgan), Baywood, Amityville, pp. 76–92.
20. Joachim C. (1986) *Chinese Religions*, Prentice Hall, Englewood Cliffs, NJ.
21. Overmyer D. (1987) *Religions of China*, Harper & Row, New York.
22. Lamm M. (1969) *The Jewish Way in Death and Mourning*, Jonathon David Publishers, Inc., New York.
23. Brener A. (1993) *Mourning and Mitzvah: A Guided Journal for Walking the Mourner's Path Through Grief to Healing*, Jewish Lights Publishing, Woodstock, VT.
24. Levine E. (1997) Jewish views and customs on death, in *Death and Bereavement Across Cultures* (eds C. Parkes, P. Laungani, B. Young), Routledge, London, pp. 98–130.
25. Ter Blanche H., Parkes C. (1997) Christianity, in *Death and Bereavement Across Cultures* (eds C. Parkes, P. Laungani, B. Young), Routledge, London, pp. 131–146.
26. Jonker G. (1997) The many facets of Islam. Death, dying and disposal between orthodox rule and historical convention, in *Death and Bereavement Across Cultures* (eds C. Parkes, P. Laungani, B. Young), Routledge, London, pp. 147–165.
27. Lanham R.A. (1983) *Literacy and the Survival of Humanism*, Yale University Press, New Haven.
28. Ross L.E., Hall I.J., Fairley T.L. *et al.* (2008) Prayer and self-reported health among cancer survivors in the United States, National Health Interview Survey, 2002. *The Journal of Alternative and Complementary Medicine*, 14, 931–938.
29. Whitford H.S., Olver I.N., Peterson M.J. (2008) Spirituality as a core domain in the assessment of quality of life in oncology. *Psycho-Oncology*, 17, 1121–1128.
30. Roberts L., Ahmed I., Hall S. *et al.* (2009) Intercessory prayer for the alleviation of ill health. *Cochrane Database of Systematic Reviews*, 15, CD000368.
31. Masters K.S., Spielmans G.I., Goodson J.T. (2006) Are there demonstrable effects of distant intercessory prayer? *Annals of Behavioral Medicine*, 32, 21–26.
32. Hodge D.R. (2007) A systematic review of the empirical literature on intercessory prayer. *Research on Social Work Practice*, 17, 174–187.
33. Thompson D.P. (2008) In *Dissertation Abstracts International: Section B: The Sciences and Engineering*, Vol. 68, ProQuest Information & Learning, USA.
34. Breslin M.J., Lewis C.A. (2008) Theoretical models of the nature of prayer and health: A review. *Mental Health, Religion & Culture*, 11, 9–21.
35. Matchim Y., Armer J.M. (2007) Measuring the psychological impact of mindfulness mediation on health among patients with cancer: A literature review. *Oncology Nursing Forum*, 34, 1059–1066.
36. Carlson L.E., Speca M., Patel K.D. *et al.* (2003) Mindfulness-based stress reduction in relation to quality of life, mood, symptoms of stress, and immune parameters in breast and prostate cancer outpatients. *Psychosomatic Medicine*, 65, 571–581.
37. Vroom P.S. (2002) Meditation as a moderator of the effect of optimism on positive coping for cancer patients, in *Dissertation Abstracts International: Section B: The Sciences and Engineering*, Vol. 63, ProQuest Information & Learning, USA, p. 129.
38. Ando M., Morita T., Akechi T. *et al.* (2009) The efficacy of mindfulness-based meditation therapy on anxiety, depression, and spirituality in Japanese patients with cancer. *Journal of Palliative Medicine*, 12, 1091–1094.
39. Speca M., Carlson L.E., Goodey E. *et al.* (2000) A randomized, wait-list controlled clinical trial: The effect of a Mindfulness Meditation-Based Stress Reduction Program on mood and symptoms of stress in cancer outpatients. *Psychosomatic Medicine*, 62, 613–622.
40. Young R.P. (1998) The experiences of cancer patients practicing mindfulness meditation, in

Dissertation Abstracts International: Section B: The Sciences and Engineering, Vol. 60, Saybrook Graduate School and Research Center, California, ProQuest Dissertations and Theses, p. 246.
41. Nelson C., Jacobson C.M., Weinberger M.I. *et al.* (2009) The role of spirituality in the relationship between religiosity and depression in prostate cancer patients. *Annals of Behavioral Medicine*, 38, 105–114.
42. Yanez B., Edmondson D., Stanton A.L. *et al.* (2009) Facets of spirituality as predictors of adjustment to cancer: Relative contributions of having faith and finding meaning. *Journal of Consulting and Clinical Psychology*, 77, 730–741.
43. Zavala M.W., Maliski S.L., Kwan L. *et al.* (2009) Spirituality and quality of life in low-income men with metastatic prostate cancer. *Psycho-Oncology*, 18, 753–761.
44. Vickberg S., DuHamel K., Smith M. *et al.* (2001) Global meaning and psychological adjustment among survivors of bone marrow transplant. *Psycho-Oncology*, 10, 29–39.
45. Bauer-Wu S., Farran C.J. (2005) Meaning in life and psycho-spiritual functioning: A comparison of breast cancer survivors and health women. *Journal of Holistic Nursing*, 23, 172–190.
46. Gall T., Guirguis-Younger M., Charbonneau C. *et al.* (2009) The trajectory of religious coping across time in response to the diagnosis of breast cancer. *Psycho-Oncology*, 18, 1165–1178.
47. Meraviglia M.G. (2001) The mediating effects of meaning in life and prayer on the physical and psychological responses of people experiencing lung cancer, in *Dissertation Abstracts International: Section B: The Sciences and Engineering*, Vol. 62, The University of Texas at Austin, Texas, ProQuest Dissertations and Theses, p. 208.
48. Lethborg C., Aranda S., Kissane D. (2007) To what extent does meaning mediate adaptation to cancer? The relationship between physical suffering, meaning in life, and connection to others in adjustment to cancer. *Palliative and Supportive Care*, 5, 377–388.
49. Richer M.C., Ezer H. (2002) Living in it and moving on: Dimensions of meaning during chemotherapy. *Oncology Nursing Forum*, 29, 113–119.
50. Tedeshi R.G., Calhoun L.G. (2004) Posttraumatic growth: Conceptual foundation and empirical evidence. *Psychological Inquiry*, 15, 1–18.
51. Neimeyer R.A. (2001) *Meaning Reconstruction and the Experience of Loss*, American Psychological Association, Washington DC.
52. Lutha S.S., Cicchetti D. (2000) The construct of resilience: Implications for interventions and social policies. *Development and Psychopathology*, 12, 857–885.
53. Park C.L., Folkman S. (1997) Meaning in the context of stress and coping. *Review of General Psychology*, 1, 115–144.
54. Moadel A., Morgan C., Fatone A. *et al.* (1999) Seeking meaning and hope: Self-reported spiritual and existential needs among an ethnically diverse cancer patient population. *Psycho-Oncology*, 8, 378–385.
55. Breitbart W., Rosenfeld B., Pessin H. *et al.* (2000) Depression, hopelessness, and desire for hastened death in terminally ill patients with cancer. *Journal of the American Medical Association*, 284, 2907–2911.
56. Nelson C., Rosenfeld B., Breitbart W. *et al.* (2002) Spirituality, religion, and depression in the terminally ill. *Psychosomatics*, 43, 213–220.
57. Moerman D.E., Jonas W.B. (2002) Deconstructing the placebo effect and finding the meaning response. *Annals of Internal Medicine*, 136, 471–476.
58. Oken B.S. (2008) Placebo effects: Clinical aspects and neurobiology. *Brain*, 131, 2812–2823.
59. Scott D.J., Stohler C.S., Egnatuk C.M. *et al.* (2008) Placebo and nocebo effects are defined by opposite opioid and dopaminergic responses. *Archives of General Psychiatry*, 65, 220–231.
60. Petrovic P., Kalso E., Petersson K.M. *et al.* (2002) Placebo and opioid analgesia – imaging a shared neuronal network. *Science*, 295, 1737–1740.
61. Khan A. *et al.* (2008) The persistence of the placebo response in antidepressant clinical trials. *Journal of Psychiatric Research*, 42, 791–796.
62. Levine J.D., Gordon N.C., Smith R. *et al.* (1981) Analgesic responses to morphine and placebo in individuals with postoperative pain. *Pain*, 10, 379–389.
63. Koenig H.G. (2005) *Faith and Mental Health*. Templeton Foundation Press, Philadelphia, PA.
64. Appelbaum P.S., Robbins P.C., Roth L.H. (1999) Dimensional approach to delusions: Comparison across types and diagnoses. *American Journal of Psychiatry*, 156, 1938–1943.
65. Taylor T. (2003) *Bernadette of Lourdes: Her Life, Death and Visions*, Burns & Oates, London.
66. Puchalski C.M., Ferrell B., Virani R. *et al.* (2009) Improving the quality of spiritual care as a dimension of palliative care: The report of the Consensus

Conference. *Journal of Palliative Medicine,* 12, 885–904.
67. Balboni T.A., Vanderwerker L.C., Block S.D. *et al.* (2007) Religiousness and spiritual support among advanced cancer patients and associations with end-of-life treatment preferences and quality of life. *Journal of Clinical Oncology,* 25, 555–560.
68. Visser A., Garssen B., Vingerhoets A. (2010) Spirituality and well-being in cancer patients: A review. *Psycho-Oncology,* 19, 565–572.
69. Chochinov H.M., Hassard T., McCLement S. *et al.* (2009) The landscape of distress in the terminally ill. *Journal of Pain Symptom Management,* 38, 641–649.
70. Surbone A., Baider L. (2010) The spiritual dimension of cancer care. *Critical Reviews in Oncology/Hematology,* 73, 228–235.
71. Chochinov H.M., Cann B.J. (2005) Interventions to enhance the spiritual aspects of dying. *Journal of Palliative Medicine,* 8, S103–S115.
72. Lo B., Ruston D., Kates L.W. *et al.* (2002) Discussing religious and spiritual issues at the end of life. *Journal of the American Medical Association,* 287, 749–754.
73. Puchalski C.M., Romer A.L. (2000) Taking a spiritual history allows clinicians to understand patients more fully. *Journal of Palliative Medicine,* 3, 129–137.
74. Kissane D.W., Grabsch B., Clarke D.M. *et al.* (2007) Supportive-expressive group therapy for women with metastatic breast cancer: Survival and psychosocial outcome from a randomized controlled trial. *Psycho-Oncology,* 16, 277–286.
75. Chochinov H.M., Hack T., Hassard T. *et al.* (2005) Dignity therapy: A novel psychotherapeutic intervention for patients near the end of life. *Journal of Clinical Oncology,* 23, 5520–5525.
76. Blazer D. (2005) *The Age of Melancholy: Major Depression and its Social Origin,* Routledge, New York.
77. Holland J., Kelly B., Weinberger M. (2010) Why psychosocial care is difficult to integrate into routine cancer care: Stigma is the elephant in the room. *Journal of NCCN,* 8, 362–366.
78. Griffith J.L., Gaby L. (2005) Brief psychotherapy at the bedside: Countering demoralization from medical illness. *Psychosomatics,* 46, 109–116.
79. Hartman D., Zimberoff M.A. (2003) The existential approach in heart-centred therapies. *Journal of Heart-Centred Therapies,* 6, 3–46.
80. Greenstein M., Breitbart W. (2000) Cancer and the experience of meaning: A group psychotherapy program for people with cancer. *American Journal of Psychotherapy,* 54, 486–500.
81. Frankl V. (1963) *Man's Search for Meaning: An Introduction to Logotherapy* [Earlier title (1959) From Death-Camp to Existentialism. Originally published in 1946 as *Ein Psycholog erlebt das Konzentrationslager*], Washington Square Press, New York.
82. Breitbart W., Rosenfeld B., Gibson C. *et al.* (2010) Meaning-centered group psychotherapy for patients with advanced cancer: A pilot randomized controlled trial. *Psycho-Oncology,* 19, 21–28.
83. Lethborg C., Aranda S., Kissane D. (2008) Meaning in adjustment to cancer: A model of care. *Palliative and Supportive Care,* 6, 61–70.
84. Viederman M. (1983) Psychodynamic life narrative in a psychotherapeutic intervention useful in crisis situations. *Psychiatry,* 46, 236–246.
85. Charon R. (2004) Narrative and medicine. *New England Journal of Medicine* 350, 862–864.
86. Zuehlke T., Watkins J. (1975) The use of psychotherapy with dying patients: An exploratory study. *Journal of Clinical Psychology,* 31, 729–732.
87. Chochinov H.M., Hack T., Hassard T. *et al.* (2005) Dignity therapy: A novel psychotherapeutic intervention for patients near the end of life. *Journal of Clinical Oncology,* 23, 5520–5525.
88. Chen L-M., Miaskowski C., Dodd M. *et al.* (2008) Chinese culture and the cancer pain experience: Implications for nursing practice. *Cancer Nursing,* 31, 103–108.
89. Chung J., Wong T., Yang J. (2000) The lens model-assessment of cancer pain in a Chinese context. *Cancer Nursing,* 23, 454–461.
90. Yeh C. (2001) Religious beliefs and practice of Taiwanese parents of pediatric patients with cancer. *Cancer Nursing,* 24, 476–482.
91. Chen Y. (1996) Conformity with nature: A theory of Chinese American elders' health promotion and illness prevention processes. *Advanced Nursing Science,* 19, 17–26.
92. Atwood M. (1991) *Spirit Healing: Native American Magic & Medicine,* Sterling Publishing, New York, NY.
93. Taylor E.J. (2005) Spiritual complementary therapies in cancer care. *Seminars in Oncology Nursing,* 21, 159–163.
94. Poloma M., Gallup G.J. (1991) *Varieties of Prayer: A Survey Report,* Trinity Press, Philadelphia, PA.
95. Woodward K. (1997) Is God listening? *Newsweek,* March 31, pp. 57–65.
96. Gallup G.J. (1996) *Religion in America,* Religion Research Center, Princeton, NJ.

97. Richards D. (1999) The phenomenology and psychological correlates of verbal prayer. *Journal of Psychology & Theology*, 19, 354–363.
98. Meraviglia M. (2002) Prayer in people with cancer. *Cancer Nursing*, 25, 326–331.
99. Taylor E., Outlaw F. (2002) Use of prayer among persons with cancer. *Holistic Nursing Practice*, 16, 46–60.
100. Galanter M. (2007) Spirituality and recovery in 12-step programs: An empirical model. *Journal of Substance Abuse Treatment*, 33, 265–272.
101. Sellman J.D., Baker M.P., Adamson S.J. *et al.* (2007) Future of God in recovery from drug addiction. *Australian and New Zealand Journal of Psychiatry*, 41, 800–808.
102. White M. (1990) *Narrative Means to Therapeutic Ends*, Norton, New York.
103. Lubrano di Ciccone B., Brown R.F., Gueguen J.A. *et al.* (2010) Interviewing patients using interpreters in an oncology setting: Initial evaluation of a communication skills module. *Annals of Oncology*, 21, 27–32.

CHAPTER 22

Psycho-oncology and Advocacy in Cancer Care: An International Perspective

Luzia Travado[1], Jan Geissler[2], Kim Thiboldeaux[3], Jeff Dunn[4], Ranjit Kaur[5] and Anne Merriman[6]

[1]Clinical Psychology Unit, Central Lisbon Hospital Centre – Hospital de S. José, Lisboa, Portugal
[2]Founder and CEO, Patvocates; Co-founder, CML Advocates Network, Chair, LeukaNET
[3]Cancer Support Community, Uniting The Wellness Community and Gilda's Club Worldwide, Washington, DC, USA
[4]Griffith Health Institute, Griffith University, Australia; School of Social Science, University of Queensland, Australia; Viertel Centre for Research in Cancer Control, Cancer Council Queensland, Australia
[5]Breast Cancer Welfare Association Malaysia, Selangor, Malaysia
[6]Department Policy and International Programmes, Hospice Africa in Uganda; Department of Internal Medicine, Makerere University, Uganda

Introduction

Advocacy in cancer care has been playing a major role in the improvement of cancer control and care all over the world. According to a formal definition, 'advocacy' is the active support of an idea or cause, especially the act of pleading or arguing for something.[1] In the case of cancer it has been particularly linked to civil society movements or organizations led by cancer survivors, which have taken on the quest and responsibility to add their voice in contributing to better treatment and care whether in their own hospitals, communities, regions, countries or worldwide.

Grassroots movements that developed in the last half of the twentieth century, like *Reach to Recovery*, joined cancer patients (breast cancer) in helping other patients in their journey 'fighting' the disease and in their coping for better adjustment and quality of life, through peer support and information, and early on also took an interest in national cancer control and care policies and in participating in their development. Patients' empowerment through better information on their disease, treatment options, and on their right to access the best possible care available, has given them the responsibility as well as the choice to participate in their own treatment as well as in influencing cancer policies. 'Nothing about us without us' – the motto of the *European Cancer Patient Coalition* (www.ecpc-online.org) – expresses well the request of cancer patient organizations to be involved as active and interested stakeholders in their own right, in the development and improvement of cancer policies, legislation and regulations, at all levels of policy-making.

Cancer patient organizations have moved from local, regional and national organizations into coalitions and federations to represent cancer patients' rights across borders, at all levels of decision-making, particularly in accessing quality cancer care, as the examples of the *European Cancer Patient Coalition* in Europe[2] and the *National Coalition for Cancer Survivorship* (www.canceradvocacy

Clinical Psycho-Oncology: An International Perspective, First Edition. Edited by Luigi Grassi and Michelle Riba.

.org) in the United States demonstrate.[3] They have raised the profile of cancer patients from recipients of care to active responsible informed partners in reaching better clinical outcomes for themselves and others with similar problems, and in doing so have achieved recognition from politicians, health care professionals and other stakeholders, as respected partners in their own right.

The psychosocial impact of cancer has received more attention since the 1970s, when Betty Ford and Happy Rockefeller publicly stated they were survivors of breast cancer. The public and the media admired them for their courage and altruism in stepping forward, confronting the cancer *taboo* by openly talking about both the cancer and its treatment and showing that a successful and satisfactory life was possible after cancer. This turning point in public attention to cancer and its treatment, along with increased survival due to new treatments and combined modalities and how it affected the person, fostered an interest in psychosocial issues and the funding of research in this area. The *American Cancer Society* began the *Psychosocial Collaborative Oncology Group*,[4] and the *National Cancer Institute* awarded the first grants for psychosocial research in breast cancer.[5]

This chapter intends to provide a brief overview of some of the main movements worldwide concerning advocacy in cancer care, by depicting some illustrative examples of some of the actions undertaken in the five continents, and how this has been translated to influence better policies in cancer care, with particular emphasis on how it has helped to move psychosocial oncology care forward. We will begin with the European perspective, followed by the United States and Australian views, and conclude with the experiences in Asia and Africa.

The European perspective

Inequalities in cancer care in Europe

Every year 3.2 million Europeans are diagnosed with cancer – a figure that is expected to further rise due to the ageing population.[6] Accounting for about one third of deaths of Europeans, cancer has become the second most common cause of death,[7] with almost every family being affected in some way by cancer. Lacking a therapeutic breakthrough in most cancers, especially in the rarer forms, cancer remains a leading cause of disability and death in Europe.

While assessment and approval of new cancer therapies has been aligned with a centralized European procedure, the provision of health care services is subject to each of the 27 European Union (EU) Member States (p.16).[8] The reasons behind these differences involve a wide range of factors from each country's health care funding, gross domestic product, reimbursement procedures, average levels of income and education, living and working conditions, organization of health care services and citizen's behaviours to access health care services. Health expenditure per capita and the share for cancer care in total health expenditure vary greatly between the 27 Members States: for example, Germany spends 7.2% of its health budget on cancer, the United Kingdom 5.6%, and Bulgaria only 4%.[9] The way health services and health information are provided shows significant inequalities across countries, with 23 official languages and 27 different national health care systems, complemented by a lack of mobility of European patients across country borders. Cancer care across Europe, from the perspective of patients, can be seen as patchwork.

Over and above the medical perspective, the psychological and societal impact of cancer on families is large but not widely acknowledged. Having cancer not only largely affects the individual, but often a whole family – in some countries even leading to their financial ruin. The impact is largest when the principal earner is affected by cancer, but also if close relatives cannot continue their job in order to provide care to the family member who has fallen ill. The family affected by cancer might be forced to sell their private assets to be able to afford cancer therapy. On average, the salary of European cancer patients falls by 25% in the first year after cancer diagnosis (p.92).[10] Furthermore, society's indirect cost of cancer, meaning lost productivity, is estimated to be around 30% higher than the direct cost being the immediate health spend on cancer treatments.[11] Employment integration of chronically ill patients as well as sickness benefit vary largely between EU countries, with the Nordic countries leading with a 30% reintegration rate, and lowest rates found in southern countries such as Greece, Malta, Italy and Spain (9–13%) (p.17).[10] In many EU countries, employment discrimination laws to protect disabled people are in place, but are mostly not suitable to support chronically sick people. This is further increased by the lack of psychosocial support, making it hard for patients to overcome the psychological hardships of a cancer diagnosis and find their way back into a performance-driven work environment. As an effect, many European cancer patients lose their job permanently.

Patient advocacy movement in Europe

By the time of the millennium, patients increasingly recognized that decisions on health care priorities were taken largely without the involvement of those affected most: the patient. The emergence of the Internet and 'social media' as an enabler of global collaboration and communication, has facilitated the appearance of both grassroots support initiatives and patient advocacy umbrella groups, providing patients with both information and emotional support on a day by day basis.

To tackle health policy issues, internationally operating patient advocacy umbrella groups like EURORDIS (www.eurordis.org), the European Cancer Patient Coalition (www.ecpc-online.org), and disease-specific networks like Europe Donna (www.europadonna.org), CML Advocates Network (www.cmladvocates.net), or Myeloma Euronet (www.myeloma-euronet.org), were founded in the early 2000s by patient advocates across Europe. Since then, cancer patients have worked hard at getting a seat at the table when health policy decisions, including ethical, societal and financial aspects, were being taken on their behalf – and for health policy to address cancer's challenges on a holistic rather than just a medical or financial level.

While in the 1990s, patient protection measures like the EU clinical trials directive or the EU regulation of information on medicinal products were introduced without prior consultation of patients, advocacy groups are today more and more accepted as an equal stakeholder. They are providing complementary expertise that cannot be provided by health care professionals, consumer groups and regulators alone.[12] They are increasingly prepared to join a fact-based debate on research priorities, reimbursement policies, multidisciplinary treatment and social inclusion, aiming to improve cancer care with an effective use of resources. Today, patient advocacy organizations have a crucial role when society, researchers and authorities need to take difficult decisions on the priorities of health care services.

Advocacy perspective on psycho-oncology

Cancer care may provide state-of-the-science medical treatment, but often fails to address the psychological and social challenges associated with the disease that the individual patient faces. Being diagnosed with cancer, or experiencing a recurrence, puts individuals and their families on an emotional roller-coaster ride. Fear and anxiety, lack of support, lack of information, stigma, physical suffering and a world full of medical terms suddenly enters the life of cancer patients. Having cancer may lead to a change in a person's priorities regarding relationships, career, or lifestyle. Taking tough decisions upon life in the downfall is already difficult enough. In cancer, treatment decisions often need to be taken within days to avoid further progression of the disease, which makes coping with disease and treatment even more difficult.

The level of psychosocial support available to cancer patients differs largely between regions and countries in the EU, increasing inequalities when informed choices between the bad and the ugly need to be made. Where it is available, psychosocial support is often not embedded into routine cancer care – despite the fact that the outcome of cancer care, including also adherence to therapies, is expected to improve significantly. As a matter of fact, due to the lack of widespread availability of professional psychosocial care, patient groups often take the role of providing emotional and social support.

In 2008, the Council of the European Union, on behalf of all 27 EU Member States, agreed in its 'Conclusions on Reducing the Burden of Cancer in Europe' to 'attain optimal results, a patient-centred comprehensive interdisciplinary approach and optimal psycho-social care should be implemented in routine cancer care, rehabilitation and post-treatment follow-up for all cancer patients'.[13] The Council also called on all EU Member States to 'take into account the psycho-social needs of patients and improve the quality of life for cancer patients through support, rehabilitation and palliative care'.

However, over and above political statements, much more needs to be done on the implementation level to make psychosocial care available to all the cancer patients in need. The requirement to offer psychosocial care for accreditation of Comprehensive Cancer Centres has at least increased the establishment of psycho-oncology services at centres of excellence, but still most patients lack access to – or awareness of availability of – professional psychosocial support.

For years, advocacy groups have been demanding multidisciplinary care, including also nurses and psycho-oncologists, to achieve multidisciplinary treatment. Although these were important achievements, to make a change, psycho-oncologist groups and patient advocacy groups need to join forces to achieve a common goal: to take policy actions as well as start joint initiatives to assure that psychosocial care and services are embedded in national cancer plans, in comprehensive treatment programmes, in treatment guidelines and in routine checklists. Professional psycho-oncology care needs to become accessible to all European cancer patients. The *European Partnership on Action Against Cancer* (www.epaac.eu) launched in 2009 is a step forward in this regard. It aims to improve cancer control and care in Europe by reducing cancer by 15% by 2020, through sharing knowledge and expertise among Member States, scientific societies, cancer patients' organizations, and cancer-related stakeholders. A Psychosocial Oncology Action promoted by Portugal, involving the International Psycho-Oncology Society and the European Cancer Patient Coalition among other organizations, is included in the health care work package of the first Joint Action project co-financed by the European Commission (2011–2014).

The US experience

The IOM Report – a turning point

The advocacy movement in cancer in the United States has evolved dramatically over the past 25 years and was strongly influenced in the 1980s and 1990s by the advocacy movement in HIV/AIDS, which prompted unprecedented federal and state funding for research and comprehensive care. While the advocacy movement in cancer saw its early roots in breast cancer and the symbol of the pink ribbon, cancer advocacy has grown steadily into other cancers, including colorectal cancer, leukaemia and lymphoma, ovarian cancer, prostate cancer and even lung cancer. The advocacy community in cancer has made great strides in achieving expanded public funding for screening and early detection, medical research, clinical trials and their associated costs, and expanded access to care.* And while the main thrust of the cancer advocacy movement has been around increases in research funding and ensuring access to quality medical care, there is now an emerging advocacy movement in psychosocial oncology in the United States, which will be discussed in greater detail here.

In 2008, the Institute of Medicine (IOM), part of the National Academies in Washington, DC, issued a report called, *Cancer Care for the Whole Patient: Meeting Psychosocial Health Needs*. The Report states that 'Today, it is not possible to deliver good-quality cancer care without using existing approaches, tools, and resources to address patients' psychosocial health needs. All patients with cancer and their families should expect and receive cancer care that ensures the provision of appropriate psychosocial health services' (p.1).[14] This critical report, truly

---

* Examples include American Cancer Society (www.cancer.org); Susan G. Komen for the Cure (www.komen.org); National Breast Cancer Coalition (www.breastcancerdeadline2020.org).

the first of its kind in the field, now provides the psychosocial oncology community in the United States with a central rallying point and a sound platform and body of data to advocate for the integration of psychosocial care into the medical standard of care for people with cancer.

The community responds

Spurred by the issuance of the IOM Report, in 2008 a number of organizations, led by the American Psychosocial Society (APOS) and the Cancer Support Community (CSC), formed the *Alliance for Quality Psychosocial Care*, a national alliance of nearly 40 organizations, united to advance the recommendations in the 2008 Report. The Alliance is led by three co-chairs from academia, community support and policy, and is driven largely by the work of five committees including: Childhood Cancer, Education and Awareness, Policy and Advocacy, Research, and Standard of Care. Notable accomplishments of the Alliance to date include the development of a comprehensive database of nationwide psychosocial resources for providers and medical institutions; the development of key collateral materials and talking points on the IOM Report and the value of psychosocial care; and, presentations at several key professional meeting such as the 2010 Sixth World Conference on the Promotion of Mental Health and Prevention of Mental and Behavioral Disorders in Washington, DC in November 2010 (http://wmhconf2010.hhd.org).[15] The Alliance is currently developing language to be used in key health care reform initiatives and in future legislation to ensure the integration of psychosocial care into quality cancer care. In fact, the President of the IOM, Dr Harvey Fineberg, in a letter to the Alliance membership dated 6 April 2010, stated, 'I was delighted and gratified that our report, *Cancer Care for the Whole Patient*, coupled with your initiative and hard work, has led to the creation of such an important new national organization devoted to the cause of higher quality care for cancer. As President of the Institute of Medicine, I would like to do what I can to be helpful to the Alliance.'

In addition, a major professional society in the United States, the American College of Surgeons (ACOS), and their specialty division, the Commission on Cancer (CoC), made an unprecedented move in 2010 by adopting a series of 'patient-centred' standards, to be added to their existing 36 standards, applied to more than 1500 hospitals and practices that see more than 70% of all new cancer diagnoses in the United States annually. The new patient-centred standards cover Patient Navigation, Survivorship Care Planning and Psychosocial Distress Screening. Importantly, in the psychosocial arena, the distress screening standard reads as follows: 'The cancer committee develops and implements a process to integrate and monitor on-site psychosocial distress screening and referral for the provision of psychosocial care as the standard for patients with cancer' (p.58).[16] The College invited three national patient support and advocacy organizations to assist with the development and implementation of the standards including the Cancer Support Community (www.cancersupportcommunity.org), LIVESTRONG (also known as the Lance Armstrong Foundation) (www.livestrong.org), and the National Coalition for Cancer Survivorship (www.canceradvocacy.org). The College has also formed a partnership with the Alliance for Quality Psychosocial Care as the Alliance strives to assist institutions and practices in the adoption of these new standards.

In addition, the American Society of Clinical Oncology (ASCO), the professional society representing oncologists in the United States, is also formally recognizing the importance of integrated psychosocial care. ASCO has incorporated distress screening and care planning into their QOPI (Quality Oncology Practice Initiative) programme (http://qopi.asco.org). QOPI is ASCO's voluntary practice-based quality improvement programme. Participating practices are assessing distress screening and awareness and making efforts to improve the identification and management of distress among patients.

The future

The release of the IOM Report, combined with the formation of a national psychosocial alliance and the adoption of new standards by professional societies, is leading to an unprecedented surge of awareness around the importance of psychosocial care in cancer. In addition, the United States will see the ageing of 77 million baby boomers in the coming years, leading to an increase in the incidence of cancer, and an increase in demand for psychological, social, emotional, spiritual and financial support. Therefore, the advocacy movement in psychosocial care must now turn to issues of reimbursement in order to achieve the full integration of these services. Psychosocial care can no longer be an 'unfunded mandate' that is 'nice to do', but not a required service. The advocacy community must now make its voice heard among policy-makers and private payers to ensure the reimbursement of psychosocial services. The IOM Report states that, 'Attending to psychosocial needs should be an integral part of quality cancer care. All components of the health care system that are involved in cancer care should explicitly incorporate attention to psychosocial needs into their policies, practices, and standards addressing clinical health care' (p.8).[14]

There is a true awakening in the United States around what can be achieved for cancer patients and their families through advocacy and through action. The belief in the possibility of better care is now being taken on by the psychosocial oncology community and will serve as a true model for other diseases.

The Australian experience

The Australian population is ageing and as the risk of cancer increases with age, the burden of cancer is increasing. On average one in two Australians will develop cancer (p.14) and one in five will die from this disease before the age of 85 years (p.25).[17] Additionally, cancer is now the leading cause of disease and injury in Australia, accounting for nearly one fifth of the disease burden (p.2).[18] To address this critical public health issue Australia has developed a National Service Improvement Framework (p.1)[19] to drive health service improvements in cancer and other chronic diseases. The Framework includes the goals of ensuring that people affected by cancer have access to the best possible level of support at all phases of the illness experience. The framework aims to articulate with evidence-based clinical practice guidelines that in the case of supportive care crosses over to disease-specific guidelines as well as guidelines that focus only on psychosocial care.[20]

Consumer advocacy for cancer in Australia has been closely linked to patient support where consumers have joined together to form peer support networks. In brief, by sharing their cancer experiences, survivors are able to provide each other with emotional, practical and informational support to build hope, reduce feelings of isolation, and learn new coping approaches.[21] In doing so, consumers both individually and as a group often come to realize their strength as advocates, and hence many such groups have dual roles, not only as support providers but also as advocates to guide the development of supportive care services and to advocate for improved treatments.

Prostate Cancer Foundation of Australia (www.prostate.org/au)

The Prostate Cancer Foundation of Australia (PCFA) was first formed in 1996 in the Australian state of New South Wales and since then has grown to become Australia's peak national consumer network for men affected by prostate cancer. The PCFA aspires to diminish the burden of prostate cancer through advocacy, research and support. The PCFA has pursued its goals through the establishment of more than 100 support groups Australia-wide and is connected to many thousands of men across the country. Each group provides support and advocacy for men affected by prostate cancer and their families. The PCFA has an extensive network of volunteers, both men and women, who have been affected by prostate cancer either directly or indirectly through their own diagnosis, or that of a partner or family member.

The PCFA network is widely recognized as one of Australia's most effective forums for advocacy on prostate cancer, raising community awareness of prostate cancer and encouraging research and service development to improve quality of life for those affected by the disease. Prostate cancer survivors in this network contribute to the development of evidence-based clinical practice guidelines, patient education materials, and scientific review committees to ensure the consumer voice is present and heard. An example of where this has been particularly powerful has been contributing to the development of clinical practice guidelines for localized and advanced prostate cancer, and then working to support the development of consumer versions for mass distribution.[22]

Breast Cancer Network Australia (BCNA) (www.bcna.org.au)

Breast Cancer Network Australia was formed in July 1999, and since then has grown to become Australia's peak national consumer organization for Australian women affected by breast cancer. BCNA's mission is to support women affected by breast cancer and their families, irrespective of their socioeconomic status and place of residence. BCNA's advocacy is focused on continuous improvement of treatment services and supportive care, as well as on providing women with all the information required to navigate the breast cancer journey.

BCNA's objectives are to inform, empower, represent and link together people affected by breast cancer. It provides women with the latest information about all aspects of breast cancer, encouraging women to actively champion their personal health care and to be active about calling for improvements in clinical treatment services and supportive care. Ultimately, BCNA serves to uphold the place of all women in guiding the development of breast cancer policies and planning. BCNA has linked women together, and with the broader community, through its member groups, and national events, such as the 'Field of Women', a fundraising event uniting Australian men, women and children in their support of women affected by breast cancer.

The organization has also established a powerful advocacy network through its website, connecting BCNA and its members with other individuals and groups to discuss common issues and experiences. BCNA representatives have a presence on committees considering breast cancer matters, and provide input into breast cancer strategies and capacity building, consulting with its members to research and analyse key breast cancer issues, with a view to contributing constructively to problem-solving in the national policy context.

Cancer Voices Australia (www.cancervoicesaustralia.org.au)

Cancer Voices Australia (CVA) was officially launched on 4 February 2007, World Cancer Day. Since its formation, CVA has developed an effective national network to provide a voice for Australians affected by cancer. Its achievements have been bolstered by the establishment of CVA chapters in all Australian states and territories, enabling Australians affected by cancer to share common issues, ideas and experiences, advocating on issues of importance to patients, survivors and their loved ones.

CVA's advocacy was particularly effective during the most recent Australian election, in 2010, calling on the Australian Government to commit to issues about access to evidence-based and best practice and emerging cancer treatments.

CVA has worked closely with Australia's peak body for clinical oncologists, the Clinical Oncological Society of Australia (COSA) to facilitate an annual forum for Australians affected by cancer that coincides with the annual scientific meeting for health professionals in cancer care. This further promotes consideration of consumer feedback in the development of integrated and multidisciplinary clinical cancer services.

The experience of '*Reach to Recovery*' in Asia

The *Reach to Recovery* experience in Asia has shown that cancer is still surrounded by social stigma, guilt and the shame of having committed a sin, being a penance or even acts as 'pay-back time'. The varying beliefs of *karma* or fate, will of God, reparation of sins committed in the past, and the disease being beyond the control of the individual and health care professionals are some ways that society in Asia deals with the impact of cancer.[23–25] The disease is regarded as a personal tragedy, associating it to cultural and religious identity and life. There is a tension in the role and the quality of relationships between the individual with cancer and loved ones, family members and the larger society. This tragedy model impacts the individual emotionally, socially, spiritually and intellectually, hence causing a disturbance in the personal, social and vocational roles of the individual. Such social attitudes are a stumbling block because society starts relating to individuals with cancer in a negative way. The cancer emanates a fear of social isolation and rejection, losing control of basic opportunities in life, and as one individual diagnosed with cancer stated, *'It is better to die than to live a life of no purpose'*.[25] Pakistan has the highest rate of breast cancer compared to other Asian countries and annually, 83 000 women get breast cancer of whom 40 000 do not survive due to the social and cultural impact.[26]

Social attitudes transcending into sympathy instead of empathy as well as hopelessness in areas where mortality rates are higher, all serve to create a vicious cycle of presentation for treatment at late stages of the disease, dying in hospital and premature deaths, which is misinterpreted as *'the death was caused due to the medical treatment'*. Hence, communities seek alternative remedies, witchcraft and other clinically unproven methods of treatment, thereby widening the gap between knowledge and ignorance.[27,28] Those who reject sympathy, adopt the social developmental model of not only changing their own identity and outlook on life but they also empower themselves to be agents of change in social attitudes. This kind of perception takes the stand that human attitudes can be improved through sharing personal cancer experiences, engaging in conversations, facilitating open public forums with stakeholders, persuasion, conviction and the enforcement of policies and legislation. As rightfully stated by someone facing social stigma *'people are nice, people are good... Human beings tend to bank on their bad experiences, rather than their good experiences...'*. Every time cancer survivors interact with the public, they have to start narrating their situation to help them understand and to alleviate the unease and prejudice facing the illness. Individuals with cancer who are unable to deal with such interactions tend to socially isolate themselves and feel rejected.

The poor quality of communication skills between the health care professional and the patient intensifies the issue further.[29] Effective communication skills are not an important component when it comes to training in medical schools in Asia, therefore there is no emphasis on ensuring that doctors are competent in breaking bad news and providing health care services in a supportive manner. Doctors are struggling with their own coping skills, as a patient commented in a gesture of humour, *'No wonder doctors wear masks'*. Psycho-oncology services do not exist in many countries in Asia because most of the treatment plans in hospital settings adopt a medical-model approach. The National Cancer Control Plans do not have any focus on psychological and social care in cancer care. While the patient is focused on the emotional and spiritual aspects of the impact of the disease, the health care professionals concentrate on the physical aspects of treating the disease. Hence, there is a divergence or discrepancy in thought, belief and action, which can lead to non-compliance of treatment by the patient.

The *Reach to Recovery* model (www.reachtorecoveryinternational.org) owes its beginnings to the quest for meaning in life by one woman, Terese Lasser, a breast cancer survivor in the 1950s who felt that her personal experience could make a positive difference in the life of other women who were at the start of a similar journey. This concept is still applicable and valid in the twenty-first century. *Reach to Recovery International* is built on a simple yet universal principle: *A woman who has lived through breast cancer and gives of her time and experience to help another woman confronting the same experience is a valuable source of support. Reach to Recovery International is committed to working to improve the quality of life for women with breast cancer and their families through a wide range of services offered worldwide.* Today, there are *Reach to Recovery* volunteers who feel committed to the cause to serve the community through their own coping experience and recovery coupled with structured training.

Social change originates from the stakeholders, namely, the individuals who are affected by the disease, the health care professionals and the immediate society. The awkward avoidance displayed by stakeholders is largely due to: (a) lack of knowledge of the disease; (b) fear of the uncertainty and consequences of the disease; (c) poor communication skills by health care professionals and the public; (d) tension between the patient and doctor in thought, belief and action.[29]

Due to the suffering and the fact that the cause of a disease like breast cancer is still unclear, people recall and relate to unpleasant experiences and premature deaths more than those who have survived and are living normal lives. The dramatization and mystification of the negative aspects of the disease experience create stereotyping, prejudice and social isolation of the newly diagnosed.[25,30] Such a vicious circle can be broken through policy changes, enforcement of clinical practice guidelines in the management of the disease, making available equitable early detection and timely treatment including psycho-oncological services by both the government and non-government sectors. For example, in Malaysia, the development of an updated edition of the clinical practice guidelines in the management of breast cancer incorporating the need for psycho-oncology services is a positive step towards a developmental approach to cancer care.[31] This change is largely due to advocacy knowledge-sharing through the *Reach to Recovery International* programme creating an urgent need to prevent suffering among women with breast cancer.[32]

Incorporating psycho-oncology in mainstream health care services can narrow the communication gap between health care professionals and patients. Listening to the patient in a supportive way and attending to the patient's emotional, spiritual and social needs can help: (a) improve the quality of life for the patient; (b) improve the patient's knowledge of the disease and its management; (c) empower the individual to be well informed and to be able to communicate with society effectively.[31]

In conclusion, a well-informed society can help prevent prejudice and discrimination towards individuals with cancer. Incorporating compulsory training and examinations for medical and nursing students in interpersonal communication skills and breaking bad news in a supportive way is indispensable to enable an improved quality of cancer services rendered. Psycho-oncology services should be an essential component of cancer treatment and rehabilitation. *Reach to Recovery International* is currently attempting to learn from the experience and knowledge of the International Psycho-Oncology Society (www.ipos-society.org) to incorporate psychosocial care and improve the quality of cancer care.

The African perspective

African reality

Almost all countries in Africa are listed within the lower third of the Human Development Index (HDI).[33] This is estimation by the United Nations (UNDP) categorizing all countries according to development in education, health and infrastructure as well as economy. In Africa large numbers of people still live below the subsistence level of $2 per day, many are subsistence farmers, so moving to the capital or out of the country for treatment is impossible. Reaching these people is a challenge to the health systems and reaching health systems a challenge to the families themselves.

It is estimated that less than 5% of African cancer patients will reach oncology services. Thirty percent of African countries do not have chemotherapy or radiotherapy available and even for those countries that do have it, there is often just one centre for the whole country. For the general population in an African country, there are always some who do not reach health care. We have noted a spectrum between 5% (in Rwanda) and 85% (in Ethiopia); in Uganda it is 57%.[34] Among these are cancer patients, who come often at an advanced stage and lie in pain with distressing disfigurements until death.

However, all patients with cancer have psychosocial problems that need to be addressed. Cultural structures do contain many support systems for those brought up within an African culture. These vary not only from country to country but from tribe to tribe. Some of their supports have better results than those of the West and there is much we can learn from them. However, many are left suffering without reference to 'Total Pain'[35] defined by Dame Cicely Saunders in 1964, and which is a part of being human.*

HIV is a problem that has increased the infectious diseases and number of deaths from infections in Africa. Governments need to concentrate resources on managing and preventing the top 10 causes of death. For the last 20 years in Uganda (143 out of 169 countries on the HDI) HIV/AIDS has been the priority, which has achieved results in that the prevalence has been reduced from 30% to 7%.[36]

Advocates for palliative care including psychosocial care

The problems of the patient must be at the forefront of how we approach using advocacy. We need to provide good listeners at village level who are knowledgeable in psychosocial issues and can refer patients to the right service, arrange for group meetings at village level for patients to meet each other and share experiences, similar to day care, and advise and explain, but most of all to listen and share. These support networks can be set up with churches and in community and church halls. This form of support is taught, as part of training for local community health volunteers attached to hospices in some countries, for example Uganda, Malawi,[37] Cameroon,[38] (pp. 230, 243).[39] In Nigeria and Cote d'Ivoire, support from similar groups is provided within the major hospitals. This is supported by funding from outside NGOs.

Spiritual issues are very high in the priorities of the dying patient in Africa. Many are battling with religions, religious rituals and at the same time their belief in animism and ancestor worship. This has to be reviewed locally and discussed with the patient early on in the encounter.[39]

Advocacy has included bringing to the attention of the government(s) the facts about the way people die from cancer, AIDS and other diseases in Africa. For cancer we need to have the evidence based on the population of each country and bring this to their notice. How many people are suffering from cancer in, for example, Uganda? We estimate that incidence since HIV is 0.2% of the population and prevalence is 0.3% (p.8).[40] Thus we can say that 99 000 in Uganda suffering from cancer NOW require palliative care including psychosocial care. In Nigeria, the most populated country in Africa, with a population of 150 million the need is for approximately 4.5 million. These statistics need to be brought to the attention of governments.

Sixty to 70% of those with cancer will require pain relief. Most require psychosocial care which cannot be started when pain is the major concern for the patient and family. Advocacy to government needs to include obtaining affordable morphine for the country, establishing safeguards for importing the powder, its preparation and storage and then ensuring that there are sufficient prescribers for this 'class A' drug. Advocacy for this was successful in Uganda.[41] Hospice Africa and more recently the African Palliative Care Association are talking to African governments, using the example of Uganda, to bring the same advocacy to other countries, which would then be taken up at local level. Fourteen out of 57 African countries now have affordable oral morphine available but most do not distribute it throughout each country, due to logistics, local myths and misunderstanding regarding its use, and the application of outdated and bureaucratic regulations. This leaves many still in need of this path to resolving their psychosocial problems.

The advocacy successes in Uganda have been attributed to the availability of morphine and to an increased number of prescribers of morphine, making it available to those in need.[41] Also there has been advocacy to allow patients to die in their own homes, as this is where most wish to die.[42–44]

* The concept of 'Total Pain' (or Total Suffering) integrates the physical, emotional, spiritual, cultural and social dimensions of the individual, which gives us a wider approach and a framework to our understanding and care for patients at the end of life (Baines M.J.: From pioneer days to implementation – lessons to be learnt. Guest lecture at EAPC conference 2011, Portugal, *Palliative Medicine;* in press).

Advocacy in Africa today, initiated by Hospice Africa in 1993 (www.hospiceafrica.or.ug; www.hospiceafrica.ie; http://hospice-africa.merseyside.org/), is very much strengthened by the efforts of the African Palliative Care Association (APCA) (www.africanpalliativecare.org) and its work with country palliative care associations, which bring together all the services in the country, and work with governments on policies and strategic planning. These organizations also promote psychosocial care through newsletters, annual reports and in the media. The African Organisation for Research and Training in Cancer (AORTIC) (www.aortic-africa.org) promotes psychosocial advocacy through publications, conferences and a network of leaders in Africa and abroad. The most rapid change has been brought about by initiatives from NGOs but they cannot move forward unless strengthened by government policies. The answer for psychosocial improvement in Africa will be through the private/public efforts of those with a heart for helping those most in need.

Psycho-oncology: to be or not to be in Africa?

Psycho-oncology is an integral part of palliative care. The problem in Africa is that palliative care is not always side by side with oncology and therefore, psycho-oncology is introduced as a separate specialty.

However, both specialties are scarce in Africa. It is more usual to find palliative care. Palliative care takes a different approach to the patient from the traditional way, which is that taken by most oncologists. The patient is no longer the tumour or the disease, but now seen as a person, a member of the family, community and tribe. Knowing him or her, they are our guest and will be entitled to all the privileges of a guest from the medical team including the oncologist. The patient will have choices in all matters pertaining to their future and their treatments. However, in order to make correct choices, they need to be fully informed of all that is going on in their body and what is available medically and psychologically, which can contribute to an improved quality of life within the cultural setting. Ideally, palliative care is introduced at diagnosis and the team is there to meet any needs that arise from the diagnosis of the disease, side-effects of treatments, the background of the patient together with addressing the support available in the family and community to sustain the patient through any eventualities including psychological.[39,45]

Palliative care is not available to most people in need in Africa. Those palliative care services that are presently functioning aim to follow the above traditions, but there are many other factors affecting the quality of a service including the level of dedication of the team members and their integrity. Thus a team that is working and moving together is very important. If the spirit and ethos is not in the team then it is difficult to give such a dedicated service. This is practised in Uganda but still only reaches 10% of those in need.[46]

Looking to the future, we need to ensure outcomes from our advocacy with time lines. Psychosocial issues as part of palliative care are moving slowly. The HIV organizations have taken this on also, which has contributed to the improvements for HIV and cancer patients. Working together, not-for-profit organizations can move mountains but need the support of the Ministry of Health especially for government policies.

In conclusion, psychosocial needs are now being addressed in Africa. If we can move forward together, working at every level of need, we will at least bring peace to the millions of patients and families affected by cancer.

Final comments

The advocacy movements throughout the world described here, illustrate well the immense and important value of having patient organizations and NGOs involved and participating in the challenges of cancer care and its improvement at policy and resource development levels. The role of psycho-oncology in cancer care is well demonstrated and supported by scientific evidence as its benefits in improving patients' clinical outcomes.[47] Recommendations and guidelines for integrating specialized psychosocial care into routine cancer care have been issued in many countries all over the world as mentioned; nevertheless its inclusion in standard cancer care remains far from optimal and in some cases absent.[48] To this end the International Psycho-Oncology Society has recently launched the *International Standard of Quality Cancer Care* (www.ipos-society.org) already endorsed by the UICC and other societies proposing: (1) Quality cancer care must integrate the psychosocial domain into routine care; (2) Distress should be measured as the Sixth Vital Sign after temperature, blood pressure, pulse, respiratory rate and pain.

As cancer treatment requires a holistic patient-centred approach for the patient's best clinical outcomes, cancer care policies also benefit from the perspective and expertise of those who have experienced the disease. To bring about change and improvement in policies, namely the inclusion and provision of psychosocial cancer care in treatment plans, requires political will. Scientific data justifies its relevance, benefits, efficiency, societal impact and cost-effectiveness. Public demand justifies its need. Together – scientists, health care professionals, policy-makers and cancer patient organizations along with other stakeholders – can do better, by sharing our knowledge and joining efforts in the quest to bring about change and improve cancer care for all.

Key points

- Advocacy in cancer care has been playing a major role in the improvement of cancer control and care all over the world.
- Cancer patients' organizations have matured and grown into national organizations, coalitions and federations representing cancer patients' rights across borders, at all levels of decision-making, having achieved significant recognition as respected partners.
- Advocacy movements throughout the world have shown the important value of having cancer patients involved and participating in the challenges of cancer care and its improvement at policy and resource development levels.
- There is a considerable lack of widespread availability of professional psychosocial care, and it varies largely between regions and countries, and across continents, being mostly linked to the country's income and health budget, and the organization of cancer care, namely the existence of an effective National Cancer Plan as well as accreditation of clinical centres.
- To bring about change and improvement in cancer policies, namely the inclusion of specialized psychosocial cancer care in treatment plans, treatment guidelines, and its provision in routine cancer care, requires political will. This can be achieved through public demand and lobbying by psycho-oncology and advocacy organizations.
- Scientists, health care professionals, policy-makers and cancer patients' NGOs along with other stakeholders – can achieve better policies and outcomes by joining efforts in the quest to bring about change and improve cancer care for all.

References

1. The Free Dictionary, http://www.thefreedictionary.com/advocacy (last accessed 25 June 2011).
2. Sundseth H., Wood L.F. (2008) Cancer patients – partners for change, in *Responding to the Challenge of Cancer in Europe* (eds M.P. Coleman, D-M. Alexe, T. Albreht, M. McKee), Slovenian Institute of Public Health, Ljubljana.
3. Stovall E. (2008) National Coalition for Cancer Survivorship: Advocacy for quality cancer care. *Journal of Oncology Practice*, 4, 145.
4. Holland J.C. (1989) Historical overview, in *Handbook of Psycho-Oncology: Psychological Care of the Patient with Cancer* (eds J.C. Holland, J.H. Rowland), Oxford University Press.
5. Taylor S.E. (1984) The developing field of health psychology, in *Handbook of Psychology and Health, Vol. IV. Social Psychological Aspects of Health* (eds A. Baum, S.E. Taylor, J. Singer), Lawrence Erlbaum Associates, New Jersey.
6. Ferlay J., Autier P., Boniol M. *et al.* (2007) Estimates of the cancer incidence and mortality in Europe in 2006. *Annals of Oncology*, 18, 581–592.
7. GLOBOCAN 2008 (IARC) Section of Cancer Information (2011).

8. Espín J., Rovira J. (2007) Analysis of differences and commonalities in pricing and reimbursement systems in Europe, Andalusian School of Public Health.
9. Health Expenditures: Eurostat (2007); Per capita health expenditures on health share WHO (2005).
10. Cancer and in general long-term illnesses at workplaces, European Parliament's Employment and Social Affairs Committee (EMPL) (2008), IP/A/EMPL/FWC/2006-05/SC3.
11. Cancerfonden, Cancerfondsrapporten, Stockholm (2006).
12. PatientPartner FP7 Project (2010), http://www.patientpartner-europe.eu (accessed January 2012).
13. The Council of the European Union (2008) Council Conclusions on reducing the burden of cancer, 2876th Employment, Social Policy, Health And Consumer Affairs Council meeting, Luxembourg, 10 June.
14. Adler N.E., Page A.E.K. (eds) (2008) *Cancer Care for the Whole Patient: Meeting Psychosocial Health Needs*, National Academies Press, Washington, DC.
15. McCorkle R., Gorman M., Thiboldeaux K., Taylor J. (2010) Developing effective partnerships to implement recommendations of the Institute of Medicine Report *Cancer Care for the Whole Patient: Meeting Psychosocial Health Needs* [Abstract]. The Sixth World Conference on the Promotion of Mental Health and Prevention of Mental and Behavioral Disorders, Washington, DC. Abstract retrieved from http://wmhconf2010.hhd.org (accessed January 2012).
16. Commission on Cancer (2011) *Cancer Program Standards 2012: Ensuring Patient-Centered Care*, 2nd edn, Edge, Chicago, IL.
17. Australian Institute of Health and Welfare & Australasian Association of Cancer Registries (2010) *Cancer in Australia: An overview, 2010.* Cancer Series No. 60, Cat. No. CAN 56, AIHW, Canberra.
18. Begg S., Vos T., Barker B. *et al.* (2007) The burden of disease and injury in Australia 2003. PHE 82, AIHW, Canberra.
19. National Health Priority Action Council (2006) National Service Improvement Framework Australian Government Department of Health and Aging, Canberra.
20. National Breast Cancer Centre, National Cancer Control Initiative (2003) *Clinical Practice Guidelines for the Psychosocial Care of Adults with Cancer.* National Health and Medical Research Council, Campesdern, NSW.
21. Dunn J., Steginga S.K., Millichap D., Rosoman, N. (2003) A review of peer support in the context of cancer. *Journal of Psychosocial Oncology*, 21, 55–67.
22. Australian Cancer Network Management of Metastatic Prostate Cancer Working Party (2010) *Clinical practice guidelines for the management of locally advanced and metastatic prostate cancer.* Cancer Council Australia and Australian Cancer Network, Sydney.
23. Yam B. (2006). *Researching the Experience of Patients with Cancer in Another Culture.* 14th International Conference on Cancer Nursing, 27 Sep – 1 Oct 2006, Toronto, Canada.
24. Sénior M., Viveash B. (1998) *Health and Illness.* Palgrave Macmillan, Hampshire, UK, pp. 166–170.
25. Coleridge P. (1993) *Disability, Liberation & Development*, Oxfam Print Unit, Oxford, pp. 27–52.
26. Rehmat K. (2009). *Asia's ultimate shock-and-awe.* Dateline Pakistan, published *Gulf Times*, 7 October 2009, Doha.
27. Lien Foundation (2010) The Quality of Death: Ranking end-of-life care across the world. *The Economist*, pp. 16–20.
28. Leong B.D.K., Chuah J.A., Kumar V.M. *et al.* (2009) Trends of breast cancer treatment in Sabah, Malaysia: A problem with lack of awareness. *Singapore Medical Journal*, 50, 772–776.
29. Taib N.A., Yip C.H., Ibrahim M. *et al.* (2007) Breast cancer in Malaysia: Are our women getting the right message? 10-year experience in a single institution in Malaysia. *Asian Pacific Journal of Cancer Prevention*, 8, 141–145.
30. Riddell S., Watcon N. (2003) *Disability, Culture and Identity*, Pearson Education Ltd, Harlow, UK, pp. 34–51.
31. Ministry of Health Malaysia (2010) *Clinical Practice Guidelines in the Management of Breast Cancer.*
32. National Coalition for Cancer Survivorship (2009) *Self-Advocacy: A Cancer Survivor's Handbook*, Silver Spring, MD, USA, pp. 9–13.
33. Indices and Data: Human Development Reports (HDR). United Nations website http://hdr.undp.org/en/statistics (last accessed 24 July 2011).
34. Ministry of Health personnel, Rwanda, Ethiopia. Personal communications on questioning (not usually in the statistics published).
35. Saunders C.S. (1964). The symptomatic treatment of incurable malignant disease. *Prescribers Journal*, 4, 68–73.
36. Ministry of Health, Uganda (2010) Second National Health Care Policy, July.

37. Hospice Africa Situational Reports: Ndi Moyo, Salima, Malawi 2001–2010. Available from Hospice Africa Uganda, www.hospiceafrica.or.ug (accessed January 2012).
38. Hospice Africa Situational Reports and Progress Reports: BBH, Bamenda, Cameroon 2008–2010. Available from Hospice Africa Uganda, www.hospice africa.or.ug (accessed January 2012).
39. Merriman A. (2010) *Audacity to Love: The Story of Hospice Africa*, Irish Hospice Foundation, ISBN 9780953488094 (pp. 34–41).
40. Merriman A. (2011) A public health issue for palliative care? Calculating PC needs for cancer and AIDS in African countries. *AORTIC News*, May, 8.
41. Merriman A., Harding R. (2010) Pain control in the African context (Uganda experience). *Philosophy, Ethics and Humanities in Medicine*, 5, 10. http://www.peh-med.com/content/5/1/10 (accessed January 2012).
42. Kikule E. (2003) A good death in Uganda: Survey of needs for palliative care for terminally ill people in urban areas. *British Medical Journal*, 327, 192–194.
43. Sepulveda C., Habiyambere V., Amandua J. *et al.* (2003) Quality care at the end of life in Africa. *British Medical Journal*, 327, 209–213.
44. Ramsay S. (2003) Leading the way in African home-based palliative care. Free oral morphine has allowed expansion of model home-based palliative care in Uganda. *Lancet*, 362, 1812–1813.
45. Merriman A. (2010) *Audacity to Love: The Story of Hospice Africa.* Irish Hospice Foundation, ISBN 9780953488094 (pp. 278–283).
46. Palliative Care Association of Uganda (2009) An Audit of PC Services in Uganda. *April.*
47. Grassi L., Travado L. (2008) The role of psychosocial oncology in cancer care, in *Responding to the Challenge of Cancer in Europe* (eds M.P. Coleman, D.-M. Alexe, T. Albreht, M. McKee), Slovenian Institute of Public Health, Ljubljana.
48. Travado L. (2012) Cancer inequalities in Europe: Access to psychosocial care. *Praxis Klinische Verhaltensmedizin und Rehabilitation (Practice of Clinical Behavior Medicine and Rehabilitation Journal*; in press).

Index

Clinical Psycho-Oncology: An International Perspective, First Edition. Edited by Luigi Grassi and Michelle Riba.